Child Maltreatment

Editors

HOWARD DUBOWITZ
JOHN M. LEVENTHAL

PEDIATRIC CLINICS OF NORTH AMERICA

www.pediatric.theclinics.com

Consulting Editor
BONITA F. STANTON

October 2014 • Volume 61 • Number 5

ELSEVIER

1600 John F. Kennedy Boulevard • Suite 1800 • Philadelphia, Pennsylvania, 19103-2899

http://www.theclinics.com

THE PEDIATRIC CLINICS OF NORTH AMERICA Volume 61, Number 5
October 2014 ISSN 0031-3955, ISBN-13: 978-0-323-32024-7

Editor: Kerry Holland
Developmental Editor: Casey Jackson

The Pediatric Clinics of North America (ISSN 0031-3955) is published bimonthly by Elsevier Inc., 360 Park Avenue South, New York, NY 10010-1710. Months of issue are February, April, June, August, October, and December. Periodicals postage paid at New York, NY and additional mailing offices. Subscription prices are $200.00 per year (US individuals), $493.00 per year (US institutions), $270.00 per year (Canadian individuals), $657.00 per year (Canadian institutions), $325.00 per year (international individuals), $657.00 per year (international institutions), $100.00 per year (US students and residents), and $165.00 per year (international and Canadian residents and students). To receive students/resident rare, orders must be accompanied by name of affiliated institution, date of term, and the signature of program/residency coordinator on institution letterhead. Orders will be billed at individual rate until proof of status is received. Foreign air speed delivery is included in all Clinics subscription prices. All prices are subject to change without notice. **POSTMASTER:** Send address changes to The Pediatric Clinics of North America, Elsevier Health Sciences Division, Subscription Customer Service, 3251 Riverport Lane, Maryland Heights, MO 63043. **Customer Service: 1-800-654-2452 (US and Canada). From outside of the US and Canada: 1-314-447-8871. Fax: 1-314-447-8029. For print support, E-mail: JournalsCustomerService-usa@elsevier.com. For online support, E-mail: JournalsOnlineSupport-usa@elsevier.com.**

Reprints. For copies of 100 or more, of articles in this publication, please contact the Commercial Reprints Department, Elsevier Inc., 360 Park Avenue South, New York, NY 10010-1710. Tel.: 212-633-3874; Fax: 212-633-3820; E-mail: reprints@elsevier.com.

The Pediatric Clinics of North America is also published in Spanish by McGraw-Hill Inter-americana Editores S.A., Mexico City, Mexico; in Portuguese by Riechmann and Affonso Editores, Rua Comandante Coelho 1085, CEP 21250, Rio de Janeiro, Brazil; and in Greek by Althayia SA, Athens, Greece.

The Pediatric Clinics of North America is covered in MEDLINE/PubMed (Index Medicus), Excerpta Medica, Current Contents, Current Contents/Clinical Medicine, Science Citation Index, ASCA, ISI/BIOMED, and BIOSIS.

PROGRAM OBJECTIVE

The goal of the *Pediatric Clinics of North America* is to keep practicing physicians and residents up to date with current clinical practice in pediatrics by providing timely articles reviewing the state-of-the-art in patient care.

TARGET AUDIENCE

All practicing pediatricians, physicians and healthcare professionals who provide patient care to pediatric patients.

LEARNING OBJECTIVES

Upon completion of this activity, participants will be able to:
1. Discuss child abuse prevention.
2. Recognize advocacy opportunities for pediatricians caring for maltreated children.
3. Review what to expect when working with child protective services and law enforcement.

ACCREDITATION

The Elsevier Office of Continuing Medical Education (EOCME) is accredited by the Accreditation Council for Continuing Medical Education (ACCME) to provide continuing medical education for physicians.

The EOCME designates this enduring material for a maximum of 15 *AMA PRA Category 1 Credit*(s) ™. Physicians should claim only the credit commensurate with the extent of their participation in the activity.

All other health care professionals requesting continuing education credit for this enduring material will be issued a certificate of participation.

DISCLOSURE OF CONFLICTS OF INTEREST

The EOCME assesses conflict of interest with its instructors, faculty, planners, and other individuals who are in a position to control the content of CME activities. All relevant conflicts of interest that are identified are thoroughly vetted by EOCME for fair balance, scientific objectivity, and patient care recommendations. EOCME is committed to providing its learners with CME activities that promote improvements or quality in healthcare and not a specific proprietary business or a commercial interest.

The planning committee, staff, authors and editors listed below have identified no financial relationships or relationships to products or devices they or their spouse/life partner have with commercial interest related to the content of this CME activity:

Carol Berkowitz, MD; Andrew M. Campbell, BS; James E. Crawford-Jakubiak, MD, FAAP; Howard Dubowitz, MD; Heather C. Forkey, MD; Nancy S. Harper, MD, FAAP; Roberta Hibbard, MD; Kerry Holland; Brynne Hunter; Kim Kaczor, MS; Nancy D. Kellogg, MD; Gauri Kolhatkar, MD, MPH, FAAP; Indu Kumari; Wendy G. Lane, MD, MPH; Antoinette L. Laskey, MD, MPH; Sandy Lavery; John Mischel Leventhal, MD; Jill McNair; John D. Melville, MD; Rebecca Moles, MD; Lindsay Parnell; Hillary W. Petska, MD; Mary Clyde Pierce, MD; Lynn K. Sheets, MD; Bonita F. Stanton, MD; John Stirling, MD; Moira Szylagi, MD, PhD; Richard Thompson, PhD; Adrienne A. Williams, PhD; Katherine S. Wright, MA; Adam J. Zolotor, MD, DrPH MD, DrPH.

The planning committee, staff, authors and editors listed below have identified financial relationships or relationships to products or devices they or their spouse/life partner have with commercial interest related to the content of this CME activity:

Andrea Asnes, MD, MSW is a paid consultant and child welfare expert to law enforcement, child welfare defense and patient attorneys.
Sandeep K. Narang, MD is a consultant/advisor in child maltreatment cases.

UNAPPROVED/OFF-LABEL USE DISCLOSURE

The EOCME requires CME faculty to disclose to the participants:
1. When products or procedures being discussed are off-label, unlabelled, experimental, and/or investigational (not US Food and Drug Administration (FDA) approved); and
2. Any limitations on the information presented, such as data that are preliminary or that represent ongoing research, interim analyses, and/or unsupported opinions. Faculty may discuss information about pharmaceutical agents that is outside of FDA-approved labelling. This information is intended solely for CME and is not intended to promote off-label use of these medications. If you have any questions, contact the medical affairs department of the manufacturer for the most recent prescribing information.

TO ENROLL

To enroll in the *Pediatric Clinics of North America* Continuing Medical Education program, call customer service at 1-800-654-2452 or sign up online at http://www.theclinics.com/home/cme. The CME program is available to subscribers for an additional annual fee of USD 290.

METHOD OF PARTICIPATION

In order to claim credit, participants must complete the following:

1. Complete enrolment as indicated above.
2. Read the activity.
3. Complete the CME Test and Evaluation. Participants must achieve a score of 70% on the test. All CME Tests and Evaluations must be completed online.

CME INQUIRIES/SPECIAL NEEDS

For all CME inquiries or special needs, please contact elsevierCME@elsevier.com.

Contributors

CONSULTING EDITOR

BONITA F. STANTON, MD
Vice Dean for Research and Professor of Pediatrics, School of Medicine, Wayne State University, Detroit, Michigan

EDITORS

HOWARD DUBOWITZ, MD, MS
Professor, Department of Pediatrics; Head, Division of Child Protection, University of Maryland School of Medicine, University of Maryland Medical Center, Baltimore, Maryland

JOHN M. LEVENTHAL, MD
Professor of Pediatrics (General Pediatrics) and in the Child Study Center and Clinical Professor of Nursing; Child Abuse Programs and Prevention Programs, Department of Pediatrics, Yale-New Haven Children's Hospital, Medical Director, Yale Medical School, New Haven, Connecticut

AUTHORS

ANDREA G. ASNES, MD, MSW
Department of Pediatrics, Yale School of Medicine, New Haven, Connecticut

CAROL BERKOWITZ, MD, FAAP, FACEP
Executive Vice Chair, Department of Pediatrics, Harbor-UCLA Medical Center; Distinguished Professor of Pediatrics, David Geffen School of Medicine at UCLA, Torrance, California

ANDREW M. CAMPBELL, BS
Research/Data Specialist, Section of Child Protection Programs, Indiana University School of Medicine, Indianapolis, Indiana

JAMES E. CRAWFORD-JAKUBIAK, MD, FAAP
Medical Director, Center for Child Protection, UCSF Benioff Children's Hospital Oakland, Oakland, California

HOWARD DUBOWITZ, MD, MS
Professor, Department of Pediatrics; Head, Division of Child Protection, University of Maryland School of Medicine, University of Maryland Medical Center, Baltimore, Maryland

HEATHER FORKEY, MD
Clinical Director, Foster Children Evaluation Service (FaCES); Assistant Professor of Pediatrics, UMass Children's Medical Center, University of Massachusetts Medical School, Worcester, Massachusetts

NANCY S. HARPER, MD
Clinical Associate Professor of Pediatrics, Texas A&M University, College Station, Texas; Children's Physician Services of South Texas, Driscoll Children's Hospital, Corpus Christi, Texas

ROBERTA HIBBARD, MD
Professor of Pediatrics and Director, Section of Child Protection Programs, Indiana University School of Medicine, Indianapolis, Indiana

KIM KACZOR, MS
Division of Emergency Medicine, Ann & Robert H. Lurie Children's Hospital of Chicago, Chicago, Illinois

NANCY D. KELLOGG, MD
Professor and Division Chief, Child Abuse, Department of Pediatrics, University of Texas Health Science Center at San Antonio; Center for Miracles, San Antonio, Texas

GAURI KOLHATKAR, MD, MPH, FAAP
Fellow, Child Abuse Pediatrics, Harbor-UCLA Medical Center, Torrance, California

WENDY GWIRTZMAN LANE, MD, MPH
Associate Professor, Department of Epidemiology and Public Health; Department of Pediatrics, University of Maryland School of Medicine, Baltimore, Maryland

ANTOINETTE L. LASKEY, MD, MPH
Associate Professor, Department of Pediatrics, Primary Children's Hospital, University of Utah School of Medicine, Salt Lake City, Utah

JOHN M. LEVENTHAL, MD
Professor of Pediatrics (General Pediatrics) and in the Child Study Center and Clinical Professor of Nursing; Child Abuse Programs and Prevention Programs, Department of Pediatrics, Yale-New Haven Children's Hospital, Medical Director, Yale Medical School, New Haven, Connecticut

JOHN D. MELVILLE, MD
Site Director, Child Advocacy Center, Akron Children's Hospital, Boardman, Ohio

REBECCA L. MOLES, MD
Department of Pediatrics, Yale School of Medicine, New Haven, Connecticut

SANDEEP K. NARANG, MD, JD
Assistant Professor, Pediatrics, UTHSC-Houston, Houston, Texas

HILLARY W. PETSKA, MD
Child Abuse Pediatrics Fellow and Instructor of Pediatrics, Children's Hospital of Wisconsin, Medical College of Wisconsin, Milwaukee, Wisconsin

MARY CLYDE PIERCE, MD
Division of Emergency Medicine, Ann & Robert H. Lurie Children's Hospital of Chicago; Department of Pediatrics, Northwestern University Feinberg School of Medicine, Chicago, Illinois

LYNN K. SHEETS, MD
Professor and Medical Director, Children's Hospital of Wisconsin, Medical College of Wisconsin, Milwaukee, Wisconsin

JOHN STIRLING, MD
Director, Center for Child Protection, Santa Clara Valley Medical Center, San Jose, California; Clinical Professor of Pediatrics (affiliated), Lucile Packard Children's Hospital Stanford, Palo Alto, California

MOIRA SZILAGYI, MD, PhD
Professor, Division of General Pediatrics, Department of Pediatrics, University of Rochester, Rochester, New York

RICHARD THOMPSON, PhD
Richard H. Calica Center for Innovation in Children and Family Services, Juvenile Protective Association, Chicago, Illinois

ADRIENNE A. WILLIAMS, PhD
Assistant Professor, Department of Family and Community Medicine, University of Maryland School of Medicine, Baltimore, Maryland

KATHERINE S. WRIGHT, MA
Doctoral Candidate, University of Maryland, Baltimore, Maryland

ADAM J. ZOLOTOR, MD, DrPH
Associate Professor, Department of Family Medicine, University of North Carolina at Chapel Hill, Chapel Hill, North Carolina

Contents

Child abuse and neglect are inherently challenging problems for pediatricians. It is hoped that this article makes this work easier, albeit not easy, and highlights the many ways that pediatricians can make a valuable difference in the lives of these vulnerable children and their families.

Pediatricians and other health care providers can play several important roles in the prevention of child maltreatment. This article aims to help pediatricians incorporate child abuse prevention into their practice. Resources for systematizing anticipatory guidance and screening for risk factors in child maltreatment are described. The modalities, strengths, and weaknesses of community-based prevention programs are discussed, and tools with which providers can identify the effectiveness of available community-based programs are offered. On a broader level, ways whereby pediatricians can advocate at the local, state, and national levels for policies and programs that support families and children are described.

The social environment of a child is a key determinant of the child's current and future health. Factors in a child's family environment, both protective and harmful, have a profound impact on a child's long-term health, brain development, and mortality. The social history may be the best all-around tool available for promoting a child's future health and well-being. It is a key first step in identifying social needs of a child and family so that they may benefit from intervention. This article focuses on key social history elements known to increase a child's risk of maltreatment and provides case examples.

Helping parents change key behaviors may reduce the risk of child maltreatment. However, traditional provider-centered approaches to working with the parents of pediatric patients may increase resistance to behavioral change. Motivational interviewing (MI) is a patient-centered communication technique that helps address problems of provider-centered approaches. In this article, evidence for use of MI to address several risk factors for child maltreatment is reviewed, including parental substance abuse, partner violence, depression treatment, harsh punishment, and parental management of children's health. Fundamental components of MI that may be incorporated into clinical practice are presented.

Injuries, other than abrasions, are rare in precruising infants. In this population, a history or observation of a sentinel skin injury, intraoral injury, or musculoskeletal injury without a plausible explanation, is concerning for physical abuse. A precruising infant with a sentinel injury should be medically evaluated for occult injury and predisposing medical conditions, as well as reported to authorities for further investigation. Early identification of sentinel injuries and appropriate interventions can prevent further abuse.

Medical providers need to monitor growth at every visit. Weight status is influenced by genetics, medical conditions, socioeconomic status, and family environment. Screening for food security and psychosocial risk factors is an integral tool to identify families at risk for nutritional deficits and child maltreatment. Nutritional rehabilitation is best accomplished in an outpatient, multidisciplinary setting. Medical neglect should be considered in failure to thrive and obesity when there is a serious risk of harm from identified medical complications, additional or worsening medical complications occurring despite a multidisciplinary approach, and/or non-adherence with the treatment plan.

Emotional maltreatment may be the most complex, prevalent, and damaging form of child maltreatment and can occur simultaneously with other forms of abuse. Children in the first few years of life seem to be at the greatest risk of suffering the most negative outcomes. Medical professionals can help identify and protect victims of emotional maltreatment by carefully observing caregiver-child interactions, paying attention to a family's social history, making referrals to community or counseling programs when necessary, and reporting any suspicions of maltreatment to Child Protective Services. A well-coordinated, multidisciplinary response must be enacted whenever emotional maltreatment is suspected or reported.

Corporal punishment is used for discipline in most homes in the United States. It is also associated with a long list of adverse developmental, behavioral, and health-related consequences. Primary care providers, as trusted sources for parenting information, have an opportunity to engage parents in discussions about discipline as early as infancy. These discussions should focus on building parents' skills in the use of other behavioral techniques, limiting (or eliminating) the use of corporal punishment and identifying additional resources as needed.

This article reviews some of the challenges and pitfalls in communicating with families when abuse is part of the differential diagnosis and offers some suggestions for improving communication with parents and children in these challenging clinical settings.

Cognitive errors have been studied in a broad array of fields, including medicine. The more that is understood about how the human mind processes complex information, the more it becomes clear that certain situations are particularly susceptible to less than optimal outcomes because of these errors. This article explores how some of the known cognitive errors may influence the diagnosis of child abuse, resulting in both false-negative and false-positive diagnoses. Suggested remedies for these errors are offered.

Cultural diversity poses challenges within the health care setting, particularly regarding the question of how health professionals can resolve the tension between respecting cultural norms or child-rearing practices and the importance of determining what constitutes harm and child maltreatment. Cultural competency and respect for cultural diversity does not imply universal tolerance of all practices. The United Nations provides a standard of universal child rights, protecting them from harmful practices. Pediatric providers must respect cross-cultural differences while maintaining legal and ethical standards of safety and wellbeing for children, promoting evidence-based prevention of maltreatment, and advocating for child wellness across all cultures.

Uncertainty in the diagnosis of abuse can have profound implications for the health and safety of the child, the emotional burden of a family, and investigative and criminal proceedings. A logical algorithm for addressing physical and sexual abuse cases that details aspects contributing to the uncertainty may aid the clinician in making a diagnosis and in communicating the crucial details to the relevant investigative agencies. This article defines and discusses uncertainty in the realms of physical and sexual abuse, and suggests an approach to managing uncertainty while still providing valuable information for the medical and child protective service systems.

Nancy D. Kellogg

The process whereby a clinician decides that child abuse is a diagnostic possibility is often marked with doubt and fear. Abusive parents can present convincing lies, and children with suspicious injuries can have unusual accidents. Personal thresholds for reporting suspected abuse vary considerably. Clinicians may mistrust or misunderstand the roles and responsibilities of the investigators and legal professionals involved. This article aims to improve understanding of the community responses to a report of child abuse, and enable the clinician to work effectively with child protective services, law enforcement agencies, and legal professionals to ensure child safety and family integrity when appropriate.

Sandeep K. Narang and John D. Melville

The most common medicolegal issues include reporting child maltreatment, the presentation of ethical and effective expert testimony, informed consent in child maltreatment cases, and various liability risks related to child maltreatment cases. The health care professional who remains knowledgeable about the laws within their jurisdiction, the mandates of their professional society and state medical board, and the local resources (eg, child abuse pediatrician and hospital counsel) available to them minimizes medicolegal risk.

Heather Forkey and Moira Szilagyi

Children enter foster care with many forms of adversity and trauma beyond maltreatment that impact their short- and long-term physical, mental, and developmental health and their adaptation to their new care environment. Applying an understanding of the impact of toxic stress on the developing brain and body allows the health care provider to understand findings in this vulnerable population. Complex trauma alters immune response, neurodevelopment, and the genome, resulting in predictable and significant cognitive, behavioral, and physical consequences. Pediatric care of children in foster care must be trauma informed to meet their medical, mental health, and developmental needs.

James E. Crawford-Jakubiak

Pediatricians are advocates for children. It is one of the central elements of the job description. In the course of their work, pediatricians have many opportunities to advocate for abused and neglected children. The most effective form of advocacy that most pediatricians will engage in with regard to child abuse and neglect is by being highly skilled doctors who provide excellent clinical care to children and families, knowing how to recognize child abuse and what to do when they encounter it, and being familiar with the resources of their communities.

PEDIATRIC CLINICS OF NORTH AMERICA

Foreword

Child Maltreatment and Prevention

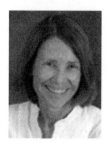

Bonita F. Stanton, MD
Consulting Editor

Child abuse is a global problem, occurring in virtually every society throughout the world.[1] Child abuse is not a product of modern society; archeological remains indicate that the practice has been present for at least many centuries.[2] In the United States, about 9 children per 1000 are victimized annually, with four-fifths of the children victimized suffering from neglect, nearly one-fifth suffering from physical abuse, one-tenth suffering from sexual abuse, and almost one-tenth suffering from psychological abuse.[3]

Most clinically active pediatricians, irrespective of their subspecialty and/or geographic or socioeconomic site of practice, are likely to encounter children who have been abused. The challenge will be in recognizing the abuse and responding appropriately, in a manner that safeguards the child and other children in the family, and offers the family support, guidance, and respect.

Drs Dubowitz and Leventhal have spent their careers working with children and impacted families and institutions. Their approach, predicated on the power of knowledge, understanding, and compassion, empowers the pediatrician to appropriately recognize, explore, refer, and remain involved with impacted children and families. While unambiguously maintaining the primacy of the impacted child in their approach, the authors of the articles in this volume empower pediatricians to recognize vulnerable children, seek information as necessary from families and children in a gentle, caring, and nonthreatening manner, and act appropriately based on this information. As this volume is written for practicing pediatricians, several articles deal explicitly with

Pediatr Clin N Am 61 (2014) xv–xvi
http://dx.doi.org/10.1016/j.pcl.2014.07.002
0031-3955/14/$ – see front matter © 2014 Published by Elsevier Inc.

pediatric.theclinics.com

preventing child abuse through appropriate counseling of families before abuse occurs and engaging with children and families in the aftermath of abuse.

Bonita F. Stanton, MD
School of Medicine
Wayne State University
1261 Scott Hall
540 East Canfield, Suite 1261
Detroit, MI 48201, USA

E-mail address:
bstanton@med.wayne.edu

REFERENCES

1. Available at: http://www.internationalcap.org. Accessed on August 5, 2014.
2. Wheeler SM, Williams L, Beauchesne P, et al. Shattered lives and broken childhoods: evidence of physical child abuse in ancient Egypt. Int J Paleopathol 2013;3:71–82.
3. U.S. Department of Health and Human Services, Administration for Children and Families, Administration on Children, Youth and Families, Children's Bureau. Child maltreatment 2012. Washington, DC: 2013. http://www.acf.hhs.gov/sites/default/files/cb/cm2012.pdf. Accessed.

Preface

Addressing Child Maltreatment: Helping Those on the Frontlines

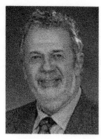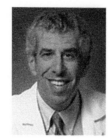

Howard Dubowitz, MD, MS   John M. Leventhal, MD
Editors

There is no doubt that child abuse and neglect are serious problems in every country. They are far too prevalent and often lead to a variety of adverse outcomes, some fatal and some lifelong. Pediatricians and other child health professionals are well-positioned to play a valuable role in helping to address this problem. But child maltreatment is inherently complex, posing difficult challenges for those on the frontlines caring for children. The goal of this volume is to effectively support pediatricians and other professionals in their roles. A priority is to offer practical information and guidance that many will find useful.

Pediatric primary care provides a unique opportunity to tackle child abuse and neglect. In the United States in particular, primary care is a well-established system, and most children have multiple visits, especially in the first few years. There is typically a very good relationship between parents and health professionals, who are respected experts on children. The interested pediatrician, thus, has a remarkable entrée into the workings of a family, its shortcomings, and its strengths. With some knowledge and skill, pediatricians can play a pivotal role, even in a few strategic minutes. We know, however, that some professionals feel very uncomfortable becoming involved in this unpleasant area and may be deterred from taking any action. Understandable as this may be, it can jeopardize a child's health and safety. Hopefully, this issue of *Pediatric Clinics of North America* will help make this work a bit easier, albeit not easy.

With training and support, pediatricians can equip themselves to be competent and more comfortable addressing child maltreatment. Aside from the possible forensic implications, the heart of this work is primarily about helping families take adequate or good care of their children. Indeed, helping address child abuse and neglect also

Pediatr Clin N Am 61 (2014) xvii–xviii
http://dx.doi.org/10.1016/j.pcl.2014.07.001
0031-3955/14/$ – see front matter © 2014 Published by Elsevier Inc.

helps promote children's health, development, and safety, and it is central to the rich mandate of Pediatrics.

Howard Dubowitz, MD, MS
Pediatrics
University of Maryland
520 W. Lombard Street
Baltimore, MD 21201, USA

John M. Leventhal, MD
Yale Medical School
Child Abuse Programs
Yale-New Haven Children's Hospital
New Haven, CT 06510, USA

E-mail addresses:
hdubowitz@peds.umaryland.edu (H. Dubowitz)
john.leventhal@yale.edu (J.M. Leventhal)

The Pediatrician and Child Maltreatment
Principles and Pointers for Practice

Howard Dubowitz, MD, MS[a],*, John M. Leventhal, MD[b]

KEYWORDS

- Child maltreatment • Pediatric practice • Principles

KEY POINTS

- An ecologic model of parenting includes risk and protective factors at the level of the child, parent, family, and community/social setting.
- Primary care clinicians have the potential to engage families and focus on prevention of abuse and neglect.
- To provide effective help to children and families, pediatricians need to partner with community agencies.
- Pediatricians need to follow the mandated reporting laws and report suspected abuse, neglect, or sexual abuse to Child Protective Services.

It is more than 50 years since Kempe and colleagues's[1] seminal report on the "battered child," and since then, much has been learned about child abuse and neglect. Despite considerable advances, however, addressing child maltreatment, including physical, sexual, and emotional abuse and neglect, remains a daunting challenge for many pediatricians. In this issue of *Pediatric Clinics of North America*, we have invited authors to help address conceptual and clinical issues facing many practitioners all too frequently.

In this introductory article, we set the stage with broad principles that guide clinical work regarding child maltreatment and offer useful pointers for practice. First, it is helpful to consider the broader context for viewing child maltreatment and significant developments in the understanding of children's health and development and pediatric practice.

Disclosures: None.
[a] Department of Pediatrics, University of Maryland School of Medicine, 520 West Lombard Street, Baltimore, MD 21201, USA; [b] Child Abuse Programs and Prevention Programs, Department of Pediatrics, Yale-New Haven Children's Hospital, Yale Medical School, 333 Cedar Street, New Haven, CT 06520, USA
* Corresponding author.
E-mail address: hdubowitz@peds.umaryland.edu

Pediatr Clin N Am 61 (2014) 865–871
http://dx.doi.org/10.1016/j.pcl.2014.06.001   pediatric.theclinics.com

IMPORTANCE OF THE FIRST FEW YEARS

For decades, pediatricians have been well aware of how critical the first few years of life are for child and brain development.[2] Exciting advances in neuroimaging have further refined this understanding. Indeed, brain architecture is found to be influenced by young children's environment and interpersonal interactions. This, in turn, influences their cognitive, social, and emotional development, perhaps for many years.[3] Although the first few years are especially important, the story hardly ends at age 3. Rather, influences during childhood, adolescence, and even into a person's 20s are also significant in shaping health and development.

TOXIC STRESS

Unfortunately, many children live with multiple adversities, the effect of which can be toxic stress. Shonkoff and colleagues[4] defined toxic stress as resulting "from strong, frequent, or prolonged activation of the body's stress response systems in the absence of the buffering protection of a supportive, adult relationship." Turner and colleagues[5] found the remarkable prevalence of adversities with which many children and youth contend and that many of them face not 1 or 2 but multiple adversities.

Different forms of child abuse and neglect can lead to toxic stress. These and other risk factors, such as parental substance abuse and depression, were found in the Adverse Childhood Experiences Study to potentially induce a toxic stress response and were linked to poor mental and physical health outcomes many years later.[6–8] It is thought that this stress response disrupts brain circuitry and other organ and metabolic systems during sensitive developmental periods. Such disruption may result in anatomic changes or physiologic dysregulations that are the precursors of later impairments in learning and behavior and are the roots of chronic, stress-related physical and mental illness. In an effort to cope with these chronic stresses and the emotional pain linked to the childhood adversities, many teens and adults turn to cigarettes, drugs, alcohol, or overeating; these maladaptive coping strategies can lead to their own serious health effects.

The potential role of toxic stress and early life adversity in the pathogenesis of health problems underscores the importance of effective surveillance for significant risk factors in the primary health care setting. There are clear implications for pediatricians: how can clinicians prevent or mitigate the toxic stress in many children's lives and help ensure their health and wellbeing well into adulthood?

A BROAD VIEW OF MALTREATMENT

The battered child report by Kempe and colleagues[1] focused on severe physical abuse. Subsequently, concerns of neglect, sexual abuse, and emotional abuse were all added as different forms of child maltreatment. As more has been learned about conditions or circumstances that harm children, other parental behaviors are increasingly viewed as maltreatment. For example, corporal punishment has long been accepted as appropriate for socializing children; some regard it as necessary. Mounting evidence, however, points to the potentially harmful physical and psychological impact of harsh punishment.[9] Arguably, this can be considered maltreatment, although most such instances are not addressed through Child Protective Services (CPS). Children's exposure to domestic (or intimate partner) violence is another example. Many studies show that exposure to domestic violence jeopardizes children's health, development, and safety—directly or indirectly.[10,11] Some CPS agencies now expect mandated reporters also to report children's exposure to domestic violence as maltreatment. Still more broadly, Gil[12] drew attention to societal neglect. Although the current focus is narrowly and conveniently on parental behavior, there are reasonable concerns regarding societal contributions to children's poor health and development. For example, poverty remains the strongest predictor of many bad child outcomes, and approximately 1 in 5 US children live in poverty.[13] Another example is the lack of health insurance, affecting 6.6 million US children in 2012[14]; the associations between health problems and limited access to health care have been well established.[15]

DEVELOPMENT OF THE FIELD OF PEDIATRICS

Twentieth century advances in public health, immunizations, antibiotics, and nutrition dramatically improved the health of many US children. These advances enabled increased attention to children's quality of life and their environment. Thus, new problems came into focus: divorce, teenage pregnancy, child abuse, and attention deficit disorder, to name a few; these were labeled the "New Morbidity."[16] Today, these and other problems such as obesity, the impact on children of the media, school violence, firearms in the home, and drug and alcohol abuse have become important concerns for pediatric practice.

Despite recognition of the new morbidity, however, medical training has been slow to adapt, and practitioners often do not feel comfortable addressing problems such as child abuse and neglect.[17] There is a clear need to better educate pediatricians in such areas and to develop models by which they can readily consult with subspecialists. The American Academy of Pediatrics' Bright Futures Project supports pediatricians in addressing the new morbidity.[18]

BEYOND THE BIOMEDICAL MODEL

Engel[19] was a psychiatrist concerned with the traditional narrow biomedical model of health and illness. Although the role of psychological and environmental influences had been recognized by the ancient Greeks, Engel[19] was concerned with modern medicine being increasingly focused on the molecular level. In a seminal report on a biopsychosocial model, Engel postulated that biological, psychological (including thoughts, emotions, and behaviors), and social factors all significantly influence human functioning, health, and illness. For example, a low-income family living in substandard housing with mold and cockroaches may trigger asthma attacks in its young child. In addition, the burdens of poverty may contribute to the mother's depression and alcohol abuse. In turn, she neglects to fill her child's prescription, aggravating the asthma. The implications for child abuse and neglect are clear.

Child maltreatment cannot simply be explained by sick or deviant parents. Rather, multiple and interacting factors are usually contributing to the problem. This understanding has been labeled the "ecological model," acknowledging the potential role of the individual child and parent, family level, and community/societal factors.[20] This model does not excuse parents from their primary responsibility to raise and protect their child. It does, however, draw attention to other factors that also deserve attention, including, for example, social policies to improve children's access to health care. Clinically, the need for collaborative interdisciplinary assessment and interventions is evident.

PROTECTIVE FACTORS

Child abuse and neglect cannot be fully understood by identifying risk factors. The role of protective factors that may buffer the impact of problems also needs consideration.[21] These may be internal, such as a child's intelligence or a father's caring for his child. They may be external, such as a supportive grandparent, a substance abuse treatment program, or a helpful pediatrician. Indeed, risk and protective factors can be found in most individuals and families. It is especially useful to identify protective factors, as they offer a constructive way to work with families. For example, rather than admonishing a parent for not filling a prescription, one can point to the father's love of his child, and say: "I can see how much you love Amy. You really don't want her back in the hospital. How can we make sure we keep her healthy?" This is not about being nice; rather, it is about being constructive and strategic in how best to engage parents and optimize children's care.

THE POTENTIAL OF PRIMARY CARE

There are several reasons why pediatric primary care offers a valuable opportunity for helping prevent child maltreatment.[22] Primary care already exists as an institution with an infrastructure. There is no need to build a whole new organization or system of care. Most children are brought in for multiple checkups, especially in the first 5 years. The focus of this care is on prevention and the early identification of problems. There has long been the understanding that it is not sufficient for health professionals to focus narrowly on just the child. Attention also needs to be paid to the home and family environments that naturally influence children's health, development, and safety.

A useful advantage of the health care system is that it does not have the stigma often associated with mental health and CPS. On the contrary, there is usually a good relationship between child health professionals and parents, with pediatricians being trusted as credible experts on children. This relationship offers health professionals an excellent opportunity to learn about the family and help address identified problems. Arguably, with such an opportunity there is a responsibility—to help.

PRACTICAL POINTERS FOR PRACTICE

Below are 8 key points to keep in mind that will enhance the care of all children and enable the appropriate recognition and management when maltreatment is suspected.

1. Prevention, which is the hallmark of pediatric care, should be a priority.[23] Each pediatric visit offers the opportunity to promote healthy and nurturing relationships between caregivers and children; to use active listening; to identify risk and protective factors; to recognize problems at the early stages; and to link families to community resources.
2. Although it is important to know when to suspect child maltreatment and follow the mandated reporting laws, it is equally important to communicate effectively about the plan to report to CPS and to help families through the crisis. When possible, the pediatrician can tell families in a forthright but kind way that one is making a report to CPS. "Whenever I see an injury (problem, child's condition) like this, I worry that Bobby may have been hurt by an adult, and I have to report this to Child Protective Services. Do you know what that agency does?"[24] It also is critical to tell the family about the process and that you will be available to provide follow-up to the child, speak with the parents by phone or at visits, and support them.
3. It is helpful to think of abuse and neglect as signs or symptoms. Thus, recognizing child maltreatment also means recognizing those critical aspects of the parent-child relationship, the family, and the social settings that are related to the maltreatment. How did the family's response to the recent stress of the father losing his job

link to the unexplained injury? Or how did the mother's depression contribute to the child's inadequate supervision and resultant injury? In each of these cases, the pediatrician might work with the caregivers to understand the underlying stresses, how the family is coping, and what services might help alleviate the stresses or help the family cope more effectively. The goal, of course, would be early recognition of the stresses before maltreatment occurs.

4. In many situations, pediatricians recognize problems that are of concern but do not necessarily rise to the level of reasonable suspicion of abuse or neglect, and reporting to CPS may not be appropriate. The challenge in these cases is to partner with the family, develop a plan to improve the situation, and offer support while monitoring the progress. It is important to work with the family to prioritize the problems to be addressed. The pediatrician can use his or her relationship with the caregivers to communicate concerns, convey useful information, express interest in helping, work with the family in developing a plan, and facilitate referrals to community resources. If at follow-up, the clinician's concern has increased, then the pediatrician needs to reevaluate the concern for maltreatment and decide whether it is necessary to report the child to CPS.

Various CPS agencies are responding to many first reports of suspected neglect using an alternative (or differential) response. This response offers a fundamentally different approach. The usual investigation aimed at finding fault is replaced with an evaluation of functioning to determine the family's needs and connect them with services. Research indicates that this promising approach has not compromised children's safety.[25] Not surprisingly, CPS workers and families are more satisfied with this alternative response.

5. To be effective at helping families address the caregiver's stresses that can impair relationships within families, including caregiver-child relationships, pediatricians need to know about and partner with community resources. Such resources might help parents (eg, mental health services, substance abuse treatment), children (eg, early intervention programs, preschool), or parent-child relationships (eg, parenting programs).

6. Although pediatricians are most used to working with mothers, engaging fathers and learning about them at health maintenance visits provide a broader perspective on the family's risk and protective factors. Also important is the understanding that serious abuse, such as fractures and head trauma, in young children is often perpetrated by men, including fathers, stepfathers, and mothers' boyfriends.[26,27] Thus, understanding the father's role in the child's life, such as how the father responds to the infant's crying or how the father who cares for the child while the mother is at work manages the 2-year-old's temper tantrums, expands the pediatrician's perspective and provides opportunities for interventions.

7. At the local, state, and federal levels, pediatricians can advocate for the development of or expansion of services for all children, especially for vulnerable children. Being actively involved in the American Academy of Pediatrics' state chapter is an excellent way of supporting services for children. Working through the American Academy of Pediatrics, pediatricians can also effectively reach state and federal legislators to advocate for specific community and regional needs.

8. Finally, it is important to recognize that child maltreatment can have a personal toll on the providers of care. Vicarious trauma refers to the impact on helping professionals that can occur from caring for children and families.[28] Seeing children's injuries and hearing about their suffering can evoke emotional pain and anger. For some who have experienced abuse or neglect themselves during childhood, this may be especially challenging. It is important for the pediatrician to be aware of

such thoughts and feelings and have constructive ways to address them. There are many options, such as talking with colleagues, a partner, or friends; exercise, music, or other activities; or seeking professional help. Keeping in mind the ecologic model may also help. Child abuse and neglect is seldom simply about bad parents who do not care. Rather, there are typically multiple and interacting factors that impair parents' wishes to see their children do well.

SUMMARY

Child abuse and neglect are inherently challenging problems for pediatricians. It is hoped that this article makes this work easier, albeit not easy, and highlights the many ways that pediatricians can make a valuable difference in the lives of these vulnerable children and their families.

REFERENCES

1. Kempe CH, Silverman FN, Steele BF, et al. The battered-child syndrome. JAMA 1962;181:17–24.
2. Piaget J. The origins of intelligence in children. New York: International Universities Press; 1952.
3. National Scientific Council on the Developing Child. Excessive Stress Disrupts the Architecture of the Developing Brain: Working Paper #3. Available at: http://developingchild.harvard.edu/resources/reports_and_working_papers/. Accessed February 12, 2014.
4. Shonkoff JP, Richter L, van der Gaag J, et al. An integrated scientific framework for child survival and early childhood development. Pediatrics 2012;129: e460–72.
5. Turner HA, Finkelhor D, Ormrod R, et al. Family context, victimization, and child trauma symptoms: variations in safe, stable, and nurturing relationships during early and middle childhood. Am J Orthopsychiatry 2012;82:209–19.
6. Felitti VJ, Anda RF, Nordenberg D, et al. Relationship of childhood abuse and household dysfunction to many of the leading causes of death in adults. The Adverse Childhood Experiences (ACE) study. Am J Prev Med 1998;14:245–58.
7. Dube SR, Anda RF, Felitti VJ, et al. Growing up with parental alcohol abuse: exposure to childhood abuse, neglect, and household dysfunction. Child Abuse Negl 2001;25:1627–40.
8. Anda RF, Felitti VJ, Bremner JD, et al. The enduring effects of abuse and related adverse experiences in childhood. A convergence of evidence from neurobiology and epidemiology. Eur Arch Psychiatry Clin Neurosci 2006;256:174–86.
9. Gershoff ET. Spanking and child development: we know enough now to stop hitting our children. Child Dev Perspect 2013;7:133–7.
10. Thackery JD, Hibbard R, Dowd MD. Committee on child abuse and neglect; committee on injury, violence, and poison prevention. intimate partner violence: the role of the pediatrician. Pediatrics 2010;125:1094–100.
11. Asnes AG, Leventhal JM. Children's experiences of IPV: time for pediatricians to take action. JAMA Pediatr 2013;167:299–300.
12. Gil D. Violence against children: physical abuse in the United States. Cambridge (England): Harvard University Press; 1970.
13. National Center for Children in Poverty. Available at: http://nccp.org/. Accessed April 19, 2014.
14. U.S. Census Bureau. Available at: http://www.census.gov/newsroom/releases/archives/income_wealth/cb13-165.html. Accessed April 19, 2014.

15. Mehta S, Nagar S, Aparasu R. Unmet prescription medication need in U.S. children. J Am Pharm Assoc 2009;49:769–76.
16. Haggerty RJ, Roghmann KJ, Pless IB. Child health and the community. 2nd edition. New Brunswick (Canada): Transaction Publishers; 1993.
17. Lane WG, Dubowitz H, Langenberg P. Primary care pediatricians' experience, comfort and competence in the evaluation and management of child maltreatment: do we need child abuse experts? Child Abuse Negl 2009;33:76–83.
18. Bright Futures. Available at: http://brightfutures.aap.org/index.html. Accessed April 19, 2014.
19. Engel GE. The need for a new medical model. Science 1977;196:129–36.
20. Belsky J. Child maltreatment: an ecological integration. Am Psychol 1980;35: 320–35.
21. National Research Council and Institute of Medicine. Risk and protective factors for mental, emotional, and behavioral disorders across the life cycle. Washington, DC: U.S. Department of Health and Human Services; 2010.
22. Dubowitz H, Feigelman S, Lane W, et al. Pediatric primary care to help prevent child maltreatment: the Safe Environment for Every Kid (SEEK) model. Pediatrics 2009;123:858–64.
23. National Center for Injury Prevention and Control at the US Centers for Disease Control and Prevention. Essentials for childhood: steps to creating safe, stable and nurturing relationships. 2013. Available at: www.cdc.gov/violenceprevention/pdf/efc-01-03-2013-a.pdf. Accessed April 27, 2014.
24. Asnes AG, Leventhal JM. Managing child abuse: general principles. Pediatr Rev 2010;31:47–55.
25. Quality Improvement Center on Differential Response in Child Protective Services. Differential response in child protective services: a literature review. Children's Bureau, US Department of Health and Human Services Administration for Children and Families; 2009. Available at: www.differentialresponseqic.org/assets/docs/quilt-review-sept-09/pdf. Accessed April 10, 2014.
26. Starling SR, Holden SR, Jenny C. Abusive head trauma: the relationship of perpetrators to their victims. Pediatrics 1995;95:259–62.
27. Starling SR, Sirotnak AP, Heisler KW, et al. Inflicted skeletal trauma: the relationship of perpetrators to their victims. Child Abuse Negl 2007;31:993–9.
28. Tabor PD. Vicarious traumatization: concept analysis. J Forensic Nurs 2011;7: 203–8.

Prevention of Child Maltreatment

Wendy Gwirtzman Lane, MD, MPH*

KEYWORDS

- Child abuse • Child neglect • Prevention • Health promotion • Primary care

KEY POINTS

- Prevention of child maltreatment can be incorporated into pediatric practice through anticipatory guidance, risk-factor screening, and referral to community-based resources.
- There is wide variation in the methods and effectiveness of community-based prevention programs. Pediatricians should therefore be knowledgable about what programs are available in their community and the evidence-based support for such programs.
- Pediatricians can be effective prevention advocates at the level of the individual patient and family, and at the local, regional, and national levels.

Prevention of child abuse needs to be explained and understood within a broad context of child well-being. A child's experiences do not occur in a vacuum but rather within the context of family, community, and society. Risk factors for maltreatment such as parental depression, substance abuse, or lack of social support may lead to other adverse outcomes in addition to maltreatment. Likewise, interventions to prevent maltreatment may have other positive effects on children and families, including improved development, improved maternal health, enhanced parent-child communication, decreased use of public assistance, and decreased involvement in the criminal justice system.[1–5] For these reasons, many organizations and experts, including the American Academy of Pediatrics (AAP), The Centers for Disease Control and Prevention (CDC), and the Harvard Center on the Developing Child directly link child maltreatment prevention to strengthening families, improving developmental outcomes, and promotion of child and family safety, stability, and nurturance.[6–8]

Disclosure Statement: The author has no financial conflicts to disclose.
Department of Pediatrics, University of Maryland School of Medicine, 660 West Redwood Street, Baltimore, MD 21201, USA
* Department of Epidemiology and Public Health, University of Maryland School of Medicine, 660 West Redwood Street, Baltimore, MD 21201.
E-mail address: wlane@epi.umaryland.edu

Pediatr Clin N Am 61 (2014) 873–888
http://dx.doi.org/10.1016/j.pcl.2014.06.002
0031-3955/14/$ – see front matter © 2014 Elsevier Inc. All rights reserved.

pediatric.theclinics.com

THE ROLE OF PEDIATRIC HEALTH CARE PROVIDERS IN CHILD MALTREATMENT PREVENTION

Pediatricians and other health care providers can play several important roles in the prevention of child maltreatment. As part of routine patient care, pediatricians can provide anticipatory guidance, screen for maltreatment risk factors, and refer parents and families to effective community-based programs. These efforts can be integrated into routine care without increasing visit length if parents complete screening questionnaires before the visit and listings of community resources are readily available. On a broader level, pediatricians can advocate at the local, state, and national level for policies and programs that support families and children. Each of these roles are discussed in this article. A summary is provided in **Box 1**.

SCREENING FOR MALTREATMENT RISK FACTORS AND IDENTIFICATION OF FAMILIES AT RISK

From an ecological perspective, interactions among and between child, parent, family, and community/society may all increase the likelihood of maltreatment.[9,10] Any characteristic that makes a child difficult to care for, including physical, emotional, behavioral, or developmental disabilities, may increase risk.[11–13] Parents with mental health problems, limited social support, limited knowledge of normal child development, low sense of parenting competence, or harsh, inattentive, or inconsistent parenting may be at higher risk of abusing or neglecting their children.[14–20] Families experiencing intimate partner violence or who have nonbiologically related adults in the home may also be at increased risk.[21,22] Several community and societal factors such as violent neighborhoods, and inadequate social welfare programs such as food and housing assistance, may increase stress on families and increase the likelihood of maltreatment.[23,24] **Table 1** summarizes major maltreatment risk factors.

Several protective factors should also be noted. Social support is an important protective factor; families with higher levels of social support have lower rates of physical abuse and greater use of discipline strategies other than corporal punishment.[25,26]

Box 1
Opportunities for child maltreatment prevention in pediatric primary care

1. Screen for child maltreatment risk factors, including parental depression, substance abuse, intimate partner violence, parental stress, harsh punishment, and food insecurity

2. Identify family protective factors (eg, social support, self-efficacy, parenting competence)

3. Provide anticipatory guidance about challenging behaviors and developmental issues that may increase the risk for maltreatment (eg, infant crying, toilet training)

4. Ask parents about discipline and help them replace corporal punishment with more effective and less harmful strategies

5. Discuss sexual development and behavior with parents. Help parents and children become more skilled in communication about sexuality and sexual abuse (see **Table 5**)

6. Become knowledgable about the availability and effectiveness of local community-based resources. Encourage families to use your expertise to identify services that meet their needs

7. Advocate for implementation and sustaining of community-based services to help families prevent maltreatment

8. Advocate for implementation and sustaining of federal, state, and local programs that ameliorate underlying maltreatment risk factors (eg, poverty, substance abuse, depression, and other mental health disorders)

Table 1
Examples of child maltreatment risk factors by ecological level

Child	Parent	Family	Community/Society
Prematurity	Teenage parent	Intimate partner violence	Violent/unsafe neighborhood
Colic/fussy baby	Depression/anxiety/ other mental health conditions	Single parent	Lack of availability of affordable, high-quality child care
Chronic illness	Substance abuse	Poverty	Absence of community activities, programs for children
Emotional/behavioral difficulties	Poor impulse control	Unemployment	Lack of government support for social welfare programs
Developmental disability	History of abuse or harsh punishment as a child	Nonbiologically related adult living in the home	
Physical disability	Lack of social support		
Unwanted child	Single parent		
Multiple gestation	Poor knowledge of normal child development and behavior Major stress		

Self-efficacy, an individual's belief in his or her ability to succeed, is another characteristic that can limit the adverse effects of risk factors. Some parents are very adept at identifying and securing helpful resources and services such as home nursing for a sick child, or a child care center that serves children with developmental disabilities. Parents' sense of competence in child rearing may enable them to better cope with the challenges of raising children.[27] Children with high intelligence, self-esteem, and/or self-efficacy, are involved with extracurricular activities or religious institutions, or who have a supportive adult involved in their lives may be less likely to suffer negative sequelae from maltreatment.[28]

A child health professional who is familiar with the risk factors of child maltreatment can work with families to identify and address these risks. Because many high-risk parents have limited health care access and do not seek out supportive services, they may have more contact with their child's primary care provider than any other professional. Child health professionals are therefore uniquely suited to identify and address the risk for child maltreatment.

As with any screening program, screening for child maltreatment risk factors should be focused on problems for which effective treatment is available, such as parental depression and substance abuse. Universal screening (ie, screening all families in a primary care practice) is recommended because it eliminates the stigma of screening selected families and reduces the likelihood of missing families at risk. Several questionnaires that screen for child maltreatment risk factors have been developed and validated.[29–37] Though brief, most identify only a single risk factor.[36]

Several screening tools identify multiple maltreatment risk factors. The SPARK (Structured Problem Analysis of Raising Kids) questionnaire identifies factors that may increase the risk of child maltreatment, such as child health, development, and behavior; parenting approach; social contacts and informal support; and family and community environment.[38,39] The 3-step model starts with detection of problems and concerns, followed by an assessment of the extent and impact of problems and the parents' perception of need for support. The final step involves making decisions about next steps. The questions are intended to be administered as part of a structured interview, which takes, on average, 29 minutes to complete. Providers are taught how to administer the SPARK in a half-day training session. A recent study has shown that the included risk factors were strongly predictive of child protective services (CPS) reports.[39] However, no data have been published on the effects of SPARK in reducing child maltreatment.

Another model that incorporates a multi–risk-factor screening questionnaire is SEEK (A Safe Environment for Every Kid). The Parent Screening Questionnaire (PSQ), a component of SEEK, is a single-page document that asks about multiple maltreatment risk factors, including parental depression, substance abuse, social support, intimate partner violence (IPV), major parental stress, and food insecurity.[36] To reduce the stigma associated with asking sensitive questions, an introductory paragraph adopts an empathetic tone and notes that parenting can be challenging for anyone. It also notes that the survey is given to all parents bringing their children for a check-up.

The SEEK model includes several other components in addition to the PSQ. Because many pediatricians may not have had training in addressing complicated issues such as IPV and parental substance abuse, training and skill building are incorporated. Motivational interviewing techniques are introduced as a means of enhancing parents' readiness to change. These techniques have proved to be effective for many types of behavior change, and pediatricians can become skilled with training and practice. With support from the Doris Duke Foundation, these training modules are now available on-line at https://theinstitute.umaryland.edu/SEEK/. The SEEK Web site also includes algorithms for further assessment and parent handouts that address each risk factor. The SEEK model ideally includes a clinical social worker or mental health professional to assist with family assessments and referrals, either in person or by phone. Alternatively, pediatricians who have been trained to briefly assess and initially address identified problems may implement the SEEK model with the help of office staff to facilitate referrals.

The effectiveness of SEEK has been studied extensively. Two studies have demonstrated the SEEK model's effectiveness in reducing child maltreatment.[40,41] One study was conducted in a pediatric resident continuity clinic based in an urban inner-city community. The other was conducted at 18 mostly suburban private primary care practices. SEEK has been endorsed as a promising practice by the federal Agency for Healthcare Research and Quality (AHRQ) Health Care Innovations Exchange, and some materials are included in the Bright Futures guidelines for anticipatory guidance. An economic analysis of SEEK demonstrated that the program would save money by reducing the need for medical and mental health expenses.[42] Of particular importance to the busy pediatrician, practices that implemented the SEEK model did not increase the average time spent with patients.

PREVENTION PROGRAMS ROOTED IN MODELS OF ANTICIPATORY GUIDANCE

Several programs use anticipatory guidance to help parents effectively manage situations that might increase the risk of maltreatment. Two programs have specifically focused on the stress associated with infant crying and preventing abusive head trauma (shaken baby syndrome). Dias and colleagues[43] developed a hospital-based postpartum intervention that taught parents the dangers of shaking babies. Equally important, it taught parents how to manage the stress that they might feel when their infant cries inconsolably. After receiving the educational materials, parents were asked to sign a commitment statement stating that they would not shake their baby and that they would teach other caregivers not to shake. An ecological study comparing change in rates of abusive head trauma in the Buffalo, New York area, where the intervention was implemented with rate changes in neighboring Pennsylvania during the same time period, showed a 47% decrease in the rate of abusive head trauma in the intervention community, but no change in rates in the control communities. Unfortunately, a case-control study of a similar intervention implemented in Utah did not show significant reductions in abusive head trauma.[44]

The Period of Purple Crying program is also focused on the parenting response to infant crying. A video and brochure provide information about infant crying behavior, with advice on how to reduce infant crying and address the associated parenting stress. Two randomized trials demonstrated significant improvement in knowledge about and response to crying. Because the incidence of abusive head trauma is relatively low (approximately 30 cases per 100,000 infants), enrollment of enough families to detect significant differences in rates of abusive head trauma between the intervention and control groups was not feasible.[45,46] Therefore, the studies were not designed to examine this outcome. The program has expanded from their original sites in Vancouver, British Columbia and Seattle, Washington to many other communities in the United States and Canada. A statewide campaign in North Carolina has incorporated in-hospital postpartum education, community-based education in primary care offices and health departments, and a media campaign.[47] To date, there have been no publications specifically examining whether the intervention leads to a reduction in the rate of abusive head trauma.

The AAP has developed 2 programs for primary prevention of child maltreatment in the clinical setting. Connected Kids: Safe, Strong, Secure is a resiliency-based educational program for parents and providers focused on managing challenging developmental stages, providing effective discipline, and other topics.[48] Although the developers have demonstrated that implementation is feasible, there has not been any evaluation of program effectiveness in reducing maltreatment rates or other benefits. Practicing Safety is another AAP-developed program that helps providers screen for and address maternal depression, and uses anticipatory guidance to help parents cope with challenging developmental stages such as infant crying, colic, and toilet training.[49] It was initially implemented as a Quality Improvement Innovation Network (QuIIN) project to increase attention to and address specific risk factors for child maltreatment. Participants demonstrated changes in practice behavior, but effects on child maltreatment were not examined.

COMMUNITY-BASED PREVENTION PROGRAMS

In addition to providing anticipatory guidance and screening for maltreatment risk factors, pediatricians can also refer families to community-based programs, and encourage them to participate. To do so, however, pediatricians must be aware of which programs are available in their communities. Gathering this information may initially require several hours of pediatrician or office staff time, followed by periodic updates. Community resource information may be available from one's local or state health department, United Way agency, and/or through an Internet search, supplemented by phone calls and requests for brochures and program information.

Identifying and communicating periodically with key contact persons at community-based agencies may also be worthwhile. Brief conversations can be helpful in learning more about the program and in collaboratively addressing the needs of referred families. In addition, families in need of services may be more willing to engage when their pediatrician is familiar with program staff and services.

Pediatricians also must be knowledgable about the quality and effectiveness of the available programs, keeping in mind that many programs have had little or no formal evaluation. Several Web sites focused on evidence-based interventions can help pediatricians acquire this knowledge by summarizing key information. Most provide program descriptions and information on program location(s), targeted populations, research outcomes, and effectiveness ratings. **Table 2** lists several useful sites.

There is a great deal of variability among programs. Whereas some explicitly focus on prevention of child abuse, the goals of others are framed in a broader context, such as enhancing parenting skills. The background and training of program staff varies considerably. Professionals such as nurses or social workers work directly with participants in some programs. These professionals may be equipped with a large fund of knowledge and years of experience. However, some programs prefer using lay persons from the intervention community because of the potential for better connections with participants. Some programs have been studied extensively with rigorous methods including randomized controlled trials, and both process and outcome evaluations; others have not been as carefully or extensively evaluated, and many have not been evaluated at all.

Table 2
On-line resources for information on Community-Based Prevention Programs

Resource	Web Site	Information Provided
Department of Health and Human Services, Administration for Children and Families—Home Visiting Evidence of Effectiveness	www.homvee.acf.hhs.gov/Default.aspx	Review of research on home-visiting programs Program descriptions Evidence of effectiveness Findings by outcome domain
California Evidence-Based Clearinghouse for Child Welfare	www.cebc4cw.org	Topic area: Home visiting for prevention of child abuse and neglect Descriptions of specific home-visiting programs Ratings of effectiveness in preventing child maltreatment
Centers for Disease Control and Prevention—Child Maltreatment: Prevention Strategies	www.cdc.gov/violence prevention/childmal treatment/prevntion.html	Listing of effective and promising programs Guidelines and planning tools
Promising Practices Network on children, families, and community	http://www.promising practices.net/programs_topic_list.asp?topicid=16	Listing and description of proven and promising programs
The Guide to Community Preventive Services: The Community Guide, What Works to Promote Health	http://www.thecommunity guide.org/violence/index.html	Systematic reviews of evidence for early childhood home visitation and other violence-prevention topics

When successful programs are replicated, fidelity to the original model becomes an important consideration. Consistency in training, implementation, and oversight may help ensure that all program components are implemented properly. However, sometimes program changes are needed with replication, particularly when they are implemented in communities that are culturally or geographically different from the original intervention community.

Keeping families engaged in community-based services can be challenging. Many families referred to community-based programs struggle with stressors such as poverty, single-parenthood, IPV, and depression, in addition to pregnancy and parenthood. High-quality interventions may better engage and retain participants than lower quality programs.[50] Engagement and retention is often more difficult in families coping with intimate partner psychological aggression, substance abuse, and depression.[50] If pediatricians screen, identify, and help families access services for these problems, they may reduce child maltreatment by both ameliorating risk factors and improving community-based program participation.

Most community-based programs fall into one of two categories: home visiting and parent training. However, some parent-training programs include a home-visiting component, and many home-visiting programs include parenting skills training. A review of 12 carefully evaluated community-based programs (including both home visiting and parent training) with control groups and measurement of child abuse outcomes demonstrated an overall positive effect of the interventions. The weighted average rate of child maltreatment was 2.9% lower in intervention families than in controls.[51] However, only 4 of the 12 programs showed a statistically significant reduction in substantiated maltreatment rates. The most effective programs had a high level of intervention and comprehensive services addressing multiple family needs. Highly trained service providers also increased program effectiveness.

Home-visiting programs assign a professional or layperson to serve families in their own environment. Services may include an assessment of needs, case management, education, emotional support, and role modeling. Home visitors assist families in accessing needed services such as health insurance, WIC (the US Women, Infants and Children Program), mental health and substance abuse treatment, and housing assistance. Most begin during pregnancy or shortly after birth.

The 2010 federal Patient Protection and Affordable Care Act included funding for evidence-based home visiting through the Maternal, Infant and Early Childhood Home Visiting Program (MIECHV). At least 75% of MIECHV community funding must be spent on evidence-based home-visiting programs. To determine which programs would be designated as evidence-based, the US Department of Health and Human Services (DHHS) conducted a systematic review, the Home Visiting Evidence of Effectiveness (HomVEE). Data from HomVEE led the DHHS to designate 12 programs as meeting evidence-based criteria (**Table 3**).[52] It must be noted that although all DHHS designated programs have shown positive outcomes for children, not all have demonstrated effectiveness in preventing child abuse and neglect. Descriptions of several widespread HomVEE designated programs with evidence of child abuse prevention are provided in **Table 4**.[53]

With the recent increases in funding for home visiting, pediatricians may find that more resources are available for their patients, particularly those living in high-risk communities. However, pediatricians should also be aware of some of the challenges of program expansion and replication. Some interventions that worked well in relatively small randomized controlled trials may be less effective when implemented on a larger scale, with different community and service provider characteristics, and with fewer resources available for oversight and evaluation. Some programs that

Table 3
Home-visiting programs meeting Department of Health and Human Services criteria for an evidence-based early childhood home-visiting model

ChildFIRST	Healthy Steps
Early Head Start—Home Visiting (EHS)	Home Instruction for Parents of Preschool Youngsters (HIPPY)
Early Intervention Program for Adolescent Mothers (EIP)	Nurse Family Partnership (NFP)
Early Start (New Zealand)	Oklahoma's Community-Based Family Resource and Support (CBFRS) Program
Family Check-Up	Parents as Teachers (PAT)
Healthy Families America (HFA)	Play and Learn Strategies (PALS) for Infants

have demonstrated effectiveness in clinical trials have not performed as well when replicated.[54,55] Pediatricians can assist families by advocating for adoption of high-quality programs, with funding for ongoing evaluation. In addition, pediatricians should develop relationships with local home visitation programs to facilitate coordination of care in addressing family needs.

Parent-training programs are intended to improve parents' comfort and competence with parenting. Program components may include child development, responsiveness, sensitivity and nurturing, positive interactions, emotional communication, and disciplinary approaches. The specific services and mode of implementation vary by program and may include individual, group, office-based, and/or home-based programs. Unfortunately, few program evaluations have directly measured child maltreatment outcomes, instead focusing on potential mediators such as child-rearing skills and emotional adjustment. A 2009 review of program reviews identified 2 meta-analyses (integration of data from multiple studies that examine similar outcomes) showing small to medium effects of parent-training programs; others showed effects on child maltreatment risk factors, but not on actual maltreatment.[56] Several meta-analyses of parent training programs have identified characteristics that may improve program effectiveness.[57–60] Programs that include multiple modalities and higher levels of intervention are more likely to be successful.

Multimodal community-based interventions have also been developed, which may include home visiting, parent training, public service announcements, and/or primary care anticipatory guidance. One of the most effective programs is Triple P – Positive Parenting Program. Triple P focuses on addressing children's behavioral, emotional, and developmental problems, enhancing family protective factors, and reducing family risk factors for maltreatment.[61]

Five tiers of Triple P services are available to families; the services received depend on family needs. Tier 1 services are universal, and include print and electronic media messages. The goals are to increase awareness of parenting challenges and reduce or eliminate the stigma associated with participation in parenting programs. Tier 2 services are intended to address discrete behavioral or developmental concerns (eg, toilet training, sleep). Trained program staff offer assistance by phone or in person in a few brief sessions (eg, two 20-minute sessions) or 60- to 90-minute seminars. More serious problems may require tier 3 services: about four 80-minute sessions that include active skills training. When parents have multiple concerns about their child or the child has more severe behavioral problems, tier 4 services may be warranted. Assistance may be provided as individual, group, or self-directed services

Table 4
Characteristics and outcomes of selected evidence-based home visitation programs

Program	Type of Home Visitor	Eligibility	Program Components	Evaluation Design	Positive Outcomes for Child Abuse and Neglect	Other Positive Outcomes
Healthy Families America[73,74]	Paraprofessional	Risk-based screening	Home visits from 3rd trimester to child age 2–3 y; biweekly to 1 y of age, then monthly	Multiple sites Randomized controlled trials	Yes: by parent report in randomized controlled trials; by substantiated child maltreatment report in quasi-experimental studies	Health care Birth outcomes Child behavior and development
Nurse Family Partnership[2,74-76]	Nurse Also nurse vs paraprofessional comparison	First-time, low-income pregnant women. Before 28 wk gestation	Home visits prenatal through 2 y Weekly to every other week to 20 mo, then monthly	Multiple sites Randomized controlled trials	Yes: decrease in substantiated child protective services (CPS) reports; not all sites	Health care Birth outcomes Child behavior and development Other
Early Head Start[77]	Educators, trained paraprofessionals	Low-income	Pregnancy to age 3 Center-based services with at least 2 home visits per year Home-based services with weekly home visits and bimonthly groups	Randomized controlled trial	Not measured Did find improvements in parenting behavior: more emotional support, fewer negative parenting behavior, less spanking at age 3	Cognitive development Child behavior Parent employment: Parent emotional support to child
Teen Parents as Teachers[78]	Nurses, teachers, social service professionals, or trained parent educators	All families pregnancy to age 5	Pregnancy to age 5 Monthly, biweekly, or weekly depending on family needs	Randomized controlled trial	Yes: fewer current suspected cases by CPS and school records (Binghampton, NY program). No difference in confirmed cases or cases remaining open with CPS	Child behavior and development

for up to 12 weeks. Tier 5 services are provided when, in addition to significant child behavior problems, parents have their own issues to address. Additional services may involve home visits and mental health services for parents.

An evaluation of Triple P implementation in 18 South Carolina counties showed promising effects in reducing child maltreatment. Counties that implemented Triple P had significantly lower rates of substantiated child maltreatment, fewer out-of-home placements, and fewer child maltreatment injuries that required inpatient or emergency department care.[62]

PREVENTION OF SEXUAL ABUSE

Prevention of child sexual abuse is addressed separately in this article because it poses unique challenges in developing effective interventions. Whereas many caregiver risk factors have been identified for physical abuse and neglect, caregiver characteristics are much less predictive of sexual abuse. There is no typical profile of a perpetrator of sexual abuse, which makes it challenging to develop prevention programs predicated on keeping children away from risky caregivers. In addition, some adults are uncomfortable with any discussion about sexuality as it pertains to their children. Therefore they may be reluctant to participate in prevention programs directed at parents, and even more reluctant to allow their children to participate in prevention programs.

Pediatricians may be uniquely suited to educating parents about preventing sexual abuse. Parents typically listen to and trust their provider's recommendations and have frequent contact with their pediatrician during the first few years of a child's life. Although there are no studies examining the effectiveness of anticipatory guidance in reducing victimization, some general concepts can be extrapolated from other interventions. Several key concepts are summarized in **Table 5**.

Education-based prevention programs became prevalent in the 1980s, and have been extensively studied and critiqued. Most are school-based, and focused on understanding and protecting personal boundaries, identifying and avoiding dangerous situations, refusing sexual approaches and invitations, and telling an adult if inappropriate behavior occurs. Evaluations of these programs show that children do learn the concepts being taught, and that they respond appropriately when challenged during simulations.[63–66] Such programs may also lead to increases in disclosure of sexual abuse and a decreased likelihood of self-blaming.[67,68]

Few studies examining whether these programs lead to reductions in sexual abuse have been published. One retrospective case-control study with college student participants did demonstrate a lower rate of sexual abuse among those students who recalled participation in a school-based program.[69] However, a prospective cohort study of 10- to 16-year-old students did not show any difference in victimization rates between those who did and did not participate in a prevention program.[67] Critics of child-focused prevention programs have argued that it is unfair to expect children to bear the responsibility for preventing sexual abuse, and that it may be harmful to tell children that someone close to them could abuse them. However, program evaluations have identified few negative consequences.[66,70]

Several public health media campaigns have been developed and disseminated in recent years. Stop It Now! is a program first introduced in Vermont that incorporated public service announcements on television and radio, newspaper articles, bus advertising, and an interactive Web site. Evaluation demonstrated greater awareness about sexual abuse and an increased number of helpline calls.[71] Darkness to Light educates parents and child-serving organizations about methods to keep children safe,

Table 5
Anticipatory guidance messages to parents and children for reducing the risk of child sexual abuse

Message	Target	Example/Context
Only the doctors and specific adult caregivers are allowed to see "private parts"	Child	Pediatrician can mention this to the child during the genital examination
	Parent	Pediatrician can ask parent to clarify which caregiver(s) are permitted to bathe/clean/dress child
It is important to maintain open channels of communication	Parent	Pediatrician can talk to parents about ways to foster good communication. For example, parents can tell children that they can and should talk to them when something is bothering them or someone's behavior is making them uncomfortable
	Child	Pediatrician can encourage children to talk to parents when something is bothering them or someone is making them uncomfortable
Parents can do some things to limit opportunity for perpetrators to access children	Parent	Parents can limit some one-adult/one-child situations through their choice of child care provider and child activities
Resources are available to help parents better understand child sexual abuse, communicate with their children about this topic, and take steps to protect them	Parent	Pediatrician can provide parents with additional resources such as those from: Enough Abuse Campaign: www.enoughabuse.org Darkness to Light: www.d2l.org Stop It Now: www.stopitnow.org

including the avoidance of one adult–one child situations. A media campaign evaluation found that the program led to increased knowledge of sexual abuse, and improvements in protective behavior on hypothetical vignettes. Unfortunately these effects did not persist 9 months after intervention.[72] The Enough Abuse campaign takes a multi-pronged approach, incorporating education of adults and children, and advocacy efforts to ensure policies and regulations that focus on child safety.

ADVOCACY

Pediatricians can be advocates for the prevention of child maltreatment in multiple ways, at the levels of the individual child, parent, community, and society. Helping parents meet their children's needs is advocacy on behalf of individual children who may be unable to communicate these needs. Acknowledging parental stress, identifying other risk factors for maltreatment, and motivating and facilitating help-seeking efforts is another form of advocacy. Pediatricians can play leadership roles in implementing hospital-based abusive head trauma prevention programs and practice-based policies for risk-factor screening and anticipatory guidance. Although pediatricians may not have direct involvement in community-based prevention programs, they can advocate for implementation and dissemination of quality home-visitation and parent-training programs in their community or state. Finally, pediatricians can advocate for increased resources to help families meet the needs of their children.

REFERENCES

1. Andrews SR, Blumenthal JB, Johnson DL, et al. The skills of mothering: a study of the Parent-Child Development Centers. Monogr Soc Res Child Dev 1982;47:1–81.
2. Olds DL, Eckenrode J, Henderson CR, et al. Long-term effects of home visitation on maternal life course and child abuse and neglect. Fifteen-year follow-up of a randomized trial. JAMA 1997;278:637–43.
3. Duggan AK, McFarlane EC, Windham AM, et al. Evaluation of Hawaii's Healthy Start Program. Future Child 1999;9:66–90.
4. Kitzman H, Olds D, Henderson R, et al. Effect of prenatal and infancy home visitation by nurses on pregnancy outcomes, childhood injuries, and repeat childbearing: a randomized controlled trial. JAMA 1997;278:644–52.
5. Olds DL, Henderson CR, Phelps C, et al. Effect of prenatal and infancy home visiting on government spending. Med Care 1993;31:155–74.
6. Flaherty EG, Stirling J. Clinical report: the pediatrician's role in child maltreatment prevention. Pediatrics 2010;126:833–41.
7. National Center for Injury Prevention and Control, Centers for Disease Control and Prevention. Strategic direction for child maltreatment prevention: preventing child maltreatment through the promotion of safe, stable, and nurturing relationships between children and caregivers. Atlanta (GA): 2013. Available at: http://www.cdc.gov/violenceprevention/pdf/cm_strategic_direction–long-a.pdf. Accessed January 21, 2014.
8. Center on the Developing Child at Harvard University. The foundations of lifelong health are built in early childhood. 2010. Available at: http://www.developingchild.harvard.edu. Accessed January 20, 2014.
9. Belsky J. Etiology of child maltreatment: a development-ecological analysis. Psychol Bull 1993;114:413–34.
10. Bronfenbrenner U. Contexts of child rearing: problems and prospects. Am Psychol 1979;34:844–50.
11. Sedlak A, Mettenburg J, Basena M, et al. Fourth National Incidence Study of Child Abuse and Neglect (NIS-4): Report to Congress. Washington, DC: 2010. Available at: http://www.acf.hhs.gov/programs/opre/abuse_neglect/natl_incid/nis4_report_congress_full_pdf_jan2010.pdf. Accessed September 8, 2010.
12. Sullivan PM, Knutson JF. Maltreatment and disabilities: a population-based epidemiological study. Child Abuse Negl 2000;24:1257–73.
13. Ammerman RT, Hersen M, Van Hasselt VB, et al. Maltreatment in psychiatrically hospitalized children and adolescents with developmental disabilities: prevalence and correlates. J Am Acad Child Adolesc Psychiatry 1994;33:567–76.
14. Chaffin M, Kelleher K, Hollenberg J. Onset of physical abuse and neglect: psychiatric, substance abuse, and social risk factors from prospective community data. Child Abuse Negl 1996;20:191–200.
15. Kelleher K, Chaffin M, Hollenberg J, et al. Alcohol and drug disorders among physically abusive and neglectful parents in a community-based sample. Am J Public Health 1994;84:1586–90.
16. Kotch JB, Browne DC, Dufort V, et al. Predicting child maltreatment in the first 4 years of life from characteristics assessed in the neonatal period. Child Abuse Negl 1999;23:305–19.
17. Bays J. Substance abuse and child abuse - impact of addiction on the child. Pediatr Clin North Am 1990;37:881–904.
18. Stringer SA, LaGreca AM. Correlates of child abuse potential. J Abnorm Child Psychol 1985;13:217–26.

19. Ellis RH, Milner JS. Child abuse and locus of control. Psychol Rep 1981;48: 507–10.
20. Nurius PS, Lovell M, Maggie E. Self-appraisals of abusive parents: a contextual approach to study and treatment. J Interpers Violence 1988;3:458–67.
21. Appel A, Holden G. The co-occurrence of spouse and physical child abuse: a review and appraisal. J Fam Psychol 1998;12:578–99.
22. Stiffman MN, Schnitzer PG, Adam P, et al. Household composition and risk of fatal child maltreatment. Pediatrics 2002;109:615–21.
23. Coulton CJ, Korbin JE, Su M. Neighborhoods and child maltreatment: a multi-level study. Child Abuse Negl 1999;23:1019–40.
24. Coulton CJ, Crampton DS, Irwin M, et al. How neighborhoods influence child maltreatment: a review of the literature and alternative pathways. Child Abuse Negl 2007;31:1117–42.
25. McCurdy K. The influence of support and stress on maternal attitudes. Child Abuse Negl 2005;29:251–68.
26. Lyons SJ, Henly JR, Schuerman JR. Informal support in maltreating families: its effect on parenting practices. Child Youth Serv Rev 2005;27:21–38.
27. Coleman PK, Karraker KH. Self-efficacy and parenting quality: findings and future applications. Dev Rev 1998;18:47–85.
28. Runyan DK, Hunter WN, Socolar R, et al. Children who prosper in unfavorable environments: the impact of social capital. Pediatrics 1998;101:12–8.
29. Ewing JA. Detecting alcoholism: The CAGE Questionnaire. JAMA 1984;252: 1905–7.
30. Feldhaus KM, Koziol-McLain J, Amsbury HL, et al. Accuracy of 3 brief screening questions for detecting partner violence in the Emergency Department. JAMA 1997;277:1357–61.
31. Weiss SJ, Ernst AA, Cham E, et al. Development of a screen for ongoing intimate partner violence. Violence Vict 2003;18:131–41.
32. Whooley MA, Avins AL, Miranda J, et al. Case-finding instruments for depression. Two questions are as good as many. J Gen Intern Med 1997;12:439–45.
33. Hinkin CH, Castellon SA, Dickson-Fuhrman E, et al. Screening for drug and alcohol abuse among older adults using a modified version of the CAGE. Am J Addict 2001;10:319–26.
34. Brown RL, Rounds LA. Conjoint screening questionnaires for alcohol and other drug abuse: criterion validity in a primary care practice. Wis Med J 1995;94: 135–40.
35. Dubowitz H, Feigelman S, Lane W, et al. Screening for depression in an urban pediatric primary care clinic. Pediatrics 2007;119:435–43.
36. Dubowitz H, Prescott L, Feigelman S, et al. Screening for intimate partner violence in an urban pediatric primary care clinic. Pediatrics 2008;121:e85–91.
37. Lane WG, Dubowitz H, Feigelman S, et al. Screening for substance abuse in pediatric primary care. Ambul Pediatr 2007;7:458–62.
38. Staal II, vandenBrink HA, Hermanns JM, et al. Assessment of parenting and developmental problems in toddlers: development and feasibility of a structured interview. Child Care Health Dev 2011;37:503–11.
39. Staal II, Hermanns JM, Schrijvers JP, et al. Risk assessment of parents' concerns at 18 months in preventive child health care predicted child abuse and neglect. Child Abuse Negl 2013;37:475–84.
40. Dubowitz H, Feigelman S, Lane W, et al. Pediatric primary care to help prevent child maltreatment: the *Safe Environment for Every Kid* (*SEEK*) Model. Pediatrics 2009;123:858–64.

41. Dubowitz H, Lane WG, Semiatin JN, et al. The SEEK model of pediatric primary care: can child maltreatment be prevented in a low-risk population? Acad Pediatr 2012;12:259–68.

42. Lane WG, Frick K, Dubowitz H, et al. Cost-effectiveness analysis of the SEEK (A Safe Environment for Every Kid) child maltreatment prevention program. American Public Health Association 139th Annual Meeting and Exposition. Washington, DC, November 1, 2011.

43. Dias MS, Smith K, DeGuehery K, et al. Preventing abusive head trauma among infants and young children: a hospital-based parent education program. Pediatrics 2005;115:e470.

44. Keenan HT, Leventhal JM. A case-control study to evaluate Utah's shaken baby prevention program. Acad Pediatr 2010;10:389–94.

45. Barr RG, Rivara FP, Barr M, et al. Effectiveness of educational materials designed to change knowledge and behaviors regarding crying and shaken-baby syndrome in mothers of newborns: a randomized controlled trial. Pediatrics 2009;123:972–80.

46. Barr RG, Barr M, Fujiwara T, et al. Do educational materials change knowledge and behavior about crying and shaken baby syndrome? A randomized controlled trial. CMAJ 2009;180:727–33.

47. Runyan DK, Hennink-Kaminski HJ, Zolotor AJ, et al. Design and testing of a shaken baby syndrome prevention program – The Period Of Purple Crying: Keeping Babies Safe in North Carolina. Soc Mar Q 2009;15:2–24.

48. Levin-Goodman R. Connected kids implementation case studies project. Final report. Elk Grove Village (IL): American Academy of Pediatrics; 2009. Available at: http://www2.aap.org/connectedkids/FinalCaseStudiesReport.pdf. Accessed February 15, 2014.

49. Practicing safety: a child abuse and neglect prevention improvement project. Available at: http://www.aap.org/en-us/professional-resources/practice-support/quality-improvement/Quality-Improvement-Innovation-Networks/Pages/Practicing-Safety-A-Child-Abuse-and-Neglect-Prevention-Improvement-Project.aspx. Accessed January 21, 2014.

50. Damashek A, Doughty D, Ware L, et al. Predictors of client engagement and attrition in home-based child maltreatment prevention services. Child Maltreat 2011;16:9–20.

51. Reynolds AJ, Mathieson LC, Topitzes JW. Do early childhood interventions prevent child maltreatment? A review of research. Child Maltreat 2009;14:182–206.

52. Avellar SA, Supplee LH. Effectiveness of home visiting for improving child health and reducing child maltreatment. Pediatrics 2013;132:S90.

53. Avellar S, Paulsen D, Sama-Miller E, et al. Home Visiting Evidence of Effectiveness review: executive summary. Washington, DC: Office of Planning, Research and Evaluation, Administration for Children and Families, U.S. Department of Health and Human Services; 2013. Available at: http://homvee.acf.hhs.gov/HomVEE_Executive_Summary_2013.pdf. Accessed February 11, 2014.

54. Matone M, O'Reilly AL, Luan X, et al. Emergency department visits and hospitalizations for injuries among infants and children following statewide implementation of a home visitation model. Matern Child Health J 2012;16:1754–61.

55. Easterbrooks MA, Jacobs FH, Bartlett JD, et al. Initial findings from a randomized controlled trial of Healthy Families Massachusetts: early program impacts on young mothers' parenting. Pew states home visitation evaluation. Available at: http://www.pewstates.org/uploadedFiles/PCS_Assets/2013/Healthy_Families_Massachusetts_report_pdf. Accessed February 11, 2014.

56. Mikton C, Butchart A. Child maltreatment prevention: a systematic review of reviews. Bull World Health Organ 2009;87:1–9.

57. MacLeod J, Nelson G. Programs for the promotion of family wellness and the prevention of child maltreatment: a meta-analytic review. Child Abuse Negl 2000;24:1127–49.

58. Lundahl BW, Nimer J, Parsons B. Preventing child abuse: a meta-analysis of parent training programs. Res Soc Work Pract 2006;16:251–62.

59. Barlow J, Coren E, Stewart-Brown SS. Parent-training programmes for improving maternal psychosocial health. Cochrane Database Syst Rev 2003;(4):CD002020. http://dx.doi.org/10.1002/14651858.CD002020.pub2.

60. Geeraert L, Van den Noortgate W, Grietens H, et al. The effects of early prevention programs for families with young children at risk for physical abuse and neglect: a meta-analysis. Child Maltreat 2004;9:277–91.

61. Sanders MR, Cann W, Markie-Dadds C. The Triple P-Positive Parenting Programme: a universal population-level approach to the prevention of child abuse. Child Abuse Rev 2003;12:155–71.

62. Prinz RJ, Sanders MR, Shapiro CJ, et al. Population-based prevention of child maltreatment: the U.S. Triple P System population trial. Prev Sci 2009;10:1–12.

63. Berrick J, Barth R. Child sexual abuse prevention training: what do they learn? Child Abuse Negl 1992;12:543–53.

64. Davis MK, Gidyez CA. Child sexual abuse prevention programs: a meta-analysis. J Clin Child Psychol 2000;29:257–65.

65. Rispens J, Aleman A, Goudena PP. Prevention of child sexual abuse victimization: a meta-analysis of school programs. Child Abuse Negl 1997;21:975–87.

66. Finkelhor D. The prevention of childhood sexual abuse. Future Child 2009;19:169–94.

67. Finkelhor D, Asdigian N, Dziuba-Leatherman J. The effectiveness of victimization prevention programs for children: a follow-up. Am J Public Health 1995;85:1684–9.

68. Zwi KJ. School-based education programs for the prevention of child sexual abuse. Cochrane Database Syst Rev 1999;(73). 281–313.

69. Gibson LE, Leitenberg H. Child sexual abuse prevention programs: do they decrease the occurrence of child sexual abuse? Child Abuse Negl 2000;24:1115–25.

70. Binder R, McNiel D. Evaluation of a school-based sexual abuse prevention program: cognitive and emotional effects. Child Abuse Negl 1987;11:497–506.

71. Chasen-Taber L, Tabachnick J. Evaluation of a child sexual abuse prevention program. Sex Abuse 1999;11:279–92.

72. Rheingold AA, Campbell C, Self-Brown S, et al. Prevention of child sexual abuse: evaluation of a community media campaign. Child Maltreat 2007;12:352–63.

73. Harding K, Galano J, Martin J, et al. Healthy Families America effectiveness: a comprehensive review of outcomes. J Prev Interv Community 2007;34:149–79.

74. Gonzalez A, MacMillan HL. Preventing child maltreatment: an evidenced-based update. J Postgrad Med 2008;54:280–6.

75. Olds DL, Henderson CR, Chamberlin R, et al. Preventing child abuse and neglect: a randomized trial of nurse home visitation. Pediatrics 1986;78:65–78.

76. Olds DL, Kitzman H, Hanks C, et al. Effects of nurse home visiting on maternal and child functioning: age-9 follow-up of a randomized trial. Pediatrics 2007;120:e832–45.

77. Love JM, Kisker EE, Ross CM, et al. Making a difference in the lives of infants and toddlers and their families: the impacts of Early Head Start. Volume I: final

technical report. Washington, DC: Office of Planning, Research and Evaluation, Administration for Children and Families, U.S. Department of Health and Human Services; 2002. Available at: http://www.acf.hhs.gov/sites/default/files/opre/impacts_vol1.pdf. Accessed February 6, 2014.

78. Drazen SM, Haust M. Raising reading readiness in low-income children by parent education. Paper presented at the annual meeting of the American Psychological Association. August 1993. Available at: http://homvee.acf.hhs.gov/Effects.aspx?rid=1&sid=16&mid=5&oid=4. Accessed February 6, 2014.

Bringing Back the Social History

Mary Clyde Pierce, MD[a,b,*], Kim Kaczor, MS[a], Richard Thompson, PhD[c]

KEYWORDS

- Adverse childhood experiences ● Child maltreatment ● Negative attributions
- Psychosocial risk factors ● Toxic stress

KEY POINTS

- The social history plays a key role in determining a child's current and future health.
- A useful social history involves asking about key elements of a child's environment, including the circumstances in which the child is being raised, adults involved in the child's life, presence of key factors associated with increased risk, and, most importantly, caregiver-child relationship and attachment.
- The social history should be obtained starting at the first well-child visit and at each visit thereafter. Children at highest risk often live in dynamic, often chaotic, environments, with frequent changes in their living situations and household compositions, increasing the importance of obtaining a social history at each visit.
- Child maltreatment (abuse or neglect) can have devastating health consequences that last for life and diminish emotional health and intellectual ability.
- Understanding each child's familial psychosocial risk and protective factors through the social history is an important link to preventing harmful parenting tactics, other threats to healthy development, and even potentially preventing child maltreatment.

WHY THE SOCIAL HISTORY MATTERS

A child's family environment is one of the most important and critical determinants of the child's health (current and future) and it is integral to the child's well-being and development.[1–4] A robust body of research has shown the role that this environment plays in brain and emotional development.[2,3,5] These environmental influences also

Financial Disclosures: None.

Conflict of Interest: None.

[a] Division of Emergency Medicine, Ann & Robert H. Lurie Children's Hospital of Chicago, 225 East Chicago Avenue, Chicago, IL 60611, USA; [b] Department of Pediatrics, Northwestern University Feinberg School of Medicine, Chicago, IL 60614, USA; [c] Richard H. Calica Center for Innovation in Children and Family Services, Juvenile Protective Association, Chicago, IL 60614, USA

* Corresponding author. Division of Emergency Medicine, Ann & Robert H. Lurie Children's Hospital of Chicago, 225 East Chicago Avenue, Box 62, Chicago, IL 60611.

E-mail address: MPierce@luriechildrens.org

have an impact on a child's physical health and play a significant role in determining future health and disease.[4–11] Thus, a social history not only is useful in identifying risk for child injury and maltreatment but also in identifying factors that might contribute to children's health problems. Strengthening families and supporting parents also promote children's health, development, and safety and help prevent child maltreatment.

A large body of research highlights the importance of environmental influences in the prenatal to early childhood period (ie, before age 2).[2,3,5] Therefore, obtaining a social history focused on the important aspects of the child's family environment is a critical component of early well-child care. The social history should be obtained at every visit because the family environment is frequently changing, and it influences child development in a dynamic way. The information obtained from social histories has the potential to contribute to a lifetime of health and well-being.

THE ILL EFFECTS OF MALTREATMENT CAN LAST A LIFETIME

Adverse childhood experiences, especially child maltreatment, are linked to risk factors for ill health as adults and early death.[6,7] Child maltreatment occurs in many forms (physical, sexual, or emotional abuse or neglect). It is not uncommon for a child to suffer from multiple forms of maltreatment at the same time.[12,13] Maltreatment is known to confer myriad deleterious health effects, both physical and mental.[6,7] In some instances, the effects of maltreatment are so severe that life ends in infancy or early childhood. In fact, 70% of deaths from maltreatment occur in children under 3 years of age.[14–16]

CHILD MALTREATMENT PREVENTION BEGINS WITH PRIMARY CARE

Problems in the family environment are often contributors to child maltreatment and indicate risk for a variety of negative outcomes (discussed previously). A social history that identifies families at risk for maltreatment has the potential to identify problems before they escalate to these most serious outcomes, in addition to helping families and children function better.

This type of prevention strategy is in line with the biopsychosocial model proposed by Engel,[17] which provides a broad view of child health and includes the psychosocial aspect when assessing children. This concept is well stated by Flaherty and colleagues[11]: "A comprehensive assessment of children's health should include a careful history of their past exposure to adverse conditions and maltreatment. Interventions aimed at reducing these exposures may result in better child health."

GOALS OF THE SOCIAL HISTORY

The goal of the social history is to assess the strengths and weaknesses in a child's environment to identify aspects of family life that can be reinforced and encouraged as well as identify potential sources of harm to the child that must be addressed. A comprehensive social history may also identify opportunities for parental education regarding parental expectations and age- and health-appropriate developmental milestones. The social history provides insight into a child's environment, which includes the circumstances in which the child is being raised, a comprehensive listing of the adults involved in the child's life, disciplinary practices, presence of key factors associated with increased risk for maltreatment, and, most importantly, caregiver-child relationship and attachment.[4,18,19] Assessing the nature of the caregiver-child relationship is important. A healthy, secure attachment between parents and children strongly predicts healthy child outcomes. The children at highest risk experience frequent changes in both their housing situations and household compositions, increasing the importance of obtaining a social history at each visit. Strengths, such as family supportiveness and concern for each other, are often ignored when focusing risk, but such strengths can buffer against even significant family risk.[20–22] Making a comprehensive social history an integral part of every visit also allows the primary care provider to follow-up on prior issues and identify any new stressors that may have arisen since the last visit.[23]

The social history also helps develop rapport; the authors have often found that thoughtfully asked questions assessing attachment have resulted in otherwise distant or suspicious parents opening up. This aspect of history taking conveys interest in the parent and family and gives the parent an opportunity to feel listened to. Thus, it strengthens the relationships between the primary care provider, parent/caregiver, and child.

Insight into family dynamics—functions and malfunctions—can be gained through a set of social history questions and should include a listing of each adult in contact with the child (including paramours, babysitters, nannies, and daycare workers as well as other adults in the home). This listing should include the ages of each adult, their relationship (to the child), and their role in the home. There is often a temptation in a social history to assume a given family structure and to focus on only the adults who are related, but unrelated adults living in the home are often associated with a higher risk for children.[24] The social history also provides a great opportunity to understand the parents' developmental expectations for their children and to educate parents about the child's needs and capabilities so that parental expectations are appropriately aligned with their child's developmental stage.

Both current and past social histories are relevant. The past history has the potential to reveal a risk for a recurrence of past problems as well as unresolved issues for the parent. The current history informs the health care provider of immediate issues. Specific questions regarding these risk factors can help identify problems to address and create opportunities to provide resources and education. Because child maltreatment entails a problem in the caregiver-child relationship, early identification of parenting problems or attachment issues is paramount. Occasionally, serious or severe problems are unearthed. By addressing the problems directly, a host of negative outcomes, including child maltreatment, can be prevented or curtailed. For example, there is a burgeoning body of research demonstrating that helping parents with mental illness get appropriate treatment can have long-term benefits for their children's health.[25] Also, the Safe Environment for Every Kid (SEEK) model, which includes training for providers on how to assess the family environment and brief screening for common psychosocial problems together with parent education resources, has been demonstrated to reduce risk of child maltreatment.[26,27] Structured social history assessments in the primary care setting are an important component in the prevention of child maltreatment.

As part of a research study of children and their families presenting to an emergency department, the authors' research team of physicians, social workers, and a psychologist developed a set of questions to assess social history. These questions, some of which are presented in **Table 1**, are typically part of social work assessments when a family is identified as at risk, but the authors have found them useful to identify risk in all families. Such social histories are useful in building rapport quickly with parents and understanding the issues that parents see as key to their child's well-being (see **Table 1**). The authors' approach to the social history is somewhat expanded in that not only are the past and current social circumstances included but also key aspects

Table 1
Topics for surveillance and sample questions to initiate discussion

Topics	Sample Questions

Child's contacts and household	1. Who lives with or is often in your child's primary home?
	2. Is there another home that your child lives in?
	  a. If yes, who lives with or is often in the child's secondary home?
	3. Has your child changed homes in the past 6 mo?
	  a. If yes, how many times?
	  b. What was the reason for each change?

Parental thoughts about child's personality and disposition	4. Describe your child's personality. 5. Provide 3 words to describe your child.
Parental expectations	6. How does your child communicate his/her wants/needs to you? 7. How do you think your child is doing compared with other children his/her age?

Understanding child's actions and parent-child interactions	8. What is your favorite thing your child does?
	  a. What do you do in response to this behavior?
	  b. Why do you think your child does this?
	9. What is your child's most frustrating behavior?
	  a. What do you do in response to this behavior?
	  b. Why do you think your child behaves this way?
	10. Have you ever been really frustrated with your child?
	  a. What were the circumstances?
	  b. What did you do?
	11. How does your child misbehave?
	  a. Why does your child misbehave?
	  b. What do you do when your child misbehaves?
	12. What's it like to take care of (insert child's name)? Easy/average/difficult—why?

Disciplinary practices	13. Do you want to raise your child the same way you were raised or differently? Why?
	14. How do you discipline your child?
	  a. Do you or have you ever spanked your child? What were the circumstances?
	  b. Do you or have you ever used an object to discipline your child? What were the circumstances?

Child care	15. What is your regular childcare arrangement? 16. Who watches your child(ren) while you run errands or shop, for example?
Child and parental literacy and education	17. Is your child in Head Start, preschool, or other early childhood enrichment? 18. How is your child doing in school? 19. Is he/she getting the help to learn what he/she needs? 20. How happy are you with how you read? 21. Do you read to your child every night?

(continued on next page)

Table 1
(continued)

Topics	Sample Questions

Household environment	22. Are there any significant life stressors in your family?
	• Death of family member or close friend
	• Major accident or illness in family
	• Separation/divorce
	• Custody battle
	• Move/relocation
	• Job change
	  ○ Job loss—who?
	  ○ New job—who?
	  ○ Mom back to work after maternity leave
	• Social isolation (local support system of family and/or friends)
	• Incarceration
	• Deployment
	• Return home from military service
	• New baby in the family
	• Excessive crying
	• Potty training
	• Other _____
	23. Do you ever have trouble making ends meet?
	24. Do you ever have a time when you don't have enough food?
	  a. Do you have WIC?
	  b. Do you have food stamps?
	25. Is your housing ever a problem for you?
	26. Do you ever have trouble paying your electric/heat/telephone bill?
	27. Do you need help accessing benefits or services for your family?
	28. Do you have questions about your immigration status?

Risk factors	29. Have you pushed, shoved, kicked, hit, and/or slapped another adult?
	30. Have you been pushed, shoved, kicked, hit, and/or slapped by another adult?
	31. Of the people in contact with your child:
	  a. Who is or has been involved with social services? Explain.
	  b. Who has or had domestic violence/interpersonal violence in his/her home? Explain.
	  c. Who has current or past police involvement, criminal activity, and/or incarceration? Explain.
	  d. Who is using or has used drugs? Explain.
	  e. Who has or had an alcohol problem/abuse? Explain.
	  f. Who has or had mental health issues, including anger or temper management issues, depression, bipolar disorder, posttraumatic stress disorder, or schizophrenia? Explain.
	  g. Who has gang involvement? Explain.

#6–13: May help identify negative attributions and parental unrealistic expectations.

#11: Suggested and used by Howard Dubowitz, MD; Professor of Pediatrics, University of Maryland.

#12: Suggested and used by Diane Baird, MSW; Instructor of Pediatrics, Kempe Center, Department of Pediatrics, University of Colorado.

#16–20, 22–27: *Data from* Social history questions incorporated from the "IHELLP" mneumonic; and *Adapted from* Kenyon C, Sandel M, Siverstein M, et al. Revisiting the social history for child health. Pediatrics 2007;120(3):e734–8.

WIC, special supplemental nutrition program for women, infants, and children.

of the parent-child relationship and the approach to parenting. This is but one sample of questions that could facilitate a discussion of family risk factors. The SEEK model is another (Appendix 1).[26,27] Also, the American Academy of Pediatrics (AAP) has a brief set of recommended questions for beginning a discussion about children's exposure to violence (**Box 1**).[28]

KEY PSYCHOSOCIAL RISK FACTORS THAT INCREASE THE RISK OF TOXIC STRESS AND CHILD MALTREATMENT

Key psychosocial factors known to increase the risk for child maltreatment include negative attributions (interpreting child behavior as malevolent, hostile, or needy), unrealistic expectations of the child, harsh disciplinary practices, and prior or current caregiver mental health problems, including anger management problems, substance abuse, prior social service involvement for abuse or neglect, and domestic violence/intimate partner violence (IPV).[29-38]

Huebner and colleagues[16] investigated fatalities and near-fatalities from child maltreatment and found that 48% of victims had been previously involved with Child Protective Services (CPS). Frequently identified risk factors in the children's family environments included caregiver substance abuse (65%), IPV (51%), and caregiver mental health problems (34%).

In addition to indicating risk for child maltreatment, each of these factors can add substantial risk of physical and psychological harm to a child apart from child maltreatment and can create a continuum of toxic stress (ie, prolonged activation of the stress response system due to frequent or prolonged exposure to stressors that results in disruption of neurobiological development and impedes future health).[2,3] Certain psychosocial risk factors are known to increase the probability of a poor outcome due to toxic stress.[2,3,6-8] The presence of multiple risk factors can be especially harmful for a child's development and, as the number increases, so does the likelihood of maltreatment.[12,38] Early identification of particular key risk factors allows more thoughtful child- and family-specific interventions and referrals for mitigating the risk and its toxic effects.[3]

PSYCHOSOCIAL RISK FACTORS
Negative Attributions and Unrealistic Expectations

When expectations are unrealistic or unreasonable, problems can ensue. Expectations affect the way the information is interpreted and can result in wrong conclusions and sometimes even harmful actions. Some parents may not have an accurate understanding of what is normal child development and thus they have unrealistic expectations regarding a child's capabilities.

Such unmet expectations may lead parents to search for explanations for why their child is not meeting expectations. These explanations are revealed in the parental attribution ascribed to a child's personality or temperament and are often negative. For example, parents may expect toilet training to be feasible before it is and assume young children have more control over the process of toilet training than they do.[39] These unrealistic expectations place the child at risk of harm when the child fails to "comply" and make the child's "failure" inevitable: "He knows how to use the potty, he's just not doing it because he knows it stresses me out." The parent may also misinterpret an action (or lack of action) as defiant or spiteful. This in turn may evoke anger in a parent.

A growing literature shows that hostile attributions toward even very young infants are common, and the authors have frequently encountered examples of such attributions.[40,41] For example, some parents attribute an infant's crying as anger or a sign of weakness (eg, "Why are you so mad?" or "Don't be a crybaby.") Some parents

Box 1
Sample questions from the American Academy of Pediatrics to help start the discussion with patients and families about exposure to violence

Violence overview

- Are there any behavior problems with the child at home and/or school?
- Has anyone come or gone from the household lately?
- Are there any problems with sleep and enuresis?
- Has your child ever witnessed anyone being harmed at home or in the community?

Bullying and cyberbullying

- Sometimes kids get picked on at school. Does this happen to you/your child? Has the child heard of or seen incidences of this?
- Have there been any problems at school with behavior?

Community violence

- Has the child had stomach pains, headaches, and other somatic complaints that seem to have no source?
- Has the child's behavior changed dramatically, seemingly without cause (eg, difficulty sleeping, avoiding people, or performance in school)?
- Has anything violence-related or frightening happened in the child's school or neighborhood since the last time you saw the child?

Child abuse and neglect

- Are there other signs or symptoms that are concerning for abuse or neglect?

Domestic and intimate partner violence

- Are you safe at home?
- Does anyone hit you or call you names?

Sexual abuse

- Has child disclosed being sexually abused?
- Has child had stomach pains, headaches, and other somatic complaints that seem to have no source?
- Has child's behavior changed dramatically, seemingly without cause (eg, difficulty sleeping, avoiding people, or performance in school)?
- Are there other signs or symptoms that are concerning for sexual abuse?

Teen dating violence

- Have there been any new boyfriends/girlfriends? How has that changed life for you? Do you feel safe with that person?

The following AAP Web site has a list of diagnostic, decision-support, and screening tools to identify children exposed to violence: http://www.aap.org/en-us/advocacy-and-policy/aap-health-initiatives/Medical-Home-for-Children-and-Adolescents-Exposed-to-Violence/Pages/Diagnostic-Tools.aspx.

Adapted from American Academy of Pediatrics. Medical Home for Children and Adolescents Exposed to Violence. Available at: http://www.aap.org/en-us/advocacy-and-policy/aap-healthinitiatives/Medical-Home-for-Children-and-Adolescents-Exposed-to-Violence/Pages/Addressing-Exposure-to-Violence-with-Families-and-Patients.aspx. Accessed on August 4, 2014.

interpret the need for frequent feedings as greed or impatience. Refusal to eat can also frustrate parents. When an infant's behavior is interpreted as stubborn, controlling, or ungrateful, the risk of harm is further increased. Another common misinterpretation that may increase the risk of maltreatment is when an infant is described as "spoiled" because the infant calms down when soothed or held by the caregiver. This positive response by the infant helps foster attachment, but when it is interpreted negatively as spoiled, it can harm caregiver-child bonding.

Different forms of maltreatment can occur as a result of caregiver misattributions and adult maladaptive responses. Sometimes a caregiver becomes frustrated to the point of yelling at and cursing an infant or child or using derogatory terms. Other mal-treating actions include withholding food "until I say we can eat" to show the infant who is in charge or to teach him/her not to be demanding or impatient or isolating the infant for extended periods of time to "teach him/her to "toughen up and stop be-ing a crybaby." A key point of risk is that when caregivers regard behavior as "bad" and/or purposeful, they are likely to believe that this behavior can and should be cor-rected. Sometime parents use physical means to "correct" or "teach a lesson," including spanking and slapping an infant or child, resulting in physical injury. Anger rather than empathy becomes the driving force, and there may be a perceived need to assert authority and use emotional intimidation, physical force, or punishment. Par-ents sometimes describe infants or children as "getting what they deserve," or "get-ting what they had coming to them." When a physical injury results, sometimes the caregiver even blames the child: "If she had not been doing ___, or if he would have just listened, then she/he wouldn't have gotten injured." The misattribution of soiling (with stool or urine) or crying may be an especially dangerous tipping point for some adults. The combination of unrealistic expectations, negative attributions, limited empathy, and use of corporal punishment to correct unwanted behaviors places a child at significant risk of harm.[42]

Guidelines on anticipatory guidance for parents regarding expected child develop-mental behaviors and emotions, such as temper tantrums or anger, may be too late for some. The problem is that the guidelines are based on age-appropriate stages of physical and emotional development, with the intent to guide parents in advance of development. Current recommendations of when to provide guidance may not be far enough in advance if a parent or caregiver is way off, with unrealistic expectations and beliefs about when and what a child can do and understand. Extremely unrealistic expectations increase risk to the child and limit the usefulness of anticipatory guid-ance that tracks normative development. Waiting to address issues until it is develop-mentally appropriate likely misses those at highest risk for maltreatment and, consequently, misses an important prevention window as well. Thus, getting a clear sense of parents' developmental expectations and attributions is important in identi-fying when to provide needed anticipatory guidance. The social history can help pri-mary care physicians identify inappropriate expectations and attributions and enable opportunities to address them. Negative attributions from case examples are illustrated in **Table 2**.

Physical Discipline

More than 90% of American families report using physical discipline at some time dur-ing a child's life, and such discipline frequently occurs with very young children.[43] In a nationally representative study, 6% of parents reported spanking their infants 4 to 9 months of age, 29% of parents reported spanking children 10 to 18 months, and 64% of parents reported spanking children 19 to 35 months of age.[44] Much research has focused on physical discipline in this early developmental period and its

Table 2
High-risk negative attributions and misinterpretations of child's actions/disposition

Child's Actions/Disposition	Parental Misinterpretation
Normal development behaviors	Bad, evil, "the devil", bitch, whore, self-centered, pouting, stubborn (especially infant), demanding, impatient
Crying	Mad, angry, weak, cry baby, titty baby, drama queen, demanding, impatient, trying to get attention
Crying, but soothes from crying when picked up/cradled	Child is spoiled
Frequent feeds	Greedy, ungrateful, selfish, self-centered, demanding, impatient
Not wanting to feed	Ungrateful, stubborn, controlling, rejection or dislike of parent
Spitting up	Ungrateful, retaliatory
Soiling (urine or stool)	Deliberate act by infant/child to control, make parent mad, or retaliate

impact.[44,45] Spanking has been significantly associated with aggression, school-age behavioral problems, and increased risk of physical abuse.[46,47] Escalation of spanking is evident in many reports of physical abuse substantiated by CPS.[45,47–49] Gershoff[50] points out that despite ample evidence that spanking is linked to undesirable outcomes, societal change around this issue has been slow in the United States. A growing list of national professional organizations have established official policy statements disavowing the use of spanking and endorsing nonpunitive discipline.

Learning a family's disciplinary approach at the first well-child visit may be important because some families report spanking as early as 2 months of age.[45] The AAP Early Brain and Child Development Leadership Workgroup recommends discussing disciplinary practices when a child is 15 months of age.[51] Although this may be appropriate for many families, it is too late for some. Waiting for the developmentally appropriate time to provide anticipatory guidance regarding disciplinary practices is especially too late for the patient population at the greatest risk for harm and maltreatment, who may not be readily identified as at risk.

Parental Mental Health

Mentally ill parents are more likely to maltreat their child, and the child is at risk for a host of other negative outcomes both in the short term and in the long term.[52–55] Parents with mental illness are also more likely to need assistance in effective parenting.[56] Research shows that mothers with mental health diagnoses, such as depression, or who ascribe negative attributions to their children were more likely to use physical discipline and to be reported for abuse.[30,34] The links between mental health and child maltreatment indicate that priority should be given to identifying mental health problems in caregivers to prevent both immediate and future harm to children. Given the chronic and recurrent nature of many forms of mental illness, asking about past problems may also provide useful information.[57]

Substance and Alcohol Abuse

Among the psychiatric disorders, substance abuse was the most common and the most powerfully associated with child maltreatment.[58] Some studies have found that the risk of violence is not increased for individuals with mental health disorders unless substance abuse is also present.[59] In a study investigating the prevalence of drug and alcohol disorders among physically abusive and neglectful parents and caregivers, 40% of adults who reported an abusive behavior and 56% who reported a neglectful behavior had a substance abuse disorder.[60] In addition, Chaffin and colleagues[59] noted, "substance abuse disorders are highly prevalent in the population at large." A Canadian study of approximately 8500 participants found that children in homes with parental substance abuse problems were at a more than 2-fold increased risk for child physical and sexual abuse."[61] Additionally, parental substance abuse increased the likelihood of re-reports to CPS.[62]

Prior Child Protective Services Involvement

Two key topics when considering CPS involvement are prior CPS involvement and intergenerational maltreatment. Unfortunately, a referral to CPS does not necessarily prevent repeat maltreatment. Thompson and Wiley[63] studied a cohort of children who were referred to CPS as infants and found that 42.3% were re-referred within 10 years of the initial report. Huebner and colleagues[16] analyzed fatalities and near-fatalities from child maltreatment, and 48% of families had prior CPS involvement. Connell and colleagues[64] found that children were at the greatest risk for re-referral to CPS in the 6-month period after case closure but that the risk continued for the next few years. Overall, research has found an alarming 40% to 70% of cases are re-referred to CPS within 5 years.[64–67] Levy and colleagues[66] found that "the greatest risk of re-abuse occurred during the first 2 years following an initial discharge diagnosis of maltreatment." The rates and time periods vary among the studies, but they all indicate a significant rate of recurrence. Thus, maltreatment seems to be a chronic problem in some families, and recurrent involvement of CPS is an ongoing risk. Asking parents about current or recent CPS involvement identifies what is likely to be a profound stressor for parents as well as markers of risk to children.

In addition to recidivism, the cycle of intergenerational abuse is of concern and places the children at increased risk for maltreatment. Estimates of intergenerational abuse rates are approximately 30%.[68,69] Despite a frequent emphasis on intergenerational abuse, the evidence indicates that most abused children do not grow up to be abusive parents. Kaufman and Ziegler[69] point out that focus should not be on the question, "Do abused children become abusive parents?" The more important question is, "Under what conditions is the transmission of abuse most likely to occur?" This new question changes the focus from inevitable to preventable.

These issues make it imperative that the primary care provider be keenly aware of a family's involvement with CPS and understand the circumstances regarding that involvement to take proactive measures against future problems and harm. This may be accomplished by anticipatory guidance and parental education or facilitating access to community-based resources and services.

Intimate Partner Violence

IPV is known to increase the risk of child maltreatment and to cause behavioral and mental health problems for children exposed to it. IPV itself is often considered a form of child maltreatment.[70–73] IPV often co-occurs with child maltreatment, and a significant proportion of children from violent families report being abused at some point in their lives.[31,37] Nationally, in 2012, 28.5% of children who had at least one substantiated or indicated maltreatment report (per state CPS agencies) were also exposed to IPV. Furthermore, 31 states were able to report whether a risk factor contributed to a child fatality; 20% did involve IPV.[14] A study of child fatalities in Florida found that men who had been violent with their partners had the highest probability of committing a fatal assault.[15] These statistics indicate that adults who have the capacity and propensity to use violence with their partners are also likely to use violence with children. A child may be physically abused directly by an aggressive adult or inadvertently harmed during an altercation between adults.[74] Additionally, lasting psychological damage to the child may occur from witnessing household violence. The well-known deleterious physical and mental effects of exposure to violence at a young age led the AAP to recommend screening for IPV at pediatric visits.[6,70] Such screening has a great deal of empirical support.[75]

SUMMARY

Understanding the environment a child is growing up in is essential to optimizing a child's developmental potential and physical health as well as the parent-child attachment and relationship. Questions that focus in a strategic way on social history and parents' attitudes and approaches to parenting can help identify positive aspects of the parent-child relationship and the family unit. The social history also can identify areas where parental anticipatory guidance is needed, including sources of frustration, challenges, physical punishment, and erroneous negative interpretations of a child's actions that heighten the risk for maltreatment.[76] The social history can help establish rapport by showing concern for the parent and family and lay the foundation necessary to screen for topics more difficult to broach, such as IPV, substance abuse/alcohol problems, or caregiver depression.

Because the social environment of a child matters greatly for the child's current and future health, it is timely to obtain a detailed social history at the start of the patient–family–medical provider relationship. Because aspects of the family environment, both protective and harmful, have such a significant impact on health and brain development for pediatric patients, screening is paramount to foster healthy parenting, help identify unhealthy factors, and, in some instances, even prevent child maltreatment.[77]

Social workers are experienced at delving into sometimes difficult areas and addressing needs with families, but, unfortunately, it is not practical for most primary care offices to have social workers on staff. The social history can be obtained in the practice setting by anyone who is medically trained. When issues in need of action are identified, referral to a specialist for further evaluation, treatment, or resources may be necessary to meet the needs of the children and families. In some instances, a report to CPS is required if maltreatment is suspected. Successful outcomes for the child and family are dependent, in part, on strategies for identifying and mitigating risk for maltreatment and collaborative efforts between the family, medical home, and social service agencies, when indicated. The social history may well be the best all-around tool available for promoting a child's future health and well-being.

REFERENCES

1. Sameroff A. A unified theory of development: a dialectic integration of nature and nurture. Child Dev 2010;81(1):6–22.
2. Shonkoff JP, Garner AS, The Committee on Psychosocial Aspects of Child and Family Health, Committee on Early Childhood Adoption, and Dependent Care, Section on Developmental and Behavioral Pediatrics. The lifelong effects of early childhood adversity and toxic stress. Pediatrics 2012;129(1):e232–46.
3. Garner AS, Shonkoff JP, Committee on Psychosocial Aspects of Child and Family Health, Committee on Early Childhood, Adoption, and Dependent Care,

Section on Developmental and Behavioral Pediatrics. Early childhood adversity, toxic stress, and the role of the pediatrician: translating developmental science into lifelong health. Pediatrics 2012;129(1):e224–31.

4. Kenyon C, Sandel M, Silverstein M, et al. Revisiting the social history for child health. Pediatrics 2007;120(3):e734–8.

5. Weder N, Zhang H, Jensen K, et al. Child abuse, depression, and methylation in genes involved with stress, neural plasticity, and brain circuitry. J Am Acad Child Adolesc Psychiatry 2014;53(4):417–24.

6. Felitti VJ, Anda RF, Nordenberg D, et al. Relationship of childhood abuse and household dysfunction to many of the leading causes of death in adults. Am J Prev Med 1998;14(4):245–58.

7. Dube SR, Anda RF, Velitti VJ, et al. Childhood abuse, household dysfunction, and the risk of attempted suicide throughout the life span. JAMA 2001;286: 3089–96.

8. Flaherty EG, Thompson R, Litrownik AJ, et al. Effect of early childhood adversity on health. Arch Pediatr Adolesc Med 2006;160:1232–8.

9. Edwards VJ, Holden GW, Felitti VJ, et al. Relationship between multiple forms of childhood maltreatment and adult mental health in community respondents: results from the adverse childhood experiences study. Am J Psychiatry 2003; 160(8):1453–60.

10. Dietz PM, Spitz AM, Anda RF, et al. Unintended pregnancy among adult women exposed to abuse or household dysfunction during their childhood. JAMA 1999; 282:1359–64.

11. Flaherty EG, Thompson R, Litrownik AJ, et al. Adverse childhood exposures and reported child health at age 12. Acad Pediatr 2009;9(3):150–6.

12. Brown J, Cohen P, Johnson JG, et al. A longitudinal analysis of risk factors for child maltreatment: findings of a 17-year prospective study of officially recorded and self-reported child abuse and neglect. Child Abuse Negl 1998;22(11): 1065–78.

13. Finkelhor D, Ormrod RK, Turner HA. Poly-victimization: a neglected component in child victimization trauma. Child Abuse Negl 2007;31:7–26.

14. US Department of Health and Human Services, Administration for Children and Families, Administration on Children, Youth and Families, Children's Bureau. Child Maltreatment. 2012. Available at: http://www.acf.hhs.gov/programs/ cb/research-data-technology/statistics-research/child-maltreatment. Accessed February 4, 2014.

15. Yampolskaya S, Greenbaum PE, Berson IR. Profiles of child maltreatment perpetrators and risk for fatal assault: a latent class analysis. J Fam Violence 2009;24:337–48.

16. Huebner RA, Webb T, Brock A, et al. Using models of lethality to enhance child welfare risk and safety assessment. Protecting Children 2010;25(3):76–89.

17. Engel GL. The need for a new medical model: a challenge for biomedicine. Science 1977;196(4286):129–36.

18. Garg A, Dworkin PM. Applying surveillance and screening to family psychosocial issues: implications for the medical home. J Dev Behav Pediatr 2011;32(5): 418–26.

19. Kemper KJ, Kelleher KJ. Rationale for family psychosocial screening. Ambul Child Health 1996;1:311–24.

20. Cyr M, Pasalich DS, McMahon RJ, et al. The longitudinal link between parenting and child aggression: the moderating effect of attachment security. Child Psychiatry Hum Dev 2013. [Epub Ahead of Print].

21. Rutter M. Psychosocial resilience and protective mechanisms. Am J Orthopsychiatry 1987;57(3):316–31.
22. Hillis SD, Anda RF, Dube SR, et al. The Protective effect of family strengths in childhood against adolescent pregnancy and its long-term psychosocial consequences. Perm J 2010;14(3):18–27.
23. Committee on Early Childhood, Adoption, and Dependent Care. The Pediatrician's role in family support and family support programs. Pediatrics 2011; 128(6):e1680–4.
24. Stiffman MN, Schnitzer PG, Adam P, et al. Household composition and risk of fatal child maltreatment. Pediatrics 2002;109(4):615–21.
25. Weissman MM, Pilowsky DJ, Wickramaratne P, et al. Remission of maternal depression is associated with reductions in psychopathology in their children: a Star*D-Child report. JAMA 2006;295(12):1389–98.
26. Dubowitz H, Feigelman S, Lane W, et al. Pediatric primary care to help prevent child maltreatment: the safe environment for every kid (SEEK) model. Pediatrics 2009;123:858–64.
27. Dubowitz H, Lane W, Semiatin JN, et al. The SEEK model of pediatric primary care: can child maltreatment be prevented in a low-risk population? Acad Pediatr 2012;12:259–68.
28. American Academy of Pediatrics. Medical home for children and adolescents exposed to violence. Available at: http://www.aap.org/en-us/advocacy-and-policy/aap-health-initiatives/Medical-Home-for-Children-and-Adolescents-Exposed-to-Violence/Pages/Addressing-Exposure-to-Violence-with-Families-and-Patients.aspx. Accessed February 26, 2014.
29. Putnam-Hornstein E. Report of maltreatment as a risk factor for injury death: a prospective birth cohort study. Child Maltreat 2011;16(3):163–74.
30. Lau AS, Valeri SM, McCarty CA, et al. Abusive parents' reports of child behavior problems: relationship to observed parent-child interactions. Child Abuse Negl 2006;30(6):639–55.
31. DiLauro MD. Psychosocial factors associated with types of child maltreatment. Child Welfare 2004;83(1):69–99.
32. Gelles RJ, Straus MA. Intimate violence: the causes and consequences of abuse in the American Family. New York: Simon & Schuster Inc; 1988.
33. Bugental DB, Happaney K. Predicting infant maltreatment in low-income families: the interactive effects of maternal attributions and Child Status at Birth. Dev Psychol 2004;40(2):234–43.
34. Paz Montes M, De Paul J, Milner JS. Evaluations, attributions, affect, and disciplinary choices in mothers at high and low risk for child physical abuse. Child Abuse Negl 2001;25:1015–36.
35. Seng AC, Prinz RJ. Parents who abuse: what are they thinking? Clin Child Fam Psychol Rev 2008;11(4):163–75.
36. Kolko DJ. Clinical monitoring of treatment course in child physical abuse: psychometric characteristics and treatment comparisons. Child Abuse Negl 1996;20(1):23–43.
37. Herrenkohl TI, Sousa C, Tajima EA, et al. Intersection of child abuse and children's exposure to domestic violence. Trauma Violence Abuse 2008;9(2):84–99.
38. Dong M, Anda RF, Felitti VJ, et al. The interrelatedness of multiple forms of childhood abuse, neglect, and household dysfunction. Child Abuse Negl 2004;28(7): 771–84.
39. Mota DM, Barros AJ. Toilet training: methods, parental expectations and related dysfunctions. J Pediatr 2008;84(1):9–17.

40. Berlin LJ, Dodge KA, Reznick J. Examining pregnant women's hostile attributions about infants as a predictor of offspring maltreatment. JAMA Pediatr 2013;167(6):549–53.

41. Milner JS, Crouch JL. Assessment of maternal attributions of infant's hostile intent and its use in child maltreatment prevention/intervention Efforts. JAMA Pediatr 2013;167(6):588–9.

42. Kolko DJ, Swenson C. Characteristics and correlates of child physical abuse. In: Assessing and treating physically abused children and their families: a cognitive-behavioral approach. Thousand Oaks (CA): Sage Publications, Inc; 2002. p. 16–21.

43. Straus MA, Stewart JH. Corporal punishment by American parents: national data on prevalence, chronicity, severity, duration, in relation to child and family characteristics. Clin Child Fam Psychol Rev 1999;2(2):55–70.

44. Regalado M, Sareen H, Inkelas M, et al. Parents' discipline of young children: results from the national survey of early childhood development. Pediatrics 2004;113(Suppl 6):1952–8.

45. Zolotor AJ, Robinson TW, Runyan DK, et al. The emergence of spanking among a representative sample of children under 2 years of age in North Carolina. Front Psychiatry 2011;2:36.

46. Slade EP, Wissow LS. Spanking in early childhood and later behavior problems: a prospective Study of Infants and Young Toddlers. Pediatrics 2004;113: 1321–30.

47. Zolotor AJ, Theodore AD, Chang JJ, et al. Speak softly-and forget the stick. Corporal punishment and child physical abuse. Am J Prev Med 2008;35(4): 364–9.

48. Gershoff ET. Corporal punishment by parents and associated child behaviors and experiences: a meta-analytic and theoretical review. Psychol Bull 2002; 128(4):539–79.

49. Kadushin A, Martin JA. Child abuse: an interactional event. New York: Columbia University Press; 1981.

50. Gershoff ET. Spanking and child development: we know enough now to stop hitting our children. Child Dev Perspect 2013;7(3):133–7.

51. American Academy of Pediatrics Early Brain and Child Development Leadership Workgroup. The First 1,000 days: Bright Futures examples for promoting Early Brain and Child Development. Available at: http://www.aap.org/en-us/advocacy-and-policy/aap-health-initiatives/EBCD/Documents/EBCD_Well_Child_Grid.pdf. Accessed January 21, 2014.

52. Trocme N, Lindsey D. What can child homicide rates tell us about the effectiveness of child welfare services? Child Abuse Negl 1996;20:171–84.

53. Lucas DR, Wezner KC, Milner JS, et al. Victim, perpetrator, family, and incident characteristics of infant and child homicide in the United States Air Force. Child Abuse Negl 2002;26:167–86.

54. Kotch JB, Browne DC, Dufort V, et al. Predicting child maltreatment in the first four years of life from characteristics assessed in the Neonatal Period. Child Abuse Negl 1999;23(4):305–19.

55. Wickramaratne PJ, Weissman MM. Onset of psychopathology in offspring by developmental phase and parental depression. J Am Acad Child Adolesc Psychiatry 1998;37(9):933–42.

56. Fisher HL, McGuffin P, Boydell J, et al. Interplay Between Childhood Physical Abuse and Familial Risk in the Onset of Psychotic Disorders. Schizophr Bull 2014. [Epub ahead of print].

57. Klinkman MS, Schwenk TL, Coyne JC. Depression in primary care–more like asthma than appendicitis: the Michigan Depression Project. Can J Psychiatry 1998;42:966–73.

58. Swanson JW, Holzer CE, Ganju VK, et al. Violence and psychiatric disorder in the community: Evidence from the Epidemiologic Catchment Area surveys. Hospital and Community. Psychiatry 1990;41:761–70.

59. Chaffin M, Kelleher K, Hollenberg J. Onset of physical abuse and neglect: psychiatric, substance abuse, and social risk factors from prospective community data. Child Abuse Negl 1996;20(3):191–203.

60. Kelleher K, Chaffin M, Hollenberg J, et al. Alcohol and drug disorders among physically abusive and neglectful parents in a community-based sample. Am J Public Health 1994;84(10):1586–90.

61. Walsh C, MacMillan HL, Jamieson E. The relationship between parental substance abuse and child maltreatment: findings from the Ontario Health Supplement. Child Abuse Negl 2003;27(12):1409–25.

62. Wolock I, Magura S. Parental substance abuse as a predictor of child maltreatment re-reports. Child Abuse Negl 1996;20(12):1183–93.

63. Thompson R, Wiley TR. Predictors of re-referral to child protective services: a longitudinal follow-up of an urban cohort maltreated as infants. Child Maltreat 2009;14(1):89–99.

64. Connell CM, Bergeron N, Katz KH, et al. Re-referral to child protective services: the influence of child, family, and case characteristics on risk status. Child Abuse Negl 2007;31(5):573–88.

65. Dakil SR, Sakai C, Lin H, et al. Recidivism in the child protection system: identifying children at greatest risk of reabuse among those remaining in the home. Arch Pediatr Adolesc Med 2011;165(11):1006–12.

66. Levy HB, Markovic J, Chaudhry U, et al. Reabuse rates in a sample of children followed for 5 years after discharge from a child abuse inpatient assessment program. Child Abuse Negl 1995;19(11):1363–77.

67. Fryer GE, Miyoshi TJ. A survival analysis of the revictimization of children: the case of Colorado. Child Abuse Negl 1994;18(12):1063–71.

68. Kolko DJ, Swenson C. Introduction and overview. In: assessing and treating physically abused children and their families: a cognitive-behavioral approach. Thousand Oaks (CA): Sage Publications, Inc; 2002. p. 1–6.

69. Kaufman J, Zigler E. Do abused children become abusive parents? Am J Orthopsychiatry 1987;57:186–92.

70. Thackeray JD, Hibbard R, Dowd D, The Committee on Child Abuse and Neglect, the Committee on Injury, Violence, and Poison Prevention. Intimate partner violence: the role of the pediatrician. Pediatrics 2010;125: 1094–100.

71. Straus MA, Gelles GT, Steinmetz SK. Behind *closed doors*: violence in the American family. Newbury Park (CA): Sage; 1980.

72. Lamers-Winkelman F, Willemen AM, Visser M. Adverse childhood experiences of referred children exposed to intimate partner violence: consequences for their wellbeing. Child Abuse Negl 2012;36(2):166–79.

73. Holmes MR. Aggressive behavior of children exposed to intimate partner violence: an examination of maternal mental health, maternal warmth and child maltreatment. Child Abuse Negl 2013;37(8):520–30.

74. Christian CW, Scribano P, Seidl T, et al. Pediatric injury resulting from family violence. Pediatrics 1997;99(2):e8.

75. Nelson HD, Bougatsos C, Blazina I. Screening Women for Intimate Partner Violence: a systematic review to update the U.S. Preventive Services Task Force Recommendation. Ann Intern Med 2012;156(11):796–808.
76. Schmitt BD. Seven deadly sins of childhood: advising parents about difficult developmental phases. Child Abuse Negl 1987;11:421–32.
77. Yelland J, Brown S. Asking women about mental health and social adversity in pregnancy: results of an Australian population-based survey. Birth 2014;41(1): 79–87.

APPENDIX 1: SAFE ENVIRONMENT FOR EVERY KID PARENT QUESTIONNAIRE

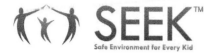

Parent Questionnaire (PQ)

Dear Parent or Caregiver: Being a parent is not always easy. We want to help families have a safe environment for kids. So, we're asking everyone these questions. They are about problems that affect many families. If there's a problem, we'll try to help.

Please answer the questions about your child being seen today for a checkup. If there's more than one child, please answer "yes" if it applies to any one of them. This is voluntary. You don't have to answer any question you prefer not to.

Today's Date: ___/___/____   Child's Name: _____

Child's Date of Birth: __/___/____

PLEASE CHECK

☐ Yes	☐ No	Do you need the phone number for Poison Control?
☐ Yes	☐ No	Do you need a smoke detector for your home?
☐ Yes	☐ No	Does anyone smoke tobacco at home?
☐ Yes	☐ No	In the last year, did you worry that your food would run out before you got money or Food Stamps to buy more?
☐ Yes	☐ No	In the last year, did the food you bought just not last and you didn't have money to get more?
☐ Yes	☐ No	Do you often feel your child is difficult to take care of?
☐ Yes	☐ No	Do you sometimes find you need to hit/spank your child?
☐ Yes	☐ No	Do you wish you had more help with your child?
☐ Yes	☐ No	Do you often feel under extreme stress?
☐ Yes	☐ No	In the past month, have you often felt down, depressed, or hopeless?
☐ Yes	☐ No	In the past month, have you felt very little interest or pleasure in things you used to enjoy?
☐ Yes	☐ No	In the past year, have you been afraid of your partner?
☐ Yes	☐ No	In the past year, have you had a problem with drugs or alcohol?
☐ Yes	☐ No	In the past year, have you felt the need to cut back on drinking or drug use?
☐ Yes	☐ No	Are there any other problems you'd like help with today?

Please give this form to the doctor or nurse you're seeing today. Thank you!

©2012, University of Maryland School of Medicine

Adapted from The SEEK Web site: www.theinstitute.umaryland.edu/SEEK; with permission from Howard Dubowitz, MD, MS, FAAP. Accessed on August 4, 2014.

Engaging Families Through Motivational Interviewing

Adrienne A. Williams, PhD[a],*, Katherine S. Wright, MA[b]

KEYWORDS

- Motivational interviewing • Health behavior change • Child maltreatment
- Risk factors • Pediatrics

KEY POINTS

- Several risk factors for child maltreatment may be addressed through successful parental behavior change.
- A primary barrier to effective behavior change intervention has been a provider-centered approach to communication about change.
- Motivational interviewing (MI) is a person-centered communication technique that helps address barriers to change.
- MI has been found to be effective in improving outcomes for multiple risk behaviors for child maltreatment.
- Implementing MI includes changing the provider's mind-set to be consistent with the patient-centered spirit of MI, and use of specific communication techniques during the medical visit.

INTRODUCTION

Several risk factors for child maltreatment may be reduced through successful parental behavior change. These risk factors include substance use, partner violence, depression, harsh punishment, and management of children's medical health.[1,2] Because the US Preventive Services Task Force concludes that there is insufficient evidence on the effectiveness of preventing child maltreatment directly among children who do not already have signs of maltreatment,[3] prevention efforts may be best aimed at addressing these risk factors that may lead to maltreatment (**Box 1**). Although health care providers may try to encourage behavior change in parents to reduce risk factors, many providers use ineffective techniques to promote behavior change.[4–7]

Disclosures: none.
[a] Department of Family and Community Medicine, University of Maryland School of Medicine, 29 South Paca Street, Lower Level, Baltimore, MD 21201, USA; [b] Department of Psychology, University of Maryland, Baltimore County, 1000 Hilltop Circle, Baltimore, MD 21250, USA
* Corresponding author.
E-mail address: awms@uic.edu

Pediatr Clin N Am 61 (2014) 907–921
http://dx.doi.org/10.1016/j.pcl.2014.06.014
0031-3955/14/$ – see front matter © 2014 Elsevier Inc. All rights reserved.

Box 1
Parental factors that increase risk of child maltreatment

- Substance use
- Partner violence
- Depression
- Inadequate parenting skills
  - Harsh punishment
  - Difficulty managing child's health care needs

EXTENT OF THE PROBLEM: HEALTH CARE PROVIDER–CENTERED APPROACH

Health care providers strive to offer the best care possible to their patients, and, in pediatrics, this may include helping parents of their patients to help themselves. This help includes encouraging changes in lifestyle or health behavior in parents, which affect how well parents care for their children, thus improving their children's health. However, it can also be frustrating to health care providers when they discover that parents have not followed through with recommendations. That frustration may grow as the provider spends another appointment telling parents the same information and hoping that they follow through.

One factor affecting the parent's adherence is not what the health care provider says, but how the provider communicates that information. Research has shown that a primary barrier to effective behavior change intervention has been a health care provider–centered, rather than a patient-centered, approach to communication about change. Provider-centered communication is often well intended and fostered by the desire to help patients or prevent suffering.[4,5,7] That is, after assessing for behaviors that can lead to poor outcomes, the health care provider may then focus on what they perceive to be the barriers to health and often elicit little input from the parents of their pediatric patients. Providers then attempt to address the barrier by telling parents that their behavior is problematic and try to persuade parents to change to what the providers see as appropriate, potentially provoking parent defensiveness or resistance.[4–7] When parents become defensive or resistant to change, providers may view them as unmotivated, unwilling, or unable to make behavior changes to improve the health of their child. However, this perception of parents may serve only to exacerbate any potential or existing problems, because it could contribute to providers feeling helpless and frustrated and could prevent providers from taking an active role in assisting parents to change.

More often, parents are not unmotivated, but instead, not yet convinced of the problem or the need for change. For instance, when a parent smokes in a car through an open window, she might believe she is protecting her child and not realize how much secondhand smoke she is exposing her child to, or how much that smoke likely contributed to her child's recent asthma attack. When parents seem unwilling, they are more likely not committed to making a change at that time. For example, a parent may see as many benefits as drawbacks to continuing to feed his diabetic child the sugary foods his child prefers to avoid battles at dinnertime, and thus exploring the pros and cons of this behavior more thoroughly with the father may help. In addition, when parents seem unable, they may need help believing in their ability to change, such as a mother who has recently relapsed who feels discouraged in her efforts to quit drinking and may feel empowered from a discussion of what worked for her the last time she was successful.[8] If providers set aside their possible assumptions about their patients' parents, and instead try to understand the parents' thoughts and feelings, the providers can both feel personally empowered to influence parents in a positive way and can help empower parents to make difficult changes in their behavior.[4,5]

SEQUELAE OF THE PROBLEM: INCREASING BARRIERS TO CHANGE

Providers may create barriers to their own goals as well as to their patients' families' goals, by failing to use parent-centered communication. Research has shown that taking a more paternalistic approach instead of a collaborative one may both distance the parent from the provider and contribute to worse health outcomes for the pediatric patient.[9,10] When parent and provider agendas or treatment goals do not align or when there is a mismatch between a provider's strategies to address a health behavior and a parent's willingness to change that behavior, the parent's resistance to change is likely to increase.

Another way that providers may be increasing barriers to change for their patients and patients' parents is by taking a more one-dimensional view of behavior change. When providers focus only on certain dimensions of change, such as concentrating solely on the parent's health education (eg, on the link between secondhand smoke and the child's asthma) and ignoring the parent's feelings (eg, she is afraid she cannot cope with stress without smoking) or how ready the parent is to try to change, the intervention is likely going to be unsuccessful.

A more multidimensional view of change is captured in the transtheoretical model, a comprehensive framework that integrates key constructs of several theories of behavior change into one. Intentional behavior change (when people actively monitor and try to modify their behavior) can be thought of as a series of stages that individuals negotiate by engaging in different behaviors and undergoing a variety of cognitive or emotional experiences.[11]

Thus, a parent may not be able to change all at once but instead moves through stages of thinking, planning, and acting to change a behavior. Parents are also at different levels of readiness to change; although they are thinking about changing, they may not be ready to actively make a change yet. Readiness is a dynamic and fluctuating state of motivation. Interacting with readiness is a person's confidence to change, or one's personal evaluation of their ability to exercise control or perform a behavior.[12] A parent may not feel ready to change because they have tried in the past without success and have little confidence in their ability to modify a behavior.

Both readiness and confidence are states that belong to the parents; providers can neither force them to be ready to change nor can providers be confident for them. However, readiness and confidence are modifiable by parents and can be influenced by providers. To influence these states, providers can help change the way parents understand or view particular risk factors or behaviors, they can increase awareness of the impact of these behaviors on their children, and they can empower parents to act. In these ways, providers can promote treatment adherence and engagement in terms of both children's and parents' health.

To decrease resistance and address other problems of provider-centered approaches, providers can learn a person/parent-centered communication technique called motivational interviewing (MI), which has 30 years of research supporting its use in health care settings. MI is not a stand-alone therapy; rather, the provider uses the MI style of interaction to empower the parent to identify their own reasons for change, perceived barriers to change, and strengths to overcome those barriers, as well as to engage the parent in collaborative goal setting. By using MI, the provider can align with the parent in achieving goals that are in the best interest of the child's health, as well as strengthen the parent-provider relationship.[4,10]

In the example given earlier, it is likely not the case that the parent learns that her smoking exacerbates her child's asthma and then quits the following day. Instead, although the educational piece has given her a reason to quit smoking, she may also need to consider ways to assist her in quitting (eg, telephone counseling, nicotine replacement therapy), what worked and did not work when she tried in the past, and what else she could do other than smoking to help her cope with stressful situations before she makes the quit attempt. Using MI techniques, the provider could help this parent to think about these other aspects of change and support her confidence to change, potentially moving her forward through the stages and increasing her likelihood of successfully quitting smoking.[13]

PREPARING FOR MI

When preparing to incorporate MI into practice, the first step is for providers to learn to approach patient interactions in a manner that encompasses the spirit of MI.[4,6] This spirit is the provider's mind-set, which informs the whole intervention and involves 3 key components: (1) collaboration, or developing a partnership that honors the patient's expertise and perspective; (2) evocation, or exploring a patient's preferences, goals and values in an effort to ignite their motivation for change; and (3) autonomy, which involves affirming a patient's right and capacity for self-direction.[4]

This MI mind-set can be different from the disease model of providing health care, in which providers focus on what they see as going wrong, and then they take actions to try to make things right.[4] For example, the provider may screen for a certain illness, and then give the patient a certain medication to treat that illness. Although this model may be effective for some illnesses, it has been found to be ineffective for behavior change. This finding is partly because the power to take action lies with the parent alone; that is, although the health care provider may affect how the parent thinks about a behavior, only the parent performs the behavior.[4] The spirit of MI focuses on the parent's agency in taking action, rather than the provider's. In pediatrics, when the provider approaches the situation with a true understanding that the parents will make their own decisions about themselves and their children, they are less likely to engage in a power struggle with parents or use techniques that contribute to parents not following through with recommendations. MI allows parents to be the more active participants, rather than providers.[6]

When MI is used effectively, the provider no longer has to shoulder the commonly perceived burden of talking patients into doing something. Instead, the provider notices that people talk themselves into changing based on their own values and goals rather than the provider's and ask for guidance when they do wish the provider to help them make decisions. The provider does not try to convince the parent to change a behavior, or make the parent see the situation from the provider's point of view; instead, the provider tries to understand the parent's thoughts, feelings, and behavior from the parent's point of view.[4] This strategy can help the provider express empathy for the patient's circumstances, emotions, and understanding of behavior and barriers, rather than simply trying to impose their perspective of what the parent needs to do.[4] This strategy also allows parents to bring up their own concerns about their own behaviors and work toward addressing them. For example, a parent may voice concern over their own occasional drunk driving, and may wish to work on ways to ensure that they do not drink and drive with their children in the car, even although they are not ready to stop drinking.

The spirit of MI also focuses on strengths, whereas the disease model focuses on weaknesses.[4] When providers concentrate on telling parents about their weaknesses, or how parents' behaviors are wrong, parents try to defend their actions and may become more resistant to change.[4] Instead, with MI, providers use the interview to help parents identify their own goals, strengths, and skills and then, how to use those strengths to achieve their goals. The parent then owns the plan.

In addition, if providers are using MI, they allow for parents to come up with their own behaviors to change, which may be different than the parental behaviors that the providers would target for change. For example, a mother in a major depressive episode may feel guilty that her depression is not allowing her to be the parent she wants to be. The provider approaches this interaction using the MI spirit and talks with the mother about her goal (ie, to be a better parent), helps her verbalize her motivation to reach that goal, explores the mother's motivations and barriers to change, and helps her identify possible solutions. Although the provider's solution (adhering to an antidepressant medication regimen) does not match the mother's solution (engaging in psychotherapy), the MI-consistent strategy is for the provider to empower the mother to try the solution in which she is motivated to engage (ie, psychotherapy) and, thus, is more likely to move the mother toward her goal of being a better parent.

By using an MI approach, providers can assess parents for risk factors for child maltreatment and build good rapport and set the stage for addressing any problems in a collaborative manner. To remain true to the MI spirit, please see **Table 1** for tips that help establish this rapport and meet parents where they are in their readiness to change their behaviors.

EFFECTIVENESS OF MI

The process to become proficient in MI typically involves rigorous training. However, it is often the case that interventions include components or adaptations of MI, and even trials of less faithful deliveries of the techniques have shown equivalency to other active treatments across health behaviors[14] and particularly positive effects on treatment engagement and retention.[15,16] In a meta-analysis of 72 MI treatment outcome studies,[17] MI was found to have small to medium effect for the improvement of health

Table 1 Tips for initiating MI		
Before You Begin the Conversation	**Starting the Conversation**	**During the Conversation**
Be aware of your own preconceptions about substance use, mental illness, and chronic health conditions Have a nonjudgmental attitude Avoid using labels (addict, alcoholic) or diagnoses	Ask permission to discuss a topic further Assure parents that you ask everyone these questions so they do not feel singled out Acknowledge that you recognize that some information is difficult to talk about Try to provide as much privacy as possible and ensure confidentiality, but be honest about limitations	Watch for nonverbal cues, such as: Eye contact Fluidity and tone of speech Posture Movements Affect

outcomes regarding alcohol, smoking, human immunodeficiency virus/AIDS, drug abuse, treatment compliance, gambling, partner violence, water purification/safety, eating disorders, and diet and exercise. In particular, MI may be used for multiple risk factors for child maltreatment, such as substance use, partner violence, depression, unbalanced discipline, and parental management of children's medical health conditions. Evidence for the effectiveness of MI when used with these risk factors is reviewed in the next sections.

Substance Use

Addressing parental substance use with MI may reduce the risk of subsequent child maltreatment. Many studies have been conducted that show the effectiveness of MI in modifying risky use or abuse of substances. Regarding the use of alcohol, a meta-analysis of 15 randomized controlled trials (RCTs)[10] concluded that MI was significantly more effective than a no-treatment control, and either as effective as or more effective than standard care or treatment as usual in reducing alcohol consumption at 3-month follow-up. Studies of MI involving abuse of other substances are also promising. Results from 1 RCT[19] for use of MI in combination with cognitive-behavioral therapy with amphetamine or stimulant users showed significantly higher reports of abstinence from participants in treatment than those in the control group. In another RCT, when providers used MI techniques during a routine medical visit with patients who used cocaine, results showed higher rates of abstinence at 6-month follow-ups.[20] Although this is a brief snapshot of the literature, the use of MI with individuals who engage in many types of substance use has been substantiated. Addressing a parent's substance use could make a significant difference, not only in reducing the risk of child maltreatment but in improving the parent's health as well.

Partner Violence

When faced with a parent of a patient who is involved in a violent relationship, health care providers may find it difficult to avoid outright telling the parent what they believe would be best for both the child and the parent. That knee-jerk reaction to be directive is likely fueled in part by the provider's genuine concern as well as in part by the strong social stigma associated with partner violence. However, this same social stigma may increase resistance to change, because the victimized parent may feel a need to defend the relationship, avoid being shamed, or fear that discussing violence may lead to their children being removed from the home or additional violence.[4]

As indicated earlier, MI is a technique that is particularly useful when the topic at hand is more stigmatized or difficult to discuss, such as substance use or partner violence. Parents experiencing partner violence have probably wrestled with many feelings about the relationship, including shame, fear, and worry, before they walk into that appointment. Because they may already be their own harshest critics, they likely assume that health care providers judge them as well, raising their resistance even before the conversation starts. By using MI, providers can meet parents where they are in weighing the pros and cons of their situation and give them a nonjudgmental space to voice their feelings. MI has been found to be effective in addressing the barriers to behavior change when used with both victims and perpetrators of partner violence.[21] Working with victims of abuse by meeting them at their stage of change and incorporating MI techniques has been found to be effective in improving safety outcomes.[22] In addition, use of MI has been proposed as a tool for helping the nonabusive parent explore their ambivalence when torn between protecting the children and saving the family unit.[23]

Depression

Motivating parents with depressive symptoms to engage in treatment can be difficult, because depressive symptoms can include decreased motivation and energy to engage in treatment. A parent's lack of motivation may be exacerbated by the need to expend energy on child care and their perception that there is little time or energy left over for self-care. Low income and culturally diverse parents may have additional barriers to engaging in treatment, such as transportation, child care, and cultural stigmas about depression or treatment.[24]

Interventions using MI in people with depressive disorders have increased engagement in treatment, increased physical activity,[25] and contributed to fewer reported depressive symptoms.[25,26] MI has also been incorporated into treatments for depression to address medication adherence, completion of therapy homework, and attendance at appointments.[26,27] MI has been effective in increasing medication adherence, especially among cultural groups who have historically had lower adherence rates, such as Latinos.[28] As with addressing parental substance use, when providers address parental depression using MI, they can contribute to parents making positive changes regarding their own physical and mental health, and in turn, may reduce the risk of child maltreatment.

Harsh Punishment

Disciplining children is a necessary part of child rearing, but the type, frequency, or extent of tactics used could modify the risk of child maltreatment. Discipline involves both reinforcing positive behaviors and punishing negative behaviors, and balanced discipline depends on the age and characteristics of the child.[29] There are many tactics that may be used to reinforce or punish children's behavior, and most of these tactics can be beneficial in moderation, but harmful to the child in the extreme.

For example, a parent may give a child a favorite food to reward a behavior; however, the use of food as a motivator can become unbalanced and harmful to the child, such as allowing a child to eat junk food all the time or withholding food for days. Similarly, nonabusive spanking as a punishment has been found to be no more harmful than other forms of discipline and has been linked to several benefits, including increased compliance, decreased fighting, increased parental affection, and enhancement of the effectiveness of other disciplinary methods (such as time-outs).[29,30] However, severe corporal punishment has been found to be harmful,[31] and using only positive forms of parenting has also been found to be problematic.[32]

Parents may be resistant to being told to change their discipline style, and MI has been suggested as a way to reduce resistance that can be exacerbated by professionals, especially when discussing child protection.[33] It has been recommended that MI be used even after other standardized forms of parent training, which include explaining or showing consequences of behaviors, have not been effective.[34] Interventions using MI have been found to be effective in improving balance in discipline, such as increasing parental structure and family management, decreasing parental permissiveness, and subsequently, decreasing problematic behavior in children.[35,36] With regard to physical punishment, MI-based intervention has been found to reduce use of physical punishment in parents who were referred for treatment after children were physically abused or at risk for abuse.[37] In addition, parents who receive MI are more likely to participate in parenting workshops.[38]

Managing Medical Health

Adhering to medical treatments is more strongly related to health outcomes among children than it is for adults,[39] and patient adherence is more than 1.5 times greater for physicians trained in communication skills such as those used in MI.[40] The effect of communication skills on adherence is even stronger among pediatricians.[40] Because nonadherance may result in poor health outcomes or harm to children, use of MI has been recommended to improve parental management of children's medical conditions.[41]

Interventions that have incorporated MI have been found to have long-term benefits for families engaging in and continuing different kinds of treatments for their children.[42] For example, when MI has been used with parents, children with obesity or diabetes have had improved weight-related behaviors, better blood glucose monitoring, and improved hemoglobin A_{1c} levels.[43,44] Similarly, parents who are given options to vaccinate their children have been found to be at different readiness levels to accept vaccination. Pediatricians may increase parents' readiness to vaccinate by using MI and meeting parents at their readiness level when communicating with them.[45]

CLINICAL ASSESSMENT

Although providers may remain in the MI spirit throughout the whole clinical encounter, MI techniques are typically used during the portion of an encounter when the provider wishes to address a specific behavior. After parents have screened positive for a risk factor for child maltreatment, the provider follows up with open-ended questions to gather more information (see section on open-ended questions) and then with more specific questions, particularly when parents provide qualified answers. It is important to pay attention to both the manner in which the parent responds as well as the content. Nonverbal behavior might indicate a positive screen or signify that the parent is holding back information (see **Table 1** for examples of nonverbal behavioral cues). If a provider notices potentially significant nonverbal behavior, acknowledging a parent's discomfort or hesitancy may provide the space for the parent to provide more information and address their feelings around the answer.[4]

Once the parent has given permission to discuss the behavior further, the MI portion of the visit begins. The provider should assess both the parent's readiness and confidence to change their behavior.[4,5] Parents' readiness to change is influenced by how important it is for them to change, or rather, their perceived need for change. Using an importance ruler, on which the numbers 0 (not important at all) to 10 (extremely important) are printed, providers can ask, "On a scale of 0 to 10, how important is it for you to change any aspect of your _____ (behavior)?" If the patient chooses any number greater than 1, the provider could follow up and ask, "What led you to choose that number and not a 0?" to elicit a parent's motivation for changing that behavior. If a parent chooses 0, the provider could ask about the parent's perceived barriers to change.[4]

After a discussion of readiness and importance, the provider should assess a parent's confidence to change, using the same ruler (a confidence ruler, in this case) and format of questioning: "On a scale of 0 to 10, how confident are you that you can change _____ (behavior)?" Once the parent has chosen a number, the provider can follow with questions about why the parent chose that number versus a number higher or lower. These questions are designed to help the provider explore the parent's previous successes, failures, and feelings about past attempts and future change.[4] In this conversation, the provider can bolster a parent's confidence by highlighting a parent's strengths or steps in the direction of change. Providers can also identify areas of skill deficits for which they could provide resources for treatment or remediation.

APPROACH

There are 4 core skills that are used during the assessment and subsequent discussion that help to make MI effective. These skills can be remembered with the mnemonic OARS: open-ended questions, affirmations, reflections, and summary statements.[4] Each of these skills contributes to a style of communicating that helps the provider elicit information from and collaborate with the parent; a style that contrasts with the provider-centered approach of trying to convince a parent to change a wrong behavior, which may increase resistance.

Open-Ended Questions

Open-ended questions gather more information as well as convey to a parent that the provider values their thoughts and feelings. Open-ended questions are the antithesis of closed-ended questions, which can convey judgment and increase resistance to change. Although providers may believe that close-ended questions are more time efficient, they sacrifice the collaborative relationship and spend more time guessing via closed-ended questions by eliciting specific information or potentially leading the parent in a certain direction. There are several types of closed questions, including multiple choice (the patient is given several options to choose from); dichotomous (question pulls for 1 of 2 answers, such as yes or no), leading (question directs the patient to 1 correct answer), or specific information questions (asking for factual information). In contrast, open-ended questions allow parents to reflect on their own emotions, thoughts, and values and to discuss them.[4] Open-ended questions often start with words like how, what, or tell me and invite the patient to provide a deeper answer and are the key to identifying the parent's perspective. In addition, open-ended questions can be used to invite parents to identify their own strategies for behavior change, which increases the likelihood that the parent tries the new behaviors (**Table 2**).

Affirmations

Affirmations are the contrast to focusing on the negative, which directs attention to the parent's weaknesses, what they need to change, have not accomplished yet, or what

Table 2
Examples of replacing closed-ended with open-ended questions

Avoid	Use Instead
Closed-Ended Questions	**Open-Ended Questions**
Multiple choice	
Will you decrease snacks, sodas, or portion sizes to help your child's weight?	What changes could you make in your child's diet to help your child's weight?
Dichotomous	
Do you want to stay in this relationship?	How do you feel about this relationship?
Leading	
You don't use corporal punishment, do you?	What forms of discipline do you use?
Specific information	
Who takes care of your daughter when you're depressed and in bed?	Tell me how your depression affects your ability to care for your daughter

misinformation the parents have. It is often difficult for providers to mention only the positive without mentioning the change that they are hoping the parent makes or correcting the misinformation. However, pulling attention to changes to be made or weaknesses is deflating rather than motivating. In addition, immediately correcting misinformation is interpreted as judgment or contradiction, rather than support. By providing affirmations, the provider can highlight the parent's strengths and what they have accomplished without drawing attention to what goals have not yet been reached or what they have done wrong.[4] This strategy can help to build the parent's self-efficacy or confidence to move forward with making changes and leaves room for the provider to provide education later (**Table 3**).

Reflections

Reflections are statements that let the parent know what the provider understands about what the parent just said. As the name suggests, reflections should mirror back only the parent's own perspective, without adding in any of the provider's values or ideas. Mirroring back does not mean that the same words need to be used; paraphrasing is sufficient, so long as the provider attempts to make a statement in which the content or meaning of what was said is reflected. Reflections are the key to ensuring that the provider understands the parent's perspective and help the provider communicate their understanding of the parent's perspective back to the parent.[4] This situation is in contrast to making statements that convey the provider's perspective, such as expressing judgment (positive or negative) or suggesting what the parent should do in the situation (**Table 4**).

Summary Statements

Summary statements help to pull together different components of the interview and can help parents develop insight into their own inner conflicts and discrepancies in their goals and actions. Summary statements are not statements that attempt to direct a parent to a specific behavior or statements that highlight only 1 side of the parent's perspective. There are several types of summary statements. They may be collective, reflecting back a list of things that the patient has said. They may form links, connecting various thoughts or experiences from different parts of the conversation, or across different conversations. Summary statements may also help transition to different

Table 3
Examples of replacing nonaffirming statements with affirmations

Avoid	Use Instead
Nonaffirming Statements	**Affirmations**
Even if you smoke outside, your child can still be exposed to smoke	You have been making good efforts to reduce your child's exposure to smoke
Asthma controller medications really need to be taken every day	Even though you have had some challenges, it sounds like you've been trying hard to give your son his medications more regularly
You're really inconsistent with your use of time-outs	You've been using time-outs when you can, and trying hard to use effective disciplining techniques
It's good that you cut down to half a pack per day, so now you can work on quitting completely	It's good that you cut down to half a pack per day. Cutting down is difficult and you've done a great job!

Table 4
Examples of replacing provider's perspective with reflections

Avoid	Use Instead
Provider's Perspective	Reflections
It really would be best for you and your kids if you got out of this violent relationship	It sounds like there are still a lot of good parts to this relationship that you don't want to lose
I really think you will only get better if you take medications	Although your depressive symptoms are upsetting and you think medication may help, you are concerned that the side effects of medication will make you feel worse
Even though the insulin shots hurt, it is important to give them to your son to prevent health problems	It is difficult to give your son shots when you know they hurt him, but you also don't want him to have the long-term effects of uncontrolled diabetes
The amount that you're drinking really could affect your children's health	Right now, you feel like the amount you're drinking won't hurt your children's health

parts of the visit, by concluding what has already been discussed and allowing the conversation to move to a different topic (**Table 5**).[4]

WHEN TO USE MI

MI is particularly effective when used across time (see **Fig. 1** for sample structure). Once a behavior that may increase the risk for child maltreatment has been identified, the behavior can be addressed at every visit. MI allows the behavior to be discussed through conversation rather than through pressure to change. The provider can start the conversation with a reflection, followed by an open-ended question.[4,6] This strategy can work well by reflecting back what was said in the summary statement at the previous visit and then asking for an update. For example, a provider may state,

Table 5
Examples of replacing directing with summarizing

Avoid	Use Instead
Directing	Summarizing
How about you try using time-outs instead of spanking?	You don't feel that your spanking will get out of control, but you'll consider using time-outs if you get really angry
So it sounds like there are a lot of reasons for you to quit drinking	On 1 hand, alcohol helps you socialize and relieve stress, and you don't want to stop drinking right now. On the other hand, you feel like it can lead to problems
The plan should be take your son to the playground for exercise and replace the processed snacks with options like cut-up vegetables and fruits	It sounds like you're interested in finding ways for your son to get more exercise through play, and you're thinking about trying healthier snacks, but you'd like to brainstorm some ways to accomplish these goals
If you don't take care of yourself, you won't be able to take care of your children	You would like to get treatment for yourself, and you will try, but you're not sure if you'll find the time

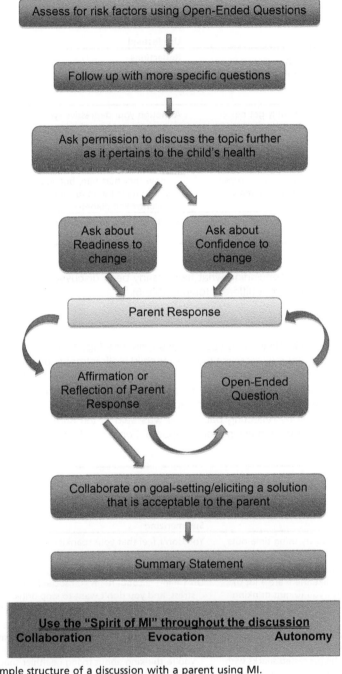

Fig. 1. Sample structure of a discussion with a parent using MI.

"At the last visit, you were telling me how you were concerned about the side effects your daughter might experience on this medication but also were concerned about not treating her condition. What are your thoughts now?"

It can be particularly helpful to make a note in the medical record about the parent's motivation to change a behavior, their primary barrier to change, and where the conversation left off. Because people do not change behaviors all at once, MI helps both the parent and provider by mirroring the process of change.[4,11,46] It allows the parent to rely on strengths and overcome barriers. It aids providers by helping them to relinquish control of a parent's behaviors, decreasing the frustration that is felt when there is a discrepancy between where the parent is in their readiness to change and where the provider wants them to be.

SUMMARY

MI helps providers to reduce the barriers to behavior change that provider-centered techniques may exacerbate. MI has been found to be effective for aiding behavior change for multiple risk factors for child maltreatment. By incorporating MI techniques, providers can collaboratively address parental risk factors, improving adherence to recommendations, decreasing provider and parent frustration, and potentially improving the health of both the parent and their child.

REFERENCES

1. Centers for Disease Control and Prevention (CDC). Child maltreatment: risk and protective factors. In: Centers for Disease Control and prevention: injury prevention & control. 2013. Available at: http://www.cdc.gov/violenceprevention/childmaltreatment/riskprotectivefactors.html. Accessed November 23, 2013.
2. US Department of Health and Human Services. Administration for Children & Families. In: Child Maltreatment 2011. Children's Bureau; 2012. Available at: http://www.acf.hhs.gov/programs/cb/resource/child-maltreatment-2011. Accessed November 23, 2013.
3. Moyer VA, US Preventive Services Task Force. Primary care interventions to prevent child maltreatment: US Preventive Services Task Force recommendation statement. Ann Intern Med 2013;159(4):289–95.
4. Miller WR, Rollnick S. Motivational interviewing: helping people change. 3rd edition. New York: Guilford Press; 2013.
5. Rollnick S, Miller WR, Butler C. Motivational interviewing in health care: helping patients change behavior. New York: Guilford Press; 2008.
6. Suarez M, Mullins S. Motivational interviewing and pediatric health behavior interventions. J Dev Behav Pediatr 2008;29(5):417–28.
7. Gance-Cleveland B. Motivational interviewing: improving patient education. J Pediatr Health Care 2007;21(2):81–8.
8. DiClemente CC. Addiction and change: how addictions develop and addicted people recover. New York: Guilford Press; 2003.
9. Eisenthal S, Emery R, Lazare A, et al. Adherence and the negotiated approach to patienthood. Arch Gen Psychiatry 1979;36:393–8.
10. Emmons KM, Rollnick S. Motivational Interviewing in health care settings: opportunities and limitations. Am J Prev Med 2001;20:68–74.
11. Prochaska JO, DiClemente CC. Transtheoretical therapy: toward a more integrative model of change. Psychotherapy 1982;19(3):276–88.
12. Bandura A. Self-efficacy: toward a unifying theory of behavioral change. Psychol Rev 1977;84(2):191–215.

13. Miller W. Motivation for treatment: a review with special emphasis on alcoholism. Psychol Bull 1985;98(1):84.
14. Burke BL, Arkowitz H, Menchola M. The efficacy of motivational interviewing: a meta-analysis of controlled clinical trials. J Consult Clin Psychol 2003;71:843–61.
15. Carroll KM, Ball SA, Nich C, et al. Motivational interviewing to improve treatment engagement and outcome in individuals seeking treatment for substance abuse: a multisite effectiveness study. Drug Alcohol Depend 2006;81:301–12.
16. Miller WR, Yahne CE, Tonigan JS. Motivational interviewing in drug abuse services: a randomized trial. J Consult Clin Psychol 2003;71:754–63.
17. Hettema J, Steele J, Miller WR. Motivational interviewing. Annu Rev Clin Psychol 2005;1:91–111.
18. Vasilaki EI, Hosier SG, Cox WM. The efficacy of motivational interviewing as a brief intervention for excessive drinking: a meta-analytic review. Alcohol Alcohol 2006;41:328–35.
19. Baker A, Lee NK, Claire M, et al. Brief cognitive behavioural interventions for regular amphetamine users: a step in the right direction. Addiction 2005;100:367–78.
20. Bernstein J, Bernstein E, Tassiopoulos K, et al. Brief motivational intervention at a clinic visit reduces cocaine and heroin use. Drug Alcohol Depend 2005;77:49–59.
21. Murphy CM, Maiuro RD. Motivational interviewing and stages of change in intimate partner violence. New York: Springer; 2009.
22. Reisenhofer S, Taft A. Women's journey to safety–the transtheoretical model in clinical practice when working with women experiencing intimate partner violence: a scientific review and clinical guidance. Patient Educ Couns 2013; 93(3):536–48.
23. Corcoran J. The transtheoretical stages of change model and motivational interviewing for building maternal supportiveness in cases of sexual abuse. J Child Sex Abus 2002;11(3):1–17.
24. Sampson M, Zayas LH, Seifert SB. Treatment engagement using motivational interviewing for low-income, ethnically diverse mothers with postpartum depression. Clin Soc Work J 2013;41(4):387–94.
25. Bombardier CH, Ehde DM, Gibbons LE, et al. Telephone-based physical activity counseling for major depression in people with multiple sclerosis. J Consult Clin Psychol 2013;81(1):89–99.
26. Westra HA, Aviram A, Doell FK. Extending motivational interviewing to the treatment of major mental health problems: current directions and evidence. Can J Psychiatry 2011;56(11):643–50.
27. Hides L, Carroll S, Lubman DI, et al. Brief motivational interviewing for depression and anxiety. In: Bennett-Levy J, Richards DA, Farrand P, et al, editors. Oxford guide to low intensity CBT interventions. New York: Oxford University Press; 2010. p. 177–85.
28. Interian A, Lewis-Fernández R, Gara MA, et al. A randomized-controlled trial of an intervention to improve antidepressant adherence among Latinos with depression. Depress Anxiety 2013;30(7):688–96.
29. Larzelere RE. Child outcomes of nonabusive and customary physical punishment by parents: an updated literature review. Clin Child Fam Psychol Rev 2000;3(4): 199–221.
30. Bernal ME, Duryee JS, Pruett HL. Behavior modification and the brat syndrome. J Consult Clin Psychol 1968;32(4):447–55.
31. Hicks-Pass S. Corporal punishment in America today: spare the rod, spoil the child? A systematic review of the literature. Best Pract Ment Health 2009;5(2): 71–88.

32. Reece H. The pitfalls of positive parenting. Ethics Educ 2013;8(1):42–54.
33. Forrester D, Westlake D, Glynn G. Parental resistance and social worker skills: towards a theory of motivational social work. Child Fam Soc Work 2012;17(2):118–29.
34. Scott S, Dadds MR. Practitioner review: when parent training doesn't work: theory-driven clinical strategies. J Child Psychol Psychiatry 2009;50(12):1441–50.
35. O'Leary CC. The early childhood family check-up: a brief intervention for at-risk families with preschool-aged children. Diss Abstr Int 2001;62(6-B):2992.
36. Rao SA. The short-term impact of the family check-up: a brief motivational intervention for at-risk families. Diss Abstr Int 1999;59(7-B):3710.
37. Runyon MK, Deblinger E, Schroeder CM. Pilot evaluation of outcomes of combined parent-child cognitive-behavioral group therapy for families at risk for child physical abuse. Cogn Behav Pract 2009;16(1):101–18.
38. Sterrett E, Jones DJ, Zalot A, et al. A pilot study of a brief motivational intervention to enhance parental engagement: a brief report. J Child Fam Stud 2010;19(6): 697–701.
39. DiMatteo MR, Giordani PJ, Lepper HS, et al. Patient adherence and medical treatment outcomes: a meta-analysis. Med Care 2002;40(9):794–811.
40. Zolnierek KB, Dimatteo MR. Physician communication and patient adherence to treatment: a meta-analysis. Med Care 2009;47(8):826–34.
41. Gance-Cleveland B. Motivational interviewing as a strategy to increase families' adherence to treatment regimens. J Spec Pediatr Nurs 2005;10(3):151–5.
42. Ingoldsby EM. Review of interventions to improve family engagement and retention in parent and child mental health programs. J Child Fam Stud 2010;19(5): 629–45.
43. Chin CN. The impact of an obesity intervention including motivational interviewing on outcomes for children and adolescents. Diss Abstr Int 2012;73(1-B):659.
44. Stanger C, Ryan SR, Delhey LM, et al. Multicomponent motivational intervention to improve adherence among adolescents with poorly controlled type 1 diabetes: a pilot study. J Pediatr Psychol 2013;38(6):629–37.
45. Leask J, Kinnersley P, Jackson C, et al. Communicating with parents about vaccination: a framework for health professionals. BMC Pediatr 2012;12:154–65.
46. Prochaska JO, DiClemente CC. Stages and processes of self-change of smoking: toward an integrative model of change. J Consult Clin Psychol 1983;51: 390–5.

Sentinel Injuries
Subtle Findings of Physical Abuse

Hillary W. Petska, MD, Lynn K. Sheets, MD*

KEYWORDS

- Sentinel injury • Child abuse • Precruising • Infants • Bruising
- Abusive head trauma • Prevention

KEY POINTS

- A sentinel injury is a visible, minor injury in a precruising infant that is poorly explained and therefore concerning for physical abuse.
- Sentinel injuries are common in abused infants and rare in nonabused infants.
- A history of a sentinel injury in an infant with suspected abuse should increase the level of concern for maltreatment.
- Identification of a sentinel injury, reporting, and intervention may prevent further abuse.

INTRODUCTION/CHARACTERIZE THE ISSUE/PROBLEM

A 7-week-old infant presented to an emergency room by ambulance after an episode of pallor, vomiting, and decreased responsiveness. Physical examination was significant for an ill-appearing infant with a weak cry. The head computed tomography (CT) showed bilateral, thin, acute, convexity subdural hemorrhages, and the skeletal survey showed acute and healing rib fractures, as well as a classic metaphyseal lesion and acute spiral fracture of the right tibia. Extensive retinal hemorrhages were also noted on dilated funduscopic examination. Following a comprehensive evaluation by the hospital-based child protection team, the child was diagnosed with abusive head trauma and fractures. In the medical history, the father reported a bruise adjacent to the infant's mouth 2 weeks before admission, which he attributed to the infant bumping her head on her pacifier while he held the infant to his chest (**Fig. 1**). The father eventually confessed to abusing the infant on multiple occasions. If this initial sentinel

Financial Disclosure: Dr L.K. Sheets has provided paid expert testimony for prosecution and defense attorneys in cases of alleged child maltreatment. Dr H.W. Petska does not have any financial relationships relevant to this article to disclose.
Conflict of Interest: The authors have no conflicts of interest.
Children's Hospital of Wisconsin, Medical College of Wisconsin, Milwaukee, WI, USA
* Corresponding author. Child Advocacy and Protection Services, Department of Pediatrics, Children's Hospital of Wisconsin, C615, PO Box 1997, Milwaukee, WI 53201.
E-mail address: lsheets@chw.org

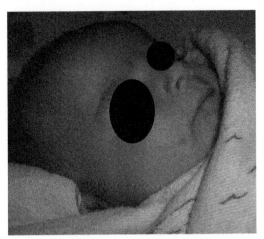

Fig. 1. Cheek bruise in a 5-week-old female infant noted by the family 2 weeks before she was admitted for abusive head trauma. (*Courtesy of* LK Sheets, MD, Milwaukee, WI.)

injury had been identified as concerning for abuse and appropriate safety measures used, the subsequent severe injuries may have been prevented.

Musculoskeletal, intraoral, and skin injuries other than superficial abrasions are not expected in the normal care and handling of infants who have not yet achieved the developmental milestone called cruising, which is pulling to a stand and taking a few steps while holding on to an object.[1–3] When such injuries occur in this population, the possibility of physical abuse should be considered because they are warning signs for abuse or sentinel injuries. A sentinel injury is a visible or detectable minor injury in a precruising infant that is poorly explained and therefore suspicious for physical abuse (**Box 1**). Sentinel injuries generally are not clinically significant from a treatment perspective because they typically heal quickly and completely without sequelae. Examples of such injuries include bruising, intraoral injury (eg, torn labial or sublingual frenum), radial head subluxation (ie, nursemaid's elbow), and minor burns (**Figs. 2** and **3**).

Occult injuries such as rib fractures are not sentinel injuries since these are not readily detectable by a caregiver. Nonspecific skin findings such as transient reddening of the skin or superficial abrasions are also excluded because these may occur in the normal care of an infant.[4] Superficial abrasions are common, unintentional injuries in infants (eg, fingernail scratches on the face of a neonate).[3]

EXTENT OF THE PROBLEM

More than 3 million reports of child maltreatment are received by child protective services every year in the United States, approximately 18% of which are for physical

---

Box 1
Definition of sentinel injuries

- Minor injuries, such as a bruise or intraoral injury (excluding skin abrasions)
- Precruising infant
- Visible or detectable to a caregiver
- Poorly explained and unexpected

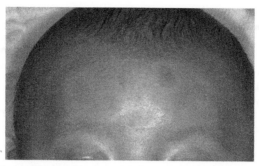

Fig. 2. Sentinel injury: 6-week-old abused infant with bruising on the forehead that had reportedly occurred from rolling into the crib slats. (*Courtesy of* LK Sheets, MD, Milwaukee, WI.)

abuse.[5] Soft tissue injury, such as bruising, is the most common presenting feature of physical abuse in children and has been studied extensively in both nonabused and abused children.[3,6–8]

Published research shows that soft tissue injuries other than abrasions are rare in normal infants who are not abused and often precede severe injuries in abused infants.[1–3,9] The prevalence of sentinel injuries in precruising infants is difficult to ascertain because caregivers may not seek medical evaluation given the minor nature of these injuries. In addition, discovery of a sentinel injury by medical professionals during a routine physical examination or through the medical history may be undocumented if the injury is incorrectly interpreted as minor or trivial. Until recently, the prevalence of sentinel injuries in infants evaluated for child maltreatment was not known.

A previous history of a sentinel injury occurs at an alarming rate in infants who are evaluated for abuse by a hospital-based child protection team. In a recent study of infants less than 12 months of age who were evaluated for maltreatment, 27.5% of those with injuries diagnostic for physical abuse (eg, abusive head trauma, abdominal trauma, fractures, or burns) had a history of previous, minor injury described by a parent during the medical history. None of the infants who were evaluated for maltreatment and ultimately diagnosed as having an accidental injury, a medical condition that could be mistaken for abuse, or a normal variant had a previous history of sentinel

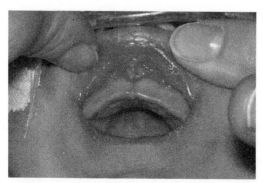

Fig. 3. A 2-month-old severely abused infant who had a healing upper labial frenum injury as well as bite wounds, a liver laceration, multiple fractures in various stages of healing, retinal hemorrhages, and subdural hemorrhages. (*Courtesy of* LK Sheets, MD, Milwaukee, WI.)

injury. The most common type of sentinel injury was bruising, followed by intraoral injury. Sentinel bruises were typically located on the head or face, and 95% occurred in infants younger than 7 months (**Box 2**).[9] Other researchers have also shown that the head and face are the most common sites for abusive injuries.[6,8,10–13] In ambulating children, the head and face may also be bruised in unintentional traumatic events, such as falls down stairs.[14–17]

Although a study by Pierce and colleagues[14] found no correlation between facial or head bruising and abuse in children less than 48 months of age, the study population included primarily mobile children admitted to an intensive care unit for trauma. However, in this study, bruising in infants less than 4 months of age was noted to be concerning for abuse.[14]

CAUSES/CONTRIBUTORY OR RISK FACTORS

Although soft tissue injuries, such as bruising, are commonly seen in mobile children, injuries in precruising infants are rare.[1–3,8,11,18,19] Before an infant is mobile, bruising does not typically occur during routine handling or normal activity. In several studies of precruising infants and infants less than 9 months of age, only 0% to 2.2% had bruising on well-child physical examinations.[1–3] In the absence of an underlying medical condition or a clear and plausible history of an unintentional event, any injury beyond superficial abrasions in infants who are not yet independently mobile is concerning for child physical abuse.[2] A plausible history should include an explanation of a discrete event in which the described mechanism is consistent with the type and severity of injury and the developmental capability of the child. For example, a forehead bruise in a 6-month-old infant who can sit independently may be plausible if the mother clearly recalls and provides a history of the child falling over and the head hitting a hard toy.

The pattern and location of bruising on the body also can be helpful in assessing the plausibility of injury in a child.[1–3,8,18,19] Unintentional bruises in mobile children typically occur over bony prominences on the anterior aspect of the body, such as the knees, shins, or forehead, although an occasional bruise over soft parts of the body, such as the cheeks, abdomen, buttocks, or upper arms, can be seen in active children (**Table 1**).[1,2,7,8,18–20] Abused children are more likely to have injuries on the soft parts of the body and on protected locations such as the neck, genitals, and inner thighs (**Fig. 4**).[8,11,12,21–24] This information on the location of suspicious bruising can be applied in practice using the TEN-4 body region–based and age-based bruising

---

Box 2
Summary of key findings

- A sentinel injury preceded severe abuse in 27.5% of cases
- A history of a sentinel injury is rare in infants evaluated for maltreatment and found to not be abused
- All sentinel injuries were observed by a parent
- Forty-two percent of the sentinel injuries were known to a medical provider but the infants were not protected from further harm
- Recognition of and appropriate response to sentinel injuries could prevent many cases of child physical abuse

Adapted from Sheets LK, Leach ME, Koszewski IJ, et al. Sentinel injuries in infants evaluated for child physical abuse. Pediatrics 2013;131:701–7.

Table 1
Characteristics of bruises that should be considered when evaluating a child for possible abuse

Characteristic	Typical	Concerning for Abuse
Age/developmental stage of the child	Independently mobile child	Precruising infant
Location (see **Fig. 4**)	Over bony prominences, especially over the knees and shins	Over soft parts of the body or unusual locations such as the cheek, ear, neck, buttock, abdomen, or hand
Pattern	Nonpatterned	Patterned (shape of an implement from high-velocity impact or from crush injury)

clinical decision rule, which states that any bruising in a precruising infant or bruising on the **T**orso, **E**ars, or **N**eck of a child 4 years of age or younger should be considered signs of possible physical abuse.[14] Multiple or clustered and patterned injuries including circumferential or linear patterns should also raise concern for inflicted injury.[3,7,8] Patterned injuries typically occur from a crushing mechanism such as a human bite or through high-velocity impact, such as a looped cord or slap (**Table 2**).

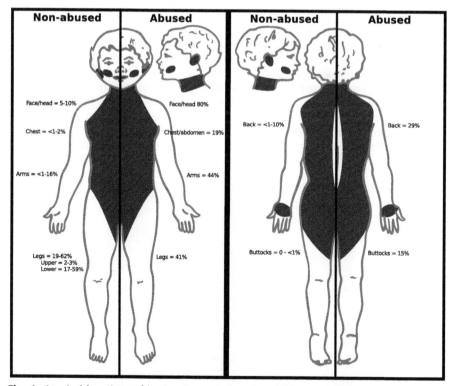

Fig. 4. Atypical locations of bruises in normal, active children. Areas in black are atypical locations for bruising in an active child. Ranges of percentages of bruising in various body locations based on published research are included for nonabused[1,2] and abused[25] children.

Table 2
Mechanisms of patterned bruising

Mechanism	Example of Injury
Crush: bruise at site of contact	Bruising from a bite (**Fig. 5**), pinch, or grab
High-velocity impact: outline of implement	Bruising impact with a hand (**Fig. 6**), looped cord (**Fig. 7**), or hanger
Pressure changes: petechiae	Hickey, facial petechiae from strangulation (**Fig. 8**)
Incised wounds (cut): bruise along edges of wound	Knife wound
Lacerations (torn skin with tissue bridges): bruise at edges of laceration	Punch to face resulting in a laceration
Indirect forces (shearing): bruise distant to contact	Vertical bruises from severe force spanking of the buttocks[26] (**Fig. 9**)
Dependent: bruise results in blood settling under the effects of gravity	Black eye from bruise on forehead

Other soft tissue and musculoskeletal injuries, such as intraoral trauma and subluxation of the radial head, are uncommon and unexpected in precruising infants.[27,28] Although an isolated finding of a torn labial or sublingual frenum is not diagnostic for abuse, intraoral injuries are found in a significant number of abused infants.[27] Unless well-explained, an intraoral injury in a precruising infant should raise serious concerns about child abuse.

Although child physical abuse occurs in all geographic, ethnic, and socioeconomic settings, there are certain risk factors that increase the likelihood of maltreatment. One of the primary variables is age of the child. Young children, especially those less than 1 year of age, have the highest rate of maltreatment, at a rate that is more than twice that of other children: 21.9 per 1000 versus 9.2 per 1000, respectively.[5] In hospitalized patients, the rate of serious physical abuse in children less than 1 year of age is 58.2 per 100,000, compared with 6.2 per 100,000 in general.[29] The high rate of infant abuse may be related to several factors, including increased needs, complete dependence

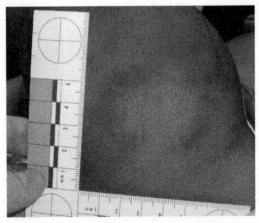

Fig. 5. Crush injury: 3-month-old fatally abused infant with human bite injury on the thigh. (*Courtesy of* LK Sheets, MD, Milwaukee, WI.)

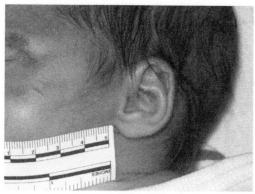

Fig. 6. High-velocity impact: 2-month-old abused twin infant with slap injury on the face. (*Courtesy of* LK Sheets, MD, Milwaukee, WI.)

on caregivers, and physical vulnerability.[30] Crying, a commonly identified trigger among perpetrators, typically peaks in duration in the second month of life, although caregiver's perception of and response to crying is a more important risk factor than the duration of crying.[9,31–33]

Other risk factors for child physical abuse include young parental age, mental health disorders, substance abuse, and domestic violence.[34] Low socioeconomic status has also been identified as a risk factor for physical abuse.[34] Differences based on race have been suggested, although this may be caused by decreased recognition in children with darker pigmentation or variation in reporting practices.[2] Bruising in abused and nonabused children does not differ by gender.[8] Although these factors have been noted to increase risk in general, the health care professional should consider each case individually to determine the level of concern for abuse.

SEQUELAE OF THE PROBLEM

Although sentinel injuries by definition are not life threatening, multiple studies have shown an association between minor abusive injuries in precruising infants and later, more severe physical abuse. Although a sentinel injury may result from an initial, isolated incident of abuse, it may also precede escalation of violence toward the infant.

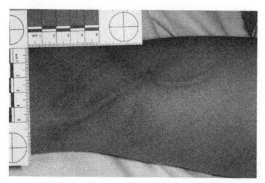

Fig. 7. High-velocity impact: abused child with looped and linear injuries on the thigh from high-velocity impacts with a belt. (*Courtesy of* LK Sheets, MD, Milwaukee, WI.)

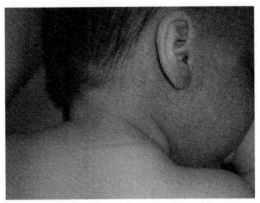

Fig. 8. Pressure change injury: infant with accidental near strangulation and facial petechiae. (*Courtesy of* A. Swenson, MD, Milwaukee, WI.)

If not appropriately addressed, more severe physical abuse may result.[4,9,26,35–42] Chronicity of infant physical abuse is also shown by perpetrator confessions in which perpetrators often admit to repetitive abuse in response to infant crying.[43] Timely intervention is critical in these cases because the interval between sentinel injury and subsequent more serious abuse can range from a day to months.[9]

CLINICAL ASSESSMENT

An accurate diagnosis of abuse may be missed by medical providers as a result of failure to consider abuse because of the subtlety of findings, perception of the injury as mild, or the presence of nonspecific symptoms.[9,34,44] Bruises can be difficult to visualize because of their location on the scalp, behind the ear, or other less visible locations, and bruises may heal quickly and be difficult to detect, especially in darkly pigmented children. Some types of abusive injuries cause symptoms such as vomiting that may be mistaken for common childhood illnesses.[36] Medical providers may misattribute bruises to self-inflicted trauma or normal care and handling in precruising infants, despite such injuries being unexpected. In the study on sentinel injuries, medical providers were reportedly aware of the sentinel injury in 41.9% of cases in which

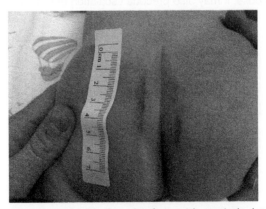

Fig. 9. Indirect forces: 10-month-old abused infant with vertical gluteal cleft bruising. (*Courtesy of* LK Sheets, MD, Milwaukee, WI.)

the infant was subsequently abused again, but in some of these cases the possibility of abuse was not considered by the medical provider.[9] Some medical providers also incorrectly assumed that abuse had been ruled out because no occult injuries were detected by injury surveillance studies, such as a skeletal survey.[9]

Even when visible injuries are present, abuse may be missed by medical providers. In a study on missed cases of abusive head trauma, 37% of the missed cases had facial or scalp injuries when they first presented for medical care with symptoms that were later attributed to abusive head trauma. When the correct diagnosis of abuse was missed at initial presentation, 27.8% of the children were reinjured before a definitive diagnosis was made.[36] Thus, the accurate identification of physical abuse in infants depends not only on thorough injury surveillance including detection of sentinel injuries and occult injuries but also on critical analysis of the diagnostic possibilities.

Given the risk of escalation and further harm or death from abuse, screening for sentinel injuries should be performed routinely during medical evaluations of infants, including well-child visits. If a sentinel injury is detected, a thorough history should be obtained, including an explanation for the injury as well as a review of birth, medical, developmental, family, and social histories. Careful physical examination also should be performed with written documentation of location, size, and pattern of any injuries as well as photodocumentation. The physical examination should include measurement of head circumference and careful inspection of the skin and oral mucosa, particularly of areas where injury is easily missed, such as the labial and sublingual frena, ears, scalp, anogenital area, hands, and feet. Furthermore, the level of concern for child abuse may be increased in the context of:

- Lack of or changing history
- History inconsistent with developmental stage
- History inconsistent with type or severity of injury
- Inappropriate delay in seeking care[34]

APPROACH/MANAGEMENT

Infants with a history or examination finding of sentinel injury should undergo an urgent, comprehensive work-up to evaluate for occult injuries and, when appropriate, predisposing conditions.[45,46] Even a single bruise in a precruising infant should prompt the medical provider to critically consider whether the history adequately explains the bruise. In precruising infants who are able to sit independently, a single bruise on the forehead and a clear and plausible history of an accident may not require further testing for occult injury unless there are other risk factors present. However, in this scenario, if there is no plausible history to explain the bruise, occult injury surveillance should be performed.

Cruising infants with bruises over bony prominences and a clear, plausible history to explain those injuries may not require injury surveillance unless there are other reasons to suspect maltreatment. However, if bruises are present in unusual or unexpected locations, are unusual in number or extent, or are patterned, occult injury surveillance should be strongly considered (**Fig. 10**).

Occult injury surveillance should include consideration of:

- Head CT in children less than 6 months of age and in those with abnormal neurologic findings
- Initial skeletal survey in children less than 2 years old
- Repeat skeletal survey 2 weeks after the initial skeletal survey
- Dilated ophthalmologic examination when abusive head trauma is suspected

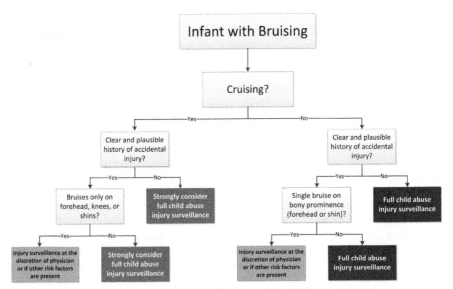

Fig. 10. Algorithm to guide management of a precruising infant with bruising.

- Laboratory studies to screen for abdominal injury
- Screening for occult drug injury[46–49]

In addition, screening for predisposing conditions should be considered; for example, testing for bleeding diatheses if bruising is present.[46,50] The medical assessment can then be formulated in the context of the reported explanation, physical examination findings, and diagnostic studies.

Sentinel injuries are often detected by the primary care provider as an incidental finding on examination or in the medical history. Evaluation for occult injuries may be completed in the primary care setting if laboratory and imaging services are available. If not, the infant may be referred to an emergency department or hospital. If no additional injury is detected on skeletal survey or head CT in an infant with a history or examination finding of a sentinel injury, abuse remains the primary diagnostic consideration because the sentinel injury may be the first and only injury from abuse. Therefore, a history or an examination finding of a sentinel injury should prompt a report to authorities for suspected abuse.

For the primary care provider, consideration of abuse as a diagnostic possibility can be extremely difficult, particularly when there is a close relationship with the family that is perceived to be at low risk of abuse. The primary care provider may also have concerns that subjecting a family to an investigation and the infant to a complete diagnostic evaluation is an excessive response to what seems to be a trivial injury. However, it is important to remember that any parent or caregiver may momentarily lose control and injure an infant, people other than the parents may have abused the child, safety of the infant is the paramount priority, the threshold for reporting suspected abuse does not require diagnostic certainty, and the risk of missing the diagnosis of abuse is potentially life threatening. Reporting a sentinel injury to authorities as suspicious for abuse and completing the diagnostic evaluation for abuse may be the only opportunity to prevent further abusive injury or even death of the infant. The approach to the family should be to inform them in a nonjudgmental style that reports for suspected abuse and further testing are required and represent standard medical care under the circumstances. The family should be informed of the results of the diagnostic studies. If primary care providers are unable to report or conduct further testing because of the close relationship with the families, they should consult with the nearest child abuse pediatrician for further guidance. Even if authorities are unable to substantiate abuse or identify a perpetrator, the diagnostic evaluation and investigation are interventions that may change the behavior of an abusive caregiver and the trajectory of abuse. In this case, primary care providers should continue to provide routine care with ongoing careful observation for additional concerning injuries. Anticipatory guidance, education, and resources should also be provided to the family.

Screening for and identification of sentinel injuries as an early sign of abuse and intervention before escalation have the potential to prevent many cases of severe injury from abuse. Education of caregivers, investigators, home visitors, daycare providers, and medical professionals regarding the significance of these injuries in precruising infants could promote secondary prevention. In this way, primary care providers can play a key role in improving child well-being and safety.

REFERENCES

1. Wedgwood J. Childhood bruising. Practitioner 1990;234:598–601.
2. Sugar NF, Taylor JA, Feldman KW, et al. Bruises in infants and toddlers: those who don't cruise rarely bruise. Arch Pediatr Adolesc Med 1999;153:399–403.
3. Labbé J, Caouette G. Recent skin injuries in normal children. Pediatrics 2001; 108:271–6.
4. Committee on Child Abuse and Neglect, American Academy of Pediatrics. When inflicted skin injuries constitute child abuse. Pediatrics 2002;110:644–5.
5. US Department of Health and Human Services, Administration for Children and Families, Administration on Children, Youth and Families, Children's Bureau. Child maltreatment 2012. 2013. Available at: http://www.acf.hhs.gov/programs/cb/research-data-technology/statistics-research/child-maltreatment. Accessed April 21, 2014.
6. O'Neill JA, Meacham WF, Griffin JP, et al. Patterns of injury in the battered child syndrome. J Trauma 1973;13:332–9.
7. Ellerstein NS. The cutaneous manifestations of child abuse and neglect. Am J Dis Child 1979;133:906–9.
8. Maguire S, Mann MK, Sibert J, et al. Are there patterns of bruising in childhood which are diagnostic or suggestive of abuse? A systematic review. Arch Dis Child 2005;90:182–6.
9. Sheets LK, Leach ME, Koszewski IJ, et al. Sentinel injuries in infants evaluated for child physical abuse. Pediatrics 2013;131:701–7.
10. Tate RJ. Facial injuries associated with the battered child syndrome. Br J Oral Surg 1971;9:41–5.
11. Roberton DM, Barbor P, Hull D. Unusual injury? Recent injury in normal children and children with suspected non-accidental injury. Br Med J (Clin Res Ed) 1982; 285:1399–401.
12. Naidoo S. A profile of the oro-facial injuries in child physical abuse at a children's hospital. Child Abuse Negl 2000;24:521–34.
13. Cairns AM, Mok JY, Welbury RR. Injuries to the head, face, mouth and neck in physical abused children in a community setting. Int J Paediatr Dent 2005;15: 310–8.
14. Pierce MC, Kaczor K, Aldridge S, et al. Bruising characteristics discriminating physical child abuse from accidental trauma. Pediatrics 2010;125:67–74.

15. Joffe M, Ludwig S. Stairway injuries in children. Pediatrics 1988;82:457–61.
16. Haney SB, Starling SP, Heisler KW, et al. Characteristics of falls and risk of injury in children younger than 2 years. Pediatr Emerg Care 2010;26:914–8.
17. Zielinski AE, Rochette LM, Smith GA. Stair-related injuries to young children treated in US emergency departments, 1999-2008. Pediatrics 2012;129: 721–7.
18. Mortimer PE, Freeman M. Are facial bruises in babies ever accidental? Arch Dis Child 1983;58:75–6.
19. Carpenter RF. The prevalence and distribution of bruising in babies. Arch Dis Child 1999;80:363–6.
20. Tush BA. Bruising in healthy 3-year-old children. Matern Child Nurs J 1982;11: 165 79.
21. Pascoe JM, Hildebrandt HM, Tarrler A, et al. Patterns of skin injury in nonaccidental and accidental injury. Pediatrics 1979;64:245–7.
22. McMahon P, Grossman W, Gaffney M, et al. Soft-tissue injury as an indication of child abuse. J Bone Joint Surg Am 1995;77:1179–83.
23. Worlock P, Stower M, Barbor P. Patterns of fractures in accidental and non-accidental injury in children: a comparative study. Br Med J (Clin Res Ed) 1986;293:100–2.
24. Atwal GS, Rutty GN, Carter N, et al. Bruising in non-accidental head injured children; a retrospective study of the prevalence, distribution and pathological associations in 24 cases. Forensic Sci Int 1998;96:215–30.
25. Dunstan FD, Guildea ZE, Kontos K, et al. A scoring system for bruise patterns: a tool for identifying abuse. Arch Dis Child 2002;86:330–3.
26. Feldman KW. Patterned abusive bruises of the buttocks and the pinnae. Pediatrics 1992;90:633–6.
27. Maguire S, Hunter B, Hunter L, et al. Diagnosing abuse: a systematic review of torn frenum and other intra-oral injuries. Arch Dis Child 2007;92:1113–7.
28. Browner EA. Nursemaid's elbow (annular ligament displacement). Pediatr Rev 2013;34:366–7.
29. Leventhal JM, Martin KD, Gaither JR. Using US data to estimate the incidence of serious physical abuse in children. Pediatrics 2012;129:458–64.
30. Johnson CF, Showers J. Injury variables in child abuse. Child Abuse Negl 1985; 9:207–15.
31. Flaherty EG. Analysis of caretaker histories in abuse: comparing initial histories with subsequent confessions. Child Abuse Negl 2006;30:789–98.
32. Lee C, Barr RG, Catherine N, et al. Age-related incidence of publicly reported shaken baby syndrome cases: is crying a trigger for shaking? J Dev Behav Pediatr 2007;28:288–93.
33. Barr RG. Preventing abusive head trauma resulting from a failure of normal interaction between infants and their caregivers. Proc Natl Acad Sci U S A 2012;109: 17294–301.
34. Jenny C, editor. Child abuse and neglect: diagnosis, treatment and evidence. 1st edition. St Louis (MO): Saunders; 2011.
35. Alexander R, Crabbe L, Sato Y, et al. Serial abuse in children who are shaken. Am J Dis Child 1990;144:58–60.
36. Jenny C, Hymel KP, Ritzen A, et al. Analysis of missed cases of abusive head trauma. JAMA 1999;281:621–6.
37. Thackeray JD. Frena tears and abusive head injury: a cautionary tale. Pediatr Emerg Care 2007;23:735–7.

38. Oral R, Yagmur F, Nashelsky M, et al. Fatal abusive head trauma cases: conse-quence of medical staff missing milder forms of physical abuse. Pediatr Emerg Care 2008;24:816–21.

39. Pierce MC, Smith S, Kaczor K. Bruising in infants: those with a bruise may be abused. Pediatr Emerg Care 2009;25:845–7.

40. Petska HW, Sheets LK, Knox BL. Facial bruising as a precursor to abusive head trauma. Clin Pediatr (Phila) 2013;52:86–8.

41. King WK, Kiesel EL, Simon HK. Child abuse fatalities: are we missing opportu-nities for intervention? Pediatr Emerg Care 2006;22:211–4.

42. Sieswerda-Hoogendoorn T, Bilo RA, van Duurling LL, et al. Abusive head trauma in young children in the Netherlands: evidence for multiple incidents of abuse. Acta Paediatr 2013;102:e497–501.

43. Adamsbaum C, Grabar S, Mejean N, et al. Abusive head trauma: judicial admis-sions highlight violent and repetitive shaking. Pediatrics 2010;126:546–55.

44. Warner-Rogers JE, Hansen DJ, Spieth LE. The influence of case and profes-sional variables on identification and reporting of physical abuse: a study with medical students. Child Abuse Negl 1996;20:851–66.

45. Livingston N. Bruising in infancy: when is it an emergency? Pediatr Ann 2010;39: 646–54.

46. Kellogg ND, American Academy of Pediatrics Committee on Child Abuse and Neglect. Evaluation of suspected child physical abuse. Pediatrics 2007;119: 1232–41.

47. Harper NS, Eddleman S, Lindberg DM, et al. The utility of follow-up skeletal surveys in child abuse. Pediatrics 2013;131:e672–8.

48. Lindberg D, Makoroff K, Harper N, et al. Utility of hepatic transaminases to recognize abuse in children. Pediatrics 2009;124:509–16.

49. Oral R, Bayman L, Assad A, et al. Illicit drug exposure in patients evaluated for alleged child abuse and neglect. Pediatr Emerg Care 2011;27:490–5.

50. Anderst JD, Carpenter SL, Abshire TC, et al. Evaluation for bleeding disorders in suspected child abuse. Pediatrics 2013;131:e1314–22.

Neglect: Failure to Thrive and Obesity

Nancy S. Harper, MD

KEYWORDS

- Failure to thrive • Medical neglect • Neglect • Obesity • Pediatrics

KEY POINTS

- Weight status and interval weight gain should be documented at every medical visit.
- Screening for psychosocial risk factors and food security is integral to prevention of nutritional deficiencies and child maltreatment.
- The etiology of FTT or obesity is seldom the result of a single causative medical, genetic or socioeconomic factor.
- The approach to nutritional rehabilitation in FTT or obesity requires multidisciplinary assessment and management.
- Weight status, in the absence of medical complications, does not necessarily constitute neglect.
- Weight status, with concern for future health, may reflect neglect, and a report to child protective services (CPS) may be needed.
- Medical neglect should be considered in both failure to thrive and obesity when there is a serious risk of harm from identified medical complications, additional or worsening medical complications occurring despite a multidisciplinary approach, and/or noncompliance with the treatment plan.

INTRODUCTION

Discussions on malnutrition in childhood and adolescence have traditionally centered on inadequate growth as well as nutrient deficiencies, such as iron or vitamin D. Malnutrition is a "cellular imbalance between nutrient requirement and intake" and should encompass both undernutrition and overnutrition.[1] Undernutrition may negatively affect both physical growth and development. Inadequate growth in weight or height, based on serial observations on a growth chart, is often referred to as failure to thrive (FTT). Whereas FTT is the result of inadequate nutrition, the focus of the

Conflicts of Interest: The author has provided paid expert testimony for prosecution and defense in cases of alleged child physical abuse.
Financial Disclosure: The author has no financial relationship relevant to this article to disclose.
Children's Physician Services of South Texas, Driscoll Children's Hospital, 3533 South Alameda, Corpus Christi, TX 78411, USA
E-mail addresses: nsharper@umn.edu; nsharper69@gmail.com

Pediatr Clin N Am 61 (2014) 937–957
http://dx.doi.org/10.1016/j.pcl.2014.06.006
0031-3955/14/$ – see front matter © 2014 Elsevier Inc. All rights reserved.

medical system often shifts to etiology (organic or nonorganic) and to determine whether there is caregiver neglect or maltreatment.[2,3] In 2013, the American Society for Parenteral and Enteral Nutrition pediatric malnutrition working group recommended defining malnutrition or FTT as illness related or non–illness related, encouraging an approach that includes the role of illness, as well as environment and behavioral factors.[1] Overnutrition, in the form of obesity, can have medical complications in childhood that predict serious morbidity in adulthood[4] with much current debate as to the role of caregiver neglect and referrals to child protective services (CPS).[5–8] Both forms of malnutrition involve a complex interaction of medical and psychosocial factors and necessitate a comprehensive, multidisciplinary approach to evaluation and treatment.

DEFINING AGE-APPROPRIATE GROWTH

The approach to malnutrition requires an understanding of normal growth in childhood. Measurements of height and weight should be obtained at serial visits and compared with growth standards for males and females as well as special populations (eg, prematurity, Down syndrome). In 2010, the Centers for Disease Control and Prevention (CDC), the National Institutes of Health, and the American Academy of Pediatrics recommended the adoption of the World Health Organization (WHO) 2006 growth charts for children ages 0 to 2 years and the CDC 2000 growth charts for children ages 2 to 19 years. The WHO 2006 growth charts include longitudinal serial data on children younger than 2 from multiple countries, whereas the CDC 2000 charts are based on cross-sectional, nonserial data from only the United States. The infants differ; 100% of WHO infants were still breastfeeding at 4 months versus only one third of CDC infants.[9] Although the CDC 2000 charts use the 5% and 95% to designate underweight and obesity, WHO 2006 utilizes z-scores of -2.0 and 2.0 translating to 2.3% and 97.7%, respectively. There are concerns that the WHO 2006 growth charts, in comparison with the CDC 2000 growth charts, underestimate the percentage of children who are underweight or stunted in height[10,11] and overestimate the percentage of children who are overweight and obese.[11] If the WHO growth chart is utilized correctly, similar results occur for height and overweight.[12] Despite these concerns, WHO 2006 charts are considered growth standards "that describe how healthy children should grow under optimal environmental and health conditions."[9]

Traditionally, FTT has been identified in children who have a weight for age that drops below 3% to 5% or who have crossed two major growth percentiles.[13–15] Crossing of major growth percentiles, however, is not uncommon in healthy children.[16] Acute malnutrition or wasting is defined as inadequate growth for fewer than 3 months and is reflected in weight for age. Chronic malnutrition, defined as inadequate growth for longer than 3 months, includes deficits in height velocity or stunting.[1] There are multiple classification strategies (**Table 1**) for determining the degree of malnutrition (mild, moderate, or severe). The use of WHO or Cole z-scores may have some benefits over other methods, because neither requires the determination of an ideal weight or ideal weight for height for the individual child. Overweight or obesity is best represented by weight for height or body mass index (BMI) with 85% to 94% defining overweight, 95% to 98% obesity, and 99% or greater severe obesity. However, caution is urged in classifying adolescents because their BMI can exceed adult criteria for obesity (BMI $\geq$30 kg/m^2).[17]

PREVALENCE

Based on WHO growth standards, it is estimated that 16% of children younger than 5 years in developing countries were underweight in 2011. This translates to more

Table 1
Definitions of malnutrition (underweight)

Classification	Definition	Severity	
Gomez[119]	% median WFA (current weight/median WFA)	Mild	75%–90% WFA
		Moderate	60%–74% WFA
		Severe	<60% WFA
Waterlow[120]	Z-score (SD) WFH	Mild	80%–90% WFH
		Moderate	70%–80% WFH
		Severe	<70% WFH
WHO[121] (wasting)	Z-score (SD) WFH	Moderate	−2 to −3
		Severe	−3 or less
WHO[121] (stunting)	Z-score (SD) HFA	Moderate	−2 to −3
		Severe	−3 or less
WHO[121]	MUAC	Severe	<115 mm
Cole[122]	Z-score for BMI for age	Mild (grade 1)	−1 to −2
		Moderate (grade 2)	−2 to −3
		Severe (grade 3)	−3 or less

Abbreviations: BMI, body mass index; HFA, height for age; MUAC, mid-upper arm circumference; WFA, weight for age; WFH, weight for height; WHO, World Health Organization.
Adapted from Grover Z, Ee LC. Protein energy malnutrition. Pediatr Clin North Am 2009;56(5):1055–68.

than 100 million children. Moderate or severe wasting was noted in 8% or 51.5 million children, with stunting occurring in 26% or an estimated 165 million children.[18] Based on data from the National Health and Nutrition Examination Survey for 2007 and 2008, it is estimated that only 3.7% of children and adolescents in the United States are underweight with a trend toward improvement from 5.1% in the National Health and Nutrition Examination Survey I (1971–1974). The prevalence of underweight among adults in the United States has also decreased from 4% of adults (20–74 years of age) in the 1960s to 1.7% in 2007 through 2010.[19] These estimates, however, include children and adults who are small but healthy.

Overweight and obesity have demonstrated an opposite trend. Worldwide, United Nations International Children Emergency Fund estimates that 7% or 43 million children are "overweight," with an increase of 54% noted over 1990.[18] The prevalence of obesity in adults in the United States has doubled as measured between National Health and Nutrition Examination Survey data from 1976 through 1980 and 2007 through 2008.[20] Weight status, as measured by BMI in childhood, is predictive of weight status and obesity in adulthood.[21] This is especially true for adolescents over 13 years of age who have a more than 50% increased risk of adult obesity if they have a BMI greater than the 95th percentile.[22] As of 2010, it is estimated that obesity affects 35.7% of US adults[23] and 16.9% of children 2 to 19 years of age, which includes 9.7% of toddlers (0–2 years) and 12.1% of preschoolers (2–5 years).[24] Most alarming, severe childhood obesity (BMI >99th percentile) affects 4% or 2.7 million children between the ages of 2 and 19 years.[25]

ETIOLOGY

The etiology of either FTT or obesity is rarely the result of a single causative factor. Nutritional status has associations with race,[26,27] sex,[24,26] and even geographic location (state-based rates of obesity).[28] Beyond these associations, there are multiple complex interactions that require a systems-based approach to both recognizing risk factors for inadequate nutrition as well as for treatment and prevention.[29,30] Contributory factors include socioeconomic status, community and health care supports, family environment and the individual child. It is not surprising that low- and middle-income countries have higher rates of malnutrition; strong negative associations exist between socioeconomic status (poverty, food security, and education), nutritional status,[25,31,32] and child development.[33,34]

Food Insecurity

Women and children in the United States have higher rates of obesity at lower income or educational levels.[31,32] In 2012, an estimated 21.8% or 16.1 million children under 18 years of age lived in poverty and 15.9 million children lived in food-insecure households.[35] As defined by the US Department of Agriculture, food security is the ability to have consistent and dependable access to enough food for an active, healthy life, food insecurity implies a reduced access to food owing to limited money. Food insecurity is associated with poor health for children and caregivers,[36] as well as risk for impaired development.[34] Growth parameters alone are not adequate screens of food insecurity; older children and adolescents may not demonstrate growth deficits.[37] Furthermore, there are also associations between food prices,[38] food insecurity, and obesity.[39]

Many food insecure families live in food deserts (urban and rural) where ready access to affordable healthy food is very limited. Food deserts occur in both low-income and low-access communities. Communities are considered "low-access" food deserts if a significant percentage of families reside more than 1 mile from a grocery in urban areas, and more than 10 miles in rural areas.[40] Food insecure families are more likely to report problems with transportation, limited income, prioritizing payment of utilities and rent over food, and a reliance on low-cost foods to feed children.[41] Although many families are eligible for participation in the Supplemental Nutritional Assistance Program, statewide access rates vary considerably.[42] Caregivers not receiving Supplemental Nutritional Assistance Program benefits such as WIC owing to access problems report higher levels of food insecurity and are more likely to have underweight and short infants.[43] Access to Supplemental Nutritional Assistance Program not only lowers rates of food insecurity, but improves academic outcomes[44] and paradoxically may reduce risk for obesity owing to less reliance on low-cost, energy-dense foods.[45]

Complex psychosocial issues challenge caregivers' abilities to nurture and feed children. Health care providers have a unique opportunity throughout childhood to interact with families with an ability to screen for nutritional and psychosocial issues, such as poverty, food insecurity, knowledge deficits, depression, substance abuse, domestic violence, and access to resources (eg, transportation, health insurance). Screening can be incorporated into health supervision utilizing questionnaires and psychosocial assessments administered before or during the appointment.[46] Food insecurity can be assessed with a sensitivity of 97% utilizing an affirmative response (true or sometimes true vs never true) to either of two following statements:

1. "Within the past 12 months we worried whether our food would run out before we got money to buy more."
2. "Within the past 12 months the food we bought just didn't last and we didn't have money to get more."[47]

Many of the risk factors for nutritional deficits such as FTT and obesity are the same risk factors associated with child maltreatment. Furthermore, the patterns of family dysfunction are quite similar between families with undernourished children and those with severely obese children.[48] Screening for psychosocial risk factors in primary care practice is an important tool in the prevention of nutritional deficits and child maltreatment.[49]

Assessment of Growth and Nutrition

Medical providers need to assess children for abnormalities in weight status. Although physicians perform similarly to parents in the identification of a child's weight status from photos,[50] calculation of BMI or weight for height does not occur at every medical visit.[51] In a large survey, few physicians calculated BMI at every visit and the majority of physicians discussed weight issues only when they identified it as a concern. Fewer than one half of the physicians knew the criteria for overweight and obesity.[51] Documentation of nutritional status, dietary history, activity level, and education provided to families also needs improvement.[52] Multiple barriers hinder physicians from addressing nutrition in daily practice, including inadequate identification of weight status, fear of offending families, a belief that families do not want weight issues addressed, as well as not having ready access to a nutritionist.[53] Because of these barriers and the demands of busy clinical practices, physicians would benefit from the development and validation of a brief screening tool for food insecurity and nutritional status.

There are syndromes, monogenic and polygenic conditions associated with FTT and obesity. Obesity genes (monogenic causes), such as LEP (leptin), LEPR (leptin receptor), proopiomelanocortin (POMC), and melanocortin 4 receptor (MC4R), are associated with early onset severe obesity.[54] Through recent advances in genetic testing, copy number variants (polygenic) have been found on almost every chromosome that are associated with obesity and concomitant developmental disorders.[55] Although there are genetic[54,56] and metabolic[57] conditions that predispose to abnormalities in weight status, the imbalance of energy intake with energy expenditure is still the most significant determinant of weight status.

SEQUELAE

Inadequate nutrition, including both FTT and obesity, is associated with medical complications affecting multiple organ systems and with serious developmental consequences, independent of socioeconomic risk factors.[58,59] Adipose tissue is an endocrine organ responsible for passive storage of excess energy and the production of leptin, a hormone integral in hunger signaling. Leptin release suppresses appetite, and ghrelin signals hunger.[60] Abnormalities of hormones in hunger signaling include low leptin levels in FTT and starvation,[60,61] and paradoxically elevated leptin and insulin levels in obesity.[60] Leptin plays a central role in metabolism through regulatory effects on the hypothalamus. High levels of leptin are seen in children with severe obesity, implying leptin resistance.[62] Published literature suggests a role for multiple other gastrointestinal hormones such as obestatin and glucagon-like peptide-1.[63] Children and adults who are underweight may have low levels of growth hormone markers (insulin-like growth factor-1, insulin-like growth factor-BP3)[61,64] and thyroid function.[64]

Nutrient deficiencies occur in children on restricted diets, in starvation, in illness-related FTT, and in obesity. Perhaps the most common nutrient deficiencies in childhood remain iron and vitamin D deficiency.[65] Vitamin D deficiency can be seen in both forms of malnutrition owing to inadequate dietary intake.[66] There are, however, numerous other nutrient deficiencies that occur with severe malnutrition, including thiamine (B_1) and other B vitamins, zinc, selenium, and fat-soluble vitamins.[65,67] Skin and oral manifestations of these nutrient deficiencies can be seen in children with moderate to severe FTT on physical examination[64] with skin lesions responding to nutritional therapy.[68]

Fluid and electrolyte abnormalities can complicate initial management of these patients, including dehydration, hypoglycemia, hyponatremia (eg, from dilution of formula, excessive water consumption) and hypernatremia (eg, from breastfeeding failure, dehydration). The most serious constellation of fluid and electrolyte abnormalities remains the refeeding syndrome (RFS). During periods of malnutrition, whether through inadequate intake of calories or intentional starvation, insulin levels decrease and glycogen stores become depleted.[69] RFS is a life-threatening complication that occurs when a child or adult with malnutrition goes from catabolism (utilization of lipids and protein for gluconeogenesis) to anabolism. As sources of energy such as carbohydrates are reintroduced, anabolism begins immediately with a release of insulin. Insulin surges drive the process of RFS with rapid cellular uptake of critical electrolytes, leading to hypokalemia, hypophosphatemia, hypomagnesemia, and hypoglycemia, as well as fluid and sodium retention owing to insulin's natriuretic effects.[69,70] RFS cannot be predicted by body habitus[70] or initial electrolytes. Clinical deficiency of electrolytes is not usually present until catabolism is reversed with initiation of nutrition.[71] Although multiple electrolytes are affected, low phosphorous levels are the hallmark of RFS and perhaps the best indicator of its occurrence.[69,70] Medical providers are urged to check phosphorous levels both as part of initial laboratory screening and after nutritional rehabilitation has been initiated. The risk factors for RFS are well outlined in the literature and include inadequate nutrition and neglect.[70]

Management of RFS requires correction of electrolyte abnormalities and hydration status before feeding,[72] as well as a targeted approach to glycemic and metabolic control.[70,71,73] Complications of RFS include vomiting, gastroparesis, ileus, diarrhea owing to villous atrophy and malabsorption, elevated liver enzymes, fatty liver disease owing to excess glycogen, brain atrophy, osteomalacia, infections, and anemia.[72] Electrolyte abnormalities and fluid shifts in RFS can lead to cardiac arrhythmia and sudden death.[74,75] Children with concerns for neglect and intentional starvation deserve special attention. There are multiple published reports on the associations among malnutrition, child fatality,[2,76–78] and blunt force injuries.[79] Mortality from RFS is difficult to predict; the literature consists primarily of case studies. A review of the literature in 2002 noted 9 deaths (33%) in 27 children with RFS.[80]

The risk of morbidity and mortality associated with a child or adolescent who is underweight or malnourished may seem obvious to the medical provider. Media reports on children dying of obesity are scant and focus on such alarming cases as the death of a 13-year-old girl in California who weighed 680 lb.[81] As noted, children with obesity have an increased risk of obesity in adulthood and face similar medical complications as obese adults. The Bogalusa Heart Study included more than 10,000 children 5 to 17 years of age who were examined for risk factors associated with cardiovascular disease, including weight status, blood pressure, insulin, and lipid panels. A nutritional status of "overweight" (defined as BMI of $\geq 95\%$) was noted in 12% of children with severe obesity occurring in 2%. Two risk factors for cardiovascular disease were found in 39% of overweight children and 59% of those considered severely obese. Four or more risk factors were noted in 11% of children with severe obesity.[82] A longitudinal cohort study of children born between 1930 and 1976 demonstrated an association between obesity in childhood and adult cardiovascular disease. For example, a 13-year-old boy with a BMI z-score of +2.0 had a 33% increased risk of a coronary event in adulthood.[4] Similar associations between obesity and earlier development of type 2 diabetes mellitus have also been observed in children and adolescents.[83]

Children and adolescents with obesity benefit from annual health surveillance for multiple medical complications, including hypertension, hyperlipidemia, insulin resistance, type 2 diabetes mellitus, nonalcoholic fatty liver disease, obstructive sleep apnea (OSA), asthma, restrictive lung disease, skin infections, and orthopedic complications (eg, Blount disease, slipped capital femoral epiphysis).[17] These medical conditions occur along a spectrum of severity progressing from complications reversible with weight management to irreversible complications and death.[84] For example, a child with snoring and OSA may have an abnormal sleep study requiring nightly continuous positive airway pressure. This would be a potentially reversible complication through weight loss, still considered the primary treatment of obesity-associated OSA.[85] Without treatment, the child can develop pulmonary hypertension, cor pulmonale, and progress to death.[84] Unfortunately, the neurocognitive deficits associated with OSA and severe obesity[86] may not be easily reversed. Additional complications of obesity whose severity and consequence are not easily estimated, treated, or reversed include diminished quality of life and psychosocial functioning,[87] weight-based victimization,[88] and bullying.[89]

CLINICAL ASSESSMENT AND APPROACH

The approach to the child with FTT or obesity starts with a detailed medical and psychosocial assessment of the caregiver–child dyad by the medical provider. Medical evaluation should include maternal pregnancy history, past medical history, review of systems, developmental history, medications, allergies (food and medications), family medical history to include parental stature and weight, feeding and physical activity history, psychosocial assessment, and physical examination. A complete review of the facets of the medical history is well outlined in the literature.[15,90]

The medical history and review of systems for FTT should focus on areas of imbalance in energy, such as (1) inadequate intake of calories (illness or non–illness related), (2) increased metabolism or requirement for calories (eg, burn injury, cancer, HIV), (3) excessive losses of calories (eg, burn injury, diarrhea, proteinuria, vomiting, protein-losing enteropathy), and (4) inadequate absorption of calories (eg, cystic fibrosis, celiac disease).[1,15] In children with obesity, additional attention is needed to identify medical complications. A separate sleep history should be performed assessing for signs and symptoms of OSA.[85] Screen time, or time spent watching television[91,92] and playing video games,[93] is a proxy measure for sedentary activity and consumption of energy-dense foods,[94] and has strong associations with weight status for children and adults.[95]

A structured approach to the feeding and physical activity history will provide the greatest understanding of the child's energy balance and weight status (**Table 2**). With infants, the history should include a step-by-step description by the caregiver on bottle preparation. Improper or dilute formula mixing as well as food fads can be seen in FTT. In obese infants, complementary foods such as cereal or jar foods may have been added to the bottle. It is also helpful to have the parent complete a food log or provide a 24-hour dietary recall. As the infant transitions to toddlerhood, the feeding approach changes from formula as the primary nutrition, to age-appropriate meals and snacks. Beverage consumption needs to be assessed, because excessive juice or sugar-sweetened beverage consumption can lead to weight loss or gain. The psychosocial assessment (**Table 3**) includes identification of risk factors with an approach focusing on the role of the child, family, environment, and personal and community resources. This assessment is ideally completed by a social worker, but can be completed by the primary care provider. Particular attention should be spent

Table 2
Elements of a detailed nutritional and activity history in malnutrition (underweight and overweight)

Age	Nutrition	History
Infant	Breast feeding	Success with latching and nursing
		Breast or pumped milk feeds
		Feeding schedule
		Amount expressed with pump
		Use of supplemental formula
		Access to lactation consultant
		Length of nursing: age at weaning
		Maternal dietary and fluid intake
	Formula feeding	Formula at birth
		Current formula
		Number of formula changes
		Feeding schedule
		Sleep schedule
		Ounces: per feed; per day
		Formula mixing history
		Have caregiver verbally or physically demonstrate bottle preparation including number of scoops of formula, number of ounces of water, which is placed in bottle first (water or scoops)
		Addition of cereal including type and amount
		Addition of supplemental foods to bottle (eg, jar foods, honey, egg, juice)
		Has parent received advice on mixing or feeding from a medical provider or relative? What type of advice were they given?
		Calculate calories per ounce
	Complementary foods	Age at introduction: jar foods; mashed table foods; cow's milk
		Feeding schedule
		Texture and amounts at meals
		Assess for food fads
		Juice and sugar-sweetened beverages (amount daily)
		Water consumption (amount daily)
		Introduction of sippy cup or straw
	Activity	Developmental history
		Physical limitations
		History of occupational or physical therapies

Child and adolescent	Liquids	Cow's milk: nonfat, 1 or 2%, whole milk, lactose-free milk (amount daily)
		Juice and sugar-sweetened beverages (amount daily)
		Water consumption (amount daily)
	Food	Schedule for meals and snacks
		Food diary or 24 h recall
		Plate and portion size (include number of servings)
		Fast food or take-out meals: number of times weekly or daily; types of meals ordered
		Advice or education: from medical provider or nutritionist, from family member or friends
	Activity	Level of physical activity (eg, sedentary, light activity, etc)
		Participation in physical education, sports, extracurricular activities
		Time spent daily in physical activity (hours)
	Screen time	Time spent daily in hours: television, video games, handheld devices (eg, Nintendo DS, cell phones), computer
	Sleep	Hours spent nightly in sleep
		Symptoms of obstructive sleep apnea: snoring, cessation of breathing or gasping during sleep, number of pillows, nighttime or daytime enuresis; daytime somnolence or napping; daytime inattention
Feeding behaviors (any age)		Drooling and swallow dysfunction
		Spit-up, vomiting, reflux
		Oral aversions (including nipples, pacifiers, spoons)
		Texture aversions
		History of speech therapy
		Does child have age-appropriate seating for meals
		Responsive feeding pattern (infants/toddlers): observation of parent–child interaction during bottle or spoon feeding including eye contact, facial expressions of caregiver and child. Does parent know when child is hungry and respond to cues? Does parent know when child is full and respond to cues?
		Child's perception of weight status
		Cooperativeness of child with nutritional plan
		Number of meals eaten as family weekly
Caregiver	Nutrition and activity	Maternal dietary history (if breastfeeding)
		Weight status (underweight, overweight)
		Vegetarian or food allergies (eg, celiac disease)
	Psychosocial	Completion of psychosocial assessment
		Screening for food security
		Eating disorder (eg, anorexia nervosa)
		Perception of child's weight status

Table 3
Elements of a detailed psychosocial assessment

Age	Temperament	Parent Perception
Child	Special health care needs	Prematurity
		Congenital abnormalities
		Severe reflux, oromotor dysfunction
		Metabolic disorder
		Allergic conditions: cow's milk protein or other food allergy, allergic gastroenteropathy
		Neurologic disorder: equipment, feeding tube
	Parent–child interaction	Attachment: response to needs (reported and observed) approach to discipline
Caregiver	Knowledge level	Level of education
		History of developmental disability
		Intellectual disability: ability to read and write; ability to count, math skills
		Understanding of nutritional plan: education on plan; cooperativeness with treatment
	Substance use	Alcohol
		Tobacco
		Prescription medications
		Illicit drugs
	Mental health	History of abuse or neglect as child
		Depression (including postpartum)
		Anxiety
		Bipolar
		Psychosis (including postpartum)
		Posttraumatic stress disorder
	Physical limitations	Medical conditions
		Sedating medications

Environment	Primary caregiver	Mother, father, relative, other
	Family composition	Single or joint parenting
		Number of children
		Number of people residing in home; caring for other children; caring for other adults
		Family health: children or adults with FTT or obesity; developmental disabilities
	Support systems	Social isolation
		Friend or family support
	Family violence	Domestic violence
		Physical abuse of children
		Child protective services involvement
		Law enforcement involvement
	Custody	Custody arrangement: court or non-court ordered; joint or primary
		Custody disputes
		Communication between caregivers
Resources: personal and community	Financial	Employment status caregivers
		Income to expenses: ability to purchase medications and supplies; ability to purchase food; ability to cover utilities, rent
	Food	WIC eligibility and enrollment
		Food stamps
		Food pantry, church food basket
	Housing	Own or rent
		Government subsidized
		Adequacy of housing: utilities functional (water, electric, gas); structure functional (leaks, safety)
	Health insurance	Insurance status of child and caregivers
		Public or private insurance
		Eligibility for Medicaid
	Transportation	Motor vehicle: personal or access to friend/family vehicle; number of vehicles; working condition
		Public transportation: consider number of changes to grocery store, clinic, hospital

Abbreviation: FTT, failure to thrive.

on the caregiver's knowledge deficits, because these deficits may interfere with the ability to prepare formula, read educational materials, and follow a treatment plan.

Physical examination needs to include measurement of growth parameters such as height and weight as well as assessment of weight for height (0–2 years) and BMI (after 2 years). The comprehensive head-to-toe examination should identify possible inflicted injury as well as the complications of inadequate nutrition as seen in the hair, skin, and extremities.[64] Skin infections occur in undernutrition (loss of protective subcutaneous fat) and obesity (skin irritation owing to maceration and friction). Velvety hyperpigmentation of acanthosis nigracans occurs in children with obesity and insulin resistance.[96] Fat distribution should be assessed; the degree of malnutrition correlates with the wasting noted on physical examination. Hepatomegaly may be present in obesity (eg, nonalcoholic fatty liver disease) and FTT (eg, metabolic disorders, RFS). Excellent reviews detail the physical examination findings in both FTT[15,64] and obesity.[17]

Prior published literature[3,15] placed little emphasis on laboratory testing in FTT. However, these articles cite a single study on laboratory evaluations in FTT from 1978.[97] Laboratory and radiologic testing in FTT should be based on medical history and physical examination findings, as well as risk for RFS and medical complications. Initial testing should include a complete blood count, chemistry panel including liver enzymes, phosphorous, magnesium, free thyroxine, thyroid-stimulating hormone, urinalysis, HIV testing, and either C-reactive protein or erythrocyte sedimentation rate (owing to the role of inflammation in energy expenditure[1]). Additional testing to consider includes hemoglobin A1C in severe starvation, skeletal survey, stool fecal elastase or sweat chloride testing, celiac panel, and stool studies with diarrheal illness. Advances in testing include genetic sequencing, such as comparative genomic hybridization (chromosome microarray analysis). This testing for copy number variants (gains and losses) may be indicated in children with FTT, dysmorphic features, or structural defects,[98] and in children with obesity and developmental delay.[55] With obesity, laboratory testing to assess for associated medical complications such as hyperlipidemia, diabetes, and fatty liver disease is well outlined in the literature.[17] In both FTT and obesity, children benefit from testing for nutrient deficiencies such as iron and vitamin D.

Most children with FTT or obesity are best managed in an outpatient setting. Hospitalization is indicated whenever there is a concern for (1) intentional starvation, (2) physical safety (eg, associated physical injuries), (3) severe malnutrition, and (4) observation and treatment for RFS. Otherwise, the approach to a child with FTT or obesity is normalization of nutrition and caloric intake. This may include estimations of ideal body weight and calculations of needed calories for catchup growth or weight loss.[17,99] Breastfeeding infants with FTT will need close coordination between the primary care provider and a lactation consultant to ensure adequate milk supply and feeding. Breast milk that is pumped can be fortified for additional calorie support. For formula-fed infants with FTT, formula preparations may require higher caloric strengths to meet calorie goals. With the assistance of a registered dietician, formula recipes can be designed for individual bottles and 24-hour containers, which can make estimates of intake easier to calculate at follow-up visits. Education for toddlers and children with obesity and FTT is similar with a focus on sleep and meal schedule, appropriate feeding chairs, and family mealtime to model responsive feeding skills. The plate method of portion control can be utilized in both weight conditions. Education using 5-2-1-0 is simple and effective[100] encouraging five servings of fruits and vegetables daily, 2-hour limits on screen time, 1 hour daily exercise, and 0 servings of sugar-sweetened beverages. Underweight children may need higher calorie toddler beverages in place of milk for catchup growth. Both underweight and overweight children benefit from incorporating healthy fats and increased fiber into the diet, as well as reduction in the amounts of sugary beverages and high-energy, low-nutrient dense foods (eg, sweet and salty snacks).[101–103]

The majority of primary care providers may not have access to multidisciplinary programs that care for children with FTT or obesity. The primary care provider is the family's medical home and the frontline in the management of child health, safety, and nutrition. Children with malnutrition, whether underweight or overweight, benefit from intensive monitoring, which may necessitate weekly to bimonthly visits for weight checks and reinforcement of the nutritional plan. Educational materials on nutrition for the provider and caregiver are available through the American Academy of Pediatrics, Let's Move (www.letsmove.gov), and through health care insurers such as Blue Cross Blue Shield (Good Health Club tip sheets). Caregivers and children may benefit from mental health screening including evaluation of the parent–child interaction through tools such as the Parent Stress Index. The primary care provider can utilize and communicate with registered dieticians available through WIC. The child younger than 36 months of age with malnutrition or developmental delays may be eligible for evaluation by early intervention services, which may provide nutritional support in addition to rehabilitation services. States and regions differ in community services available to support families. Primary care providers should identify programs in their communities that provide additional parenting education and support to families.

THE ROLE OF NEGLECT

Child neglect should be considered whenever a caregiver fails to meet a child's basic needs, such as adequate food, shelter, clothing, education, health care, and supervision. In 2012, more than 78% of the 686,000 US children substantiated for maltreatment were considered victims of neglect. Data on medical neglect (reported by only 40 states), as defined as a "failure by a caregiver to provide appropriate health care of the child although financially able to do so," occurred in 2.3% of children.[104] This is an underestimate of the true prevalence of medical neglect because the diagnosis is not straightforward. Because neglect occurs along a continuum from optimal to grossly inadequate care,[105] additional factors need to be considered including whether (1) the child has been harmed or is at risk of harm owing to a lack of health care, (2) the recommended treatment plan offers significant benefit to the child, (3) the benefit of treatment outweighs the risk, (4) access to health care is available and has not been utilized, and (5) the caregiver has an understanding of the medical problem, complications, and treatment plan.[106]

Medical providers may be relatively willing to diagnose medical neglect in conditions with a tangible risk of harm, such as severe asthma, congenital heart disease, or cancer. Pediatricians are less comfortable considering medical neglect in FTT, with a tendency to consider neglect only if overt psychosocial risk factors are present.[3] A caregiver's inability to provide adequate nutrition to a child is by definition neglect. However, improper mixing of formula, too few feedings of an infant, or excessive juice consumption in a toddler do not necessitate referrals to CPS, but rather a more intensive response and education from the primary care provider. There is even greater confusion in understanding when to consider medical neglect in obesity with the worry that a child's weight status alone is triggering the referral to CPS[7] and a deepening concern that the community is not equipped to provide services to these families.[6] Weight status, in the absence of medical complications, does not necessarily constitute neglect. If a child's basic needs such as nutrition are not adequately met and result in actual or potential harm, this does constitute neglect. The health care provider and community need to be concerned about the potential for long-term complications and adverse health consequences of inadequate nutrition. There is a need for a tailored approach to the individual child and a public health initiative tackling food insecurity and malnutrition nationally.

Diagnoses of neglect and involvement of CPS however should not be considered "moral judgments, but rather...a means to protect children from harm."[84] Referrals to CPS are imperative when concerns are identified for the child's safety such as concomitant physical injuries, intentional starvation, intentional noncompliance with dietary plans, and with unusual dietary beliefs or food fads that place the child in medical jeopardy. Detailed psychosocial assessments (see **Table 3**) should be completed for all children to access the role of financial stressors and access to resources, family environment, and caregiver knowledge needs. A comprehensive medical evaluation is necessary to identify medical complications that carry a risk of harm for the child such as stunting or poor brain growth (in FTT), RFS, OSA (in obesity or FTT), type 2 diabetes mellitus, hypertension, hyperlipidemia, and fatty liver disease.

Referrals to CPS for medical neglect should be considered in both FTT and obesity when there is a serious risk of harm from documented medical complications, additional or worsening medical complications occurring despite a multidisciplinary approach, and/or noncompliance with the treatment plan. Note that this is not a dissimilar approach to initiating referrals to CPS for medical neglect in other metabolic and nutritional conditions, such as inborn errors of metabolism or insulin-dependent diabetes mellitus, when there are concerns for nonadherence with medical recommendations. CPS may be able to provide a more complete assessment of the role of the environment and family dysfunction and address comorbidities in the home, including child maltreatment, substance abuse, family violence, caregiver mental health, and parenting skills. Effective parenting skills are also essential in the prevention of health disparities and obesity.[107] More coercive interventions, such as relative or foster care, may be needed in FTT or obesity when there is (1) "high likelihood for serious and imminent harm," (2) a likelihood that state intervention will be effective, and (3) alternative options for addressing the problem have not succeeded (eg, multidisciplinary management, inpatient hospitalization, family-based support services).[5]

PREVENTION

Prevention of FTT and obesity as well as child neglect requires a comprehensive approach that includes the child, family, community, health care system, and state and national policy development.[29,30] With associations noted between obesity in childhood and adulthood,[21] promotion of healthy eating and physical activity needs to start in pregnancy and early childhood.[108,109] Communities need to encourage and support breastfeeding and healthy feeding practices as a means of obesity prevention.[101,110] Health care providers need to review weight status and interval weight gain at every visit[111] using the proper growth chart (WHO 2006, CDC 2000), screen for food insecurity, and provide education on nutrition and physical activity. Likewise, hospitals that care for children need to screen for weight status at visits providing health promotion and treatment.[112] Children and adolescents at nutritional risk (underweight or overweight) need access to a medical home, dietary education, and multidisciplinary treatment programs.[17]

Nutritional education of both children who are underweight and overweight is approached with the same goal of normalizing nutritional intake. Physical activity promotion is also important in maintaining a healthy weight status.[113] The education needs to be simple and easily shared in the health care provider's office, family, and community as demonstrated by the effectiveness of the "Let's Go" program in Maine. This multisite, community-based obesity prevention program shared the four components of "5-2-1-0" message at child care programs, schools, afterschool programs, community sites, health care practices, and worksites with parent recognition of the message increasing from 10% in 2007 to 47% in 2011, and in increased fruit and vegetable consumption and decreased sugar sweetened beverage consumption.[100] This message has already been incorporated into the nutritional programs of many communities, hospitals, and states and could easily become a national message incorporated into nutritional programs such as WIC.

The cornerstone of healthy nutrition is healthy feeding and parenting practices. Mothers who are educated on healthy eating are more likely to reduce unhealthy behaviors associated with obesity in infants, such as excessive juice consumption.[114] Children whose families promote habits, such as adequate nighttime sleep, limited screen time, and family meals, are more likely to have a healthy weight status.[115] There are associations between neglect in childhood and abnormal weight status in adolescence[116] and adulthood.[117] Screening for psychosocial risk factors in the health care provider's office will improve identification of families at risk for child maltreatment[49] who would benefit from community services and parenting education. In a longitudinal study of youth at risk for behavior problems, children whose parents received education on effective parenting were more likely to have a lower BMI and demonstrate healthy nutritional and physical activity behaviors.[107] Evidence-based programs such as SEEK (Safe Environment for Every Kid) provide education and training modules to assist health care providers in identifying and addressing these risk factors.[118] Supporting and empowering families, health care providers, and communities will affect feeding practices, nutrition, physical activity, and parenting practices ultimately placing our children on a growth curve toward a healthy adulthood.

REFERENCES

1. Mehta NM, Corkins MR, Lyman B, et al. Defining pediatric malnutrition: a paradigm shift toward etiology-related definitions. JPEN J Parenter Enteral Nutr 2013;37:460–81.
2. Berkowitz CD. Fatal child neglect. Adv Pediatr 2001;48:331–61.
3. Block RW, Krebs NF, American Academy of Pediatrics Committee on Child Abuse and Neglect, et al. Failure to thrive as a manifestation of child neglect. Pediatrics 2005;116:1234–7.
4. Baker JL, Olsen LW, Sorensen TI. Childhood body-mass index and the risk of coronary heart disease in adulthood. N Engl J Med 2007;357:2329–37.
5. Allen DB, Fost N. Obesity and neglect: it's about the child. J Pediatr 2012;160: 898–9.
6. Cheng JK. Confronting the social determinants of health–obesity, neglect, and inequity. N Engl J Med 2012;367:1976–7.
7. Jones DJ, Gonzalez M, Ward DS, et al. Should child obesity be an issue for child protective services? A call for more research on this critical public health issue. Trauma Violence Abuse 2014;15:113–25.
8. Siegel RM, Inge TH. Life-threatening childhood obesity and legal intervention. JAMA 2011;306:1763.
9. Grummer-Strawn LM, Reinold C, Krebs NF, Centers for Disease Control and Prevention (CDC). Use of World Health Organization and CDC growth charts for children aged 0-59 months in the United States. MMWR Recomm Rep 2010;59:1–15.

10. Meyers A, Joyce K, Coleman SM, et al. Health of children classified as underweight by CDC reference but normal by WHO standard. Pediatrics 2013;131: E1780–7.
11. Nash A, Secker D, Corey M, et al. Field testing of the 2006 World Health Organization growth charts from birth to 2 years: assessment of hospital undernutrition and overnutrition rates and the usefulness of BMI. JPEN J Parenter Enteral Nutr 2008;32:145–53.
12. Mei Z, Grummer-Strawn LM. Comparison of changes in growth percentiles of US children on CDC 2000 growth charts with corresponding changes on WHO 2006 growth charts. Clin Pediatr (Phila) 2011;50:402–7.
13. Bithoney WG, Dubowitz H, Egan H. Failure to thrive/growth deficiency. Pediatr Rev 1992;13:453–60.
14. Jaffe AC. Failure to thrive: current clinical concepts. Pediatr Rev 2011;32:100–7.
15. Krugman SD, Dubowitz H. Failure to thrive. Am Fam Physician 2003;68:879–84.
16. Mei Z, Grummer-Strawn LM, Thompson D, et al. Shifts in percentiles of growth during early childhood: analysis of longitudinal data from the California Child Health and Development Study. Pediatrics 2004;113:E617–27.
17. Barlow SE. Expert committee recommendations regarding the prevention, assessment, and treatment of child and adolescent overweight and obesity: summary report. Pediatrics 2007;120:S164–92.
18. United Nations Children's Fund, World Health Organization, The World Bank. UNICEF-WHO-World Bank joint child malnutrition estimates. New York; Washington (DC); Geneva (Switzerland): UNICEF; WHO; The World Bank; 2012.
19. Fryar CD, Ogden CL. Division of Health and Nutrition Examination Surveys. Prevalence of underweight among adults aged 20 and over: United States, 1960-1962 through 2007-2010. Health E-Stat 2012. Available at: http://www.cdc.gov/nchs/data/hestat/underweight_adult_07_10/underweight_adult_07_10.pdf. Accessed January 22, 2014.
20. Ogden CL, Carroll MD. Division of Health and Nutrition Examination Surveys. Prevalence of overweight, obesity, and extreme obesity among adults: United States, trends 1960-1962 through 2007-2008. Atlanta (GA): Centers for Disease Control and Prevention; 2010. Available at: http://www.cdc.gov/nchs/data/hestat/obesity_adult_07_08/obesity_adult_07_08.pdf. Accessed January 23, 2014.
21. Whitaker RC, Wright JA, Pepe MS, et al. Predicting obesity in young adulthood from childhood and parental obesity. N Engl J Med 1997;337:869–73.
22. Whitlock EP, Williams SB, Gold R, et al. Screening and interventions for childhood overweight: a summary of evidence for the US Preventive Services Task Force. Pediatrics 2005;116:E125–44.
23. Flegal KM, Carroll MD, Kit BK, et al. Prevalence of obesity and trends in the distribution of body mass index among US adults, 1999-2010. JAMA 2012;307: 491–7.
24. Ogden CL, Carroll MD, Kit BK, et al. Prevalence of obesity and trends in body mass index among US children and adolescents, 1999-2010. JAMA 2012;307: 483–90.
25. Skelton JA, Cook SR, Auinger P, et al. Prevalence and trends of severe obesity among US children and adolescents. Acad Pediatr 2009;9:322–9.
26. Ogden CL, Carroll MD, Flegal KM. High body mass index for age among US children and adolescents, 2003-2006. JAMA 2008;299:2401–5.
27. Park MK, Menard SW, Schoolfield J. Prevalence of overweight in a triethnic pediatric population of San Antonio, Texas. Int J Obes Relat Metab Disord 2001;25: 409–16.

28. Division of Nutrition Physical Activity and Obesity. National Center for Chronic Disease Prevention and Health Promotion. Overweight and obesity. 2013. Available at: http://www.cdc.gov/obesity/data/adult.html. Accessed January 23, 2014.

29. Black MM, Hager ER. Commentary: pediatric obesity: systems science strategies for prevention. J Pediatr Psychol 2013;38:1044–50.

30. Nader PR, Huang TT, Gahagan S, et al. Next steps in obesity prevention: altering early life systems to support healthy parents, infants, and toddlers. Child Obes 2012;8:195–204.

31. Ogden CL, Lamb MM, Carroll MD, et al. Obesity and socioeconomic status in adults: United States, 2005-2008. NCHS Data Brief 2010;(50):1–8.

32. Ogden CL, Lamb MM, Carroll MD, et al. Obesity and socioeconomic status in children and adolescents: United States, 2005-2008. NCHS Data Brief 2010;(51):1–8.

33. Luby J, Belden A, Botteron K, et al. The effects of poverty on childhood brain development: the mediating effect of caregiving and stressful life events. JAMA Pediatr 2013;167:1135–42.

34. Rose-Jacobs R, Black MM, Casey PH, et al. Household food insecurity: associations with at-risk infant and toddler development. Pediatrics 2008;121:65–72.

35. Hunger in American. Hunger & poverty statistics. Available at: http://feedingamerica.org/hunger-in-america/hunger-facts/hunger-and-poverty-statistics.aspx. Accessed December 27, 2013.

36. Cook JT, Black M, Chilton M, et al. Are food insecurity's health impacts underestimated in the U.S. population? Marginal food security also predicts adverse health outcomes in young U.S. children and mothers. Adv Nutr 2013;4:51–61.

37. Cook JT, Frank DA, Casey PH, et al. A brief indicator of household energy security: associations with food security, child health, and child development in US infants and toddlers. Pediatrics 2008;122:E867–75.

38. Morrissey TW, Jacknowitz A, Vinopal K. Local food prices and their associations with children's weight and food security. Pediatrics 2014;133:422–30.

39. Casey PH, Simpson PM, Gossett JM, et al. The association of child and household food insecurity with childhood overweight status. Pediatrics 2006;118:E1406–13.

40. United States Department of Agriculture. Food deserts. Available at: http://apps.ams.usda.gov/fooddeserts/foodDeserts.aspx. Accessed December 27, 2013.

41. DeMartini TL, Beck AF, Kahn RS, et al. Food insecure families: description of access and barriers to food from one pediatric primary care center. J Community Health 2013;38:1182–7.

42. Newman C, Scherpf E. Supplemental Nutrition Assistance Program (SNAP) access at the state and county levels: evidence from Texas SNAP administrative records and the American Community Survey, ERR-156. Washington, DC: US Department of Agriculture, Economic Research Service; 2013.

43. Black MM. Special Supplemental Nutrition Program for Women, Infants, and children participation and infants' growth and health: a Multisite Surveillance Study. Pediatrics 2004;114:169–76.

44. Frongillo EA, Jyoti DF, Jones SJ. Food Stamp Program participation is associated with better academic learning among school children. J Nutr 2006;136:1077–80.

45. Leung CW, Blumenthal SJ, Hoffnagle EE, et al. Associations of food stamp participation with dietary quality and obesity in children. Pediatrics 2013;131:463–72.

46. Dubowitz H, Giardino A, Gustavson E. Child neglect: guidance for pediatricians. Pediatr Rev 2000;21:111–6.
47. Hager ER, Quigg AM, Black MM, et al. Development and validity of a 2-item screen to identify families at risk for food insecurity. Pediatrics 2010;126:E26–32.
48. Christoffel KK, Forsyth BW. Mirror image of environmental deprivation: severe childhood obesity of psychosocial origin. Child Abuse Negl 1989;13:249–56.
49. Dubowitz H, Kim J, Black MM, et al. Identifying children at high risk for a child maltreatment report. Child Abuse Negl 2011;35:96–104.
50. Huang JS, Becerra K, Oda T, et al. Parental ability to discriminate the weight status of children: results of a survey. Pediatrics 2007;120:E112–9.
51. Huang JS, Donohue M, Golnari G, et al. Pediatricians' weight assessment and obesity management practices. BMC Pediatr 2009;9:19.
52. O'Brien SH, Holubkov R, Reis EC. Identification, evaluation, and management of obesity in an academic primary care center. Pediatrics 2004;114:E154–9.
53. Klein JD, Sesselberg TS, Johnson MS, et al. Adoption of body mass index guidelines for screening and counseling in pediatric practice. Pediatrics 2010;125:265–72.
54. Sabin MA, Werther GA, Kiess W. Genetics of obesity and overgrowth syndromes. Best Pract Res Clin Endocrinol Metab 2011;25:207–20.
55. D'Angelo CS, Koiffmann CP. Copy number variants in obesity-related syndromes: review and perspectives on novel molecular approaches. J Obes 2012;2012:1–15.
56. Manco M, Dallapiccola B. Genetics of pediatric obesity. Pediatrics 2012;130:123–33.
57. Ficicioglu C, An Haack K. Failure to thrive: when to suspect inborn errors of metabolism. Pediatrics 2009;124:972–9.
58. Liu J, Raine A, Venables PH, et al. Malnutrition at age 3 years and lower cognitive ability at age 11 years: independence from psychosocial adversity. Arch Pediatr Adolesc Med 2003;157:593–600.
59. Krombholz H. Motor and cognitive performance of overweight preschool children. Percept Mot Skills 2013;116:40–57.
60. Klok MD, Jakobsdottir S, Drent ML. The role of leptin and ghrelin in the regulation of food intake and body weight in humans: a review. Obes Rev 2007;8:21–34.
61. Korbonits M, Blaine D, Elia M, et al. Metabolic and hormonal changes during the refeeding period of prolonged fasting. Eur J Endocrinol 2007;157:157–66.
62. Kelly AS, Metzig AM, Schwarzenberg SJ, et al. Hyperleptinemia and hypoadiponectinemia in extreme pediatric obesity. Metab Syndr Relat Disord 2012;10:123–7.
63. Bascietto C, Giannini C, D'Adamo E, et al. Implications of gastrointestinal hormones in the pathogenesis of obesity in prepubertal children. J Pediatr Endocrinol Metab 2012;25:255–60.
64. Grover Z, Ee LC. Protein energy malnutrition. Pediatr Clin North Am 2009;56:1055–68.
65. Suskind DL. Nutritional deficiencies during normal growth. Pediatr Clin North Am 2009;56:1035–53.
66. Misra M, Pacaud D, Petryk A, et al. Vitamin D deficiency in children and its management: review of current knowledge and recommendations. Pediatrics 2008;122:398–417.
67. Kirby M, Danner E. Nutritional deficiencies in children on restricted diets. Pediatr Clin North Am 2009;56:1085–103.

68. Lee BY, Hogan DJ, Ursine S, et al. Personal observation of skin disorders in malnutrition. Clin Dermatol 2006;24.222–7.
69. Crook MA, Hally V, Panteli JV. The importance of the refeeding syndrome. Nutrition 2001;17:632–7.
70. Fuentebella J, Kerner JA. Refeeding syndrome. Pediatr Clin North Am 2009;56: 1201–10.
71. Stanga Z, Brunner A, Leuenberger M, et al. Nutrition in clinical practice-the refeeding syndrome: illustrative cases and guidelines for prevention and treatment. Eur J Clin Nutr 2008;62:687–94.
72. Boateng AA, Sriram K, Meguid MM, et al. Refeeding syndrome: treatment considerations based on collective analysis of literature case reports. Nutrition 2010;26:156–67.
73. Panteli JV, Crook MA. Refeeding syndrome still needs to be recognized and managed appropriately. Nutrition 2009;25:130–1.
74. Kohn MR, Golden NH, Shenker IR. Cardiac arrest and delirium: presentations of the refeeding syndrome in severely malnourished adolescents with anorexia nervosa. J Adolesc Health 1998;22:239–43.
75. Isner JM, Roberts WC, Heymsfield SB, et al. Anorexia nervosa and sudden death. Ann Intern Med 1985;102:49–52.
76. Kellogg ND, Lukefahr JL. Criminally prosecuted cases of child starvation. Pediatrics 2005;116:1309–16.
77. Knight LD, Collins KA. A 25-year retrospective review of deaths due to pediatric neglect. Am J Forensic Med Pathol 2005;26:221–8.
78. Solarino B, Grattagliano I, Catanesi R, et al. Child starvation and neglect: a report of two fatal cases. J Forensic Leg Med 2012;19:171–4.
79. Trokel M, Discala C, Terrin NC, et al. Patient and injury characteristics in abusive abdominal injuries. Pediatr Emerg Care 2006;22:700–4.
80. Afzal NA, Addai S, Fagbemi A, et al. Refeeding syndrome with enteral nutrition in children: a case report, literature review and clinical guidelines. Clin Nutr 2002;21:515–20.
81. La Ganga M. For obese girl, battle of blame comes too late. Los Angeles Times 1997. Available at: http://articles.latimes.com/1997/dec/26/news/mn-2357. Accessed April 22, 2014.
82. Freedman DS, Mei Z, Srinivasan SR, et al. Cardiovascular risk factors and excess adiposity among overweight children and adolescents: the Bogalusa Heart Study. J Pediatr 2007;150:12–7.
83. Nguyen QM, Srinivasan SR, Xu JH, et al. Changes in risk variables of metabolic syndrome since childhood in pre-diabetic and type 2 diabetic subjects: the Bogalusa Heart Study. Diabetes Care 2008;31:2044–9.
84. Varness T, Allen DB, Carrel AL, et al. Childhood obesity and medical neglect. Pediatrics 2009;123:399–406.
85. Marcus CL, Brooks LJ, Draper KA, et al. Diagnosis and management of childhood obstructive sleep apnea syndrome. Pediatrics 2012;130:576–84.
86. Rhodes SK, Shimoda KC, Waid LR, et al. Neurocognitive deficits in morbidly obese children with obstructive sleep apnea. J Pediatr 1995;127:741–4.
87. Schwimmer JB, Burwinkle TM, Varni JW. Health-related quality of life of severely obese children and adolescents. JAMA 2003;289:1813–9.
88. Puhl RM, Peterson JL, Luedicke J. Weight-based victimization: bullying experiences of weight loss treatment-seeking youth. Pediatrics 2013;131:E1–9.
89. Lumeng JC, Forrest P, Appugliese DP, et al. Weight status as a predictor of being bullied in third through sixth grades. Pediatrics 2010;125:E1301–7.

90. Lowen DE. Failure to thrive. In: Jenny C, editor. Child abuse and neglect: diagnosis, treatment and evidence. St Louis (MO): Elsevier Saunders; 2011. p. 547–62.
91. Council on Communications and Media, Strasburger VC. Children, adolescents, obesity, and the media. Pediatrics 2011;128:201–8.
92. Gortmaker SL, Must A, Sobol AM, et al. Television viewing as a cause of increasing obesity among children in the United States, 1986-1990. Arch Pediatr Adolesc Med 1996;150:356–62.
93. Vandewater EA, Shim MS, Caplovitz AG. Linking obesity and activity level with children's television and video game use. J Adolesc 2004;27:71–85.
94. Phillips SM, Bandini LG, Naumova EN, et al. Energy-dense snack food intake in adolescence. longitudinal relationship to weight and fatness. Obes Res 2004; 12:461–72.
95. Fulton JE, Wang X, Yore MM, et al. Television viewing, computer use, and BMI among U.S. children and adolescents. J Phys Act Health 2009;6:S28–35.
96. Kong AS, Williams RL, Smith M, et al. Acanthosis nigricans and diabetes risk factors: prevalence in young persons seen in southwestern US primary care practices. Ann Fam Med 2007;5:202–8.
97. Sills RH. Failure to thrive. The role of clinical and laboratory evaluation. Am J Dis Child 1978;132:967–9.
98. Southard AE, Edelmann LJ, Gelb BD. Role of copy number variants in structural birth defects. Pediatrics 2012;129:755–63.
99. American Society for Parenteral and Enteral Nutrition. The A.S.P.E.N. Pediatric nutrition support core curriculum. Silver Spring (MD): American Society for Parental and Enteral Nutrition; 2010.
100. Rogers VW, Hart PH, Motyka E, et al. Impact of let's go! 5-2-1-0: a community-based, multisetting childhood obesity prevention program. J Pediatr Psychol 2013;38:1010–20.
101. May AL, Dietz WH. The Feeding Infants and Toddlers Study 2008: opportunities to assess parental, cultural, and environmental influences on dietary behaviors and obesity prevention among young children. J Am Diet Assoc 2010;110: S11–5.
102. Butte NF, Fox MK, Briefel RR, et al. Nutrient intakes of US infants, toddlers, and preschoolers meet or exceed dietary reference intakes. J Am Diet Assoc 2010; 110:S27–37.
103. Dwyer JT, Butte NF, Deming DM, et al. Feeding Infants and Toddlers Study 2008: progress, continuing concerns, and implications. J Am Diet Assoc 2010;110: S60–7.
104. U.S. Department of Health and Human Services, Administration for Children and Families, Administration on Children, Youth and Families, Children's Bureau. Child maltreatment 2012. Available at: http://www.acf.hhs.gov/programs/cb/research-data-technology/statistics-research/child-maltreatment. Accessed April 23, 2014.
105. Dubowitz H. Neglect in children. Pediatr Ann 2013;42:73–7.
106. Jenny C. Recognizing and responding to medical neglect. Pediatrics 2007;120: 1385–9.
107. Brotman LM, Dawson-McClure S, Huang KY, et al. Early childhood family intervention and long-term obesity prevention among high-risk minority youth. Pediatrics 2012;129:E621–8.
108. Nader PR, O'Brien M, Houts R, et al. Identifying risk for obesity in early childhood. Pediatrics 2006;118:E594–601.

109. Cunningham SA, Kramer MR, Narayan KM. Incidence of childhood obesity in the United States. N Engl J Med 2014;370:403 11.
110. Gibbs BG, Forste R. Socioeconomic status, infant feeding practices and early childhood obesity. Pediatr Obes 2014;9(2):135–46.
111. Institute of Medicine. Early childhood obesity prevention policies. Washington, DC: The National Academies Press; 2011.
112. Young KL, Demeule M, Stuhlsatz K, et al. Identification and treatment of obesity as a standard of care for all patients in children's hospitals. Pediatrics 2011;128: S47–50.
113. Perez A, Reininger BM, Aguirre Flores MI, et al. Physical activity and overweight among adolescents on the Texas-Mexico border. Rev Panam Salud Publica 2006;19:244–52.
114. French GM, Nicholson L, Skybo T, et al. An evaluation of mother-centered anticipatory guidance to reduce obesogenic infant feeding behaviors. Pediatrics 2012;130:E507–17.
115. Anderson SE, Whitaker RC. Household routines and obesity in US preschool-aged children. Pediatrics 2010;125:420–8.
116. Shin SH, Miller DP. A longitudinal examination of childhood maltreatment and adolescent obesity: results from the National Longitudinal Study of Adolescent Health (AddHealth) Study. Child Abuse Negl 2012;36:84–94.
117. Bentley T, Widom CS. A 30-year follow-up of the effects of child abuse and neglect on obesity in adulthood. Obesity (Silver Spring) 2009;17:1900–5.
118. Dubowitz H, Lane WG, Semiatin JN, et al. The safe environment for every kid model: impact on pediatric primary care professionals. Pediatrics 2011;127: E962–70.
119. Gomez F, Galvan RR, Cravioto J, et al. Malnutrition in infancy and childhood, with special reference to kwashiorkor. Adv Pediatr 1955;7:131–69.
120. Waterlow JC. Classification and definition of protein-calorie malnutrition. Br Med J 1972;3(5826):566–9.
121. World Health Organization (WHO). WHO child growth standards and the identification of severe acute malnutrition in infants and children. Geneva (Switzerland): World Health Organization and UNICEF; 2009.
122. Cole TJ, Flegal KM, Nicholls D, et al. Body mass index cut offs to define thinness in children and adolescents: international survey. BMJ 2007;335(7612):194.

More than Words
The Emotional Maltreatment of Children

Andrew M. Campbell, BS*, Roberta Hibbard, MD

KEYWORDS

- Emotional maltreatment • Child abuse • Child maltreatment • Psychological abuse
- Domestic violence • Emotional abuse

KEY POINTS

- Children who experience emotional maltreatment in the first few years of life seem to be at the greatest risk of suffering the most negative and damaging outcomes.
- Emotional maltreatment can cause permanent damage to a child's developing brain and often leads to a wide range of damaging social, cognitive, and behavioral symptoms.
- Medical professionals can identify children at risk of emotional maltreatment by noting difficult or inappropriate caregiver-child interactions, paying attention to the facial expressions and language used by the caregiver when describing his or her child, and by being aware of specific risk factors for emotional maltreatment that may be present in the family's social history.
- A wide range of factors, including domestic violence, caregiver mental health concerns, and caregiver history of abuse put a child at an increased risk of being emotionally maltreated.
- Prevention/intervention techniques must focus on improving life circumstances of the child and caregivers.

INTRODUCTION

Emotional maltreatment, although often overlooked and underappreciated, may be the most complex, prevalent, and damaging form of child abuse or neglect. Difficulties in understanding and defining emotional maltreatment have resulted, in part, from varying terminology used to refer to this form of maltreatment over the last 30 years: psychological abuse, emotional abuse, psychological maltreatment, and emotional neglect are terms that have been used interchangeably but inconsistently. The purpose of this article is to focus on what is known about emotional maltreatment.

Disclosures: None.
Section of Child Protection Programs, Indiana University School of Medicine, 705 Riley Hospital Drive, Room 3038 C, Indianapolis, IN 46202, USA
* Corresponding author.
E-mail address: campbela@iu.edu

Emotional maltreatment likely affects, either directly or indirectly, a large portion of the population, and its victims often suffer from a constellation of damaging cognitive, emotional, and behavioral symptoms. If these symptoms remain untreated, childhood victims of emotional maltreatment become adults with a wide range of behavioral and emotional difficulties that often put their own children at risk of emotional maltreatment. Medical professionals are in a unique position to identify children who may be at risk of emotional maltreatment and direct the child and his or her family to community programs and social service providers that can work to improve the quality of life for the family.

WHAT IS EMOTIONAL MALTREATMENT?

Emotional maltreatment may include a single traumatic event or a repeated pattern of behavior that harms a child's emotional, developmental, or psychological well-being.[1] It includes acts of omission or commission and can be verbal or nonverbal, active or passive, and perpetrated with or without actual intent to harm the child. This harm can be manifested as emotional distress or maladaptive behavior in the child resulting from the impact on cognitive, social, emotional or physical development. Emotional maltreatment (encompassing both emotional abuse and emotional neglect) requires no physical contact and occurs within the interactions between the perpetrator and child. These negative interactions characterize the relationship[2] and may leave the child feeling deficient, unimportant, or unloved.[3]

Emotional maltreatment can take several forms, including spurning; terrorizing; exploiting/corrupting; denying emotional responsiveness; isolating; and mental health, medical, and educational neglect (**Fig. 1**)—all negative and potentially degrading

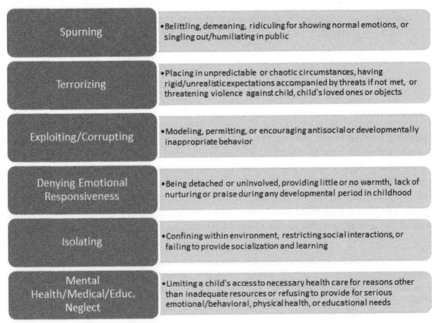

Fig. 1. Forms of emotional maltreatment. (*Data from* Hart SN, Brassard MR, Binggeli NJ, et al. Psychological maltreatment. In: Myers JE, Berliner L, Briere J, editors. The APSAC handbook on child maltreatment. 2nd edition. Thousand Oaks (CA): Sage Publications; 2002. p. 79–104.)

interactions.[1,3] Single incidents may, but do not necessarily, constitute maltreatment; repeated caregiver behaviors in these categories undermine development and socialization and are clearly harmful. Mental, medical, and educational neglect may become emotional maltreatment when the omission of such care and nurturance makes the child feel unworthy and not deserving. Differentiating suboptimal parenting from emotional maltreatment is often difficult because of a lack of societal consensus. Key in the determination of maltreatment is the harm to the child.

Emotional maltreatment can stand alone as the sole form of maltreatment experienced by the victim or coexist with any of the other forms of child abuse or neglect.[4] Many of the lasting and most damaging effects of physical abuse, sexual abuse, and neglect are psychological in nature and may be a manifestation of the underlying emotional maltreatment. The broken bone can heal, the sexually transmitted infection can be treated, but the fear, uncertainty, and emotional component of not knowing when or if it may happen again often has a longer-lasting, damaging effect on the child. The overlapping nature of the various types of child maltreatment make it imperative to consider all other forms whenever any one of them is suspected, as failure to do so could lead to an inadequate intervention plan.[5] Emotional maltreatment is often the greatest predictor of potential psychological problems later in the victim's life.[6,7]

HOW EMOTIONAL MALTREATMENT AFFECTS CHILDREN

Emotional maltreatment comprises the most damaging and consequential components of child abuse and neglect[1] and is often the most substantive threat to the victim's mental health.[8] Emotional maltreatment affects a child's mental and physical development and may lead to deficits in academic performance, IQ, memory, learning capacity, and brain volume.[9] Children who are victims of emotional maltreatment also suffer from a wide range of social and behavior difficulties including depression, personality disorders, anxiety, and aggression.[10]

Emotional maltreatment can begin to negatively affect children from the earliest stages of infancy. The human brain possesses a great deal of adaptability after birth, allowing for the growth and development of the areas of the brain most used by the child during the early years of life.[11,12] This important process enables the brain to adapt itself to best suit the environment of the child. With attuned, responsive parenting and healthy and appropriate stimulation, the child's developing brain can flourish in an environment that promotes growth and stability.[13,14] However, when a child does not receive this healthy stimulus, which is often the case in an abusive or neglectful home environment, development of specific areas of the brain, for example those responsible for caring behavior and cognitive abilities, are damaged in a manner that becomes increasingly irreversible with age.[12]

The elevated levels of stress, often experienced by victims of emotional maltreatment, can also put the child's developing brain at an increased risk of structural changes.[15,16] When a child experiences stress, his or her body's physiologic response kicks in. Designed to be simply a temporary response, these changes (eg, elevated blood pressure, increased heart rate) are regulated by cortisol, a hormone released from the adrenal cortex to contain the effects of the body's stress response and restore equilibrium.[17] Chronic elevations of cortisol, which result from regular exposure to high-stress situations, can cause great harm to a child's developing brain and lead to an alteration in the body's stress response for future events.[18,19]

When children live in an abusive or neglectful environment, they begin to internalize the concept that the world is a dangerous and unstable place. The development of emotional and social skills, often dependent on the strength and quality of the child's interactions within his or her early relationships, suffer, and the child may experience an overwhelming sense of helplessness. The child becomes more likely to overestimate danger and adversity, experience a decreased sense of self-worth, suffer from anxiety and depression, and experience emotional numbing or hyperarousal (symptoms of posttraumatic stress disorder).[18,20–23]

Perhaps the most complete examination of the overall emotional, behavioral, and social effects of abuse and neglect on a child's functioning is the work of Egeland and his colleagues[24] with the Minnesota Mother-Child Interaction Project. This longitudinal study followed the development of 267 children born to first-time mothers who were identified as being at risk of parenting problems based on several factors including age, lack of education, low income, lack of support, and instability. The study examined several different forms of child maltreatment, but the children who were identified as having experienced emotional neglect or "psychologically unavailable parenting" suffered the most dramatic consequences. Many of these children experienced a wide range of negative symptoms that were present throughout their childhood and extended into their teen years (**Fig. 2**). Participants who suffered from maltreatment in the first 2 years of life seemed to exhibit more negative outcomes than those who were victimized after they had reached the age of 2 years.[25]

THE LINGERING EFFECTS OF EMOTIONAL MALTREATMENT

Children who are victims of emotional maltreatment often grow up to be adults with several psychological, social, and behavioral difficulties. Research suggests they are often at increased risk for both mental and physical illness, including eating disorders, deficits in psychological functioning, depression, and low self-esteem.[1] They may be unable to appropriately cope with stress or anxiety, more likely to exhibit violent or aggressive behavior, and more likely to abuse alcohol or drugs[1]—all characteristics often identified as risk factors for perpetrating emotional maltreatment.

The negative effects of emotional maltreatment are not simply limited to the victim; everyone connected to the victim may also be affected in some way. The negative behavioral and social symptoms often experienced by victims of emotional maltreatment may make forming strong and healthy relationships with those around them difficult (**Fig. 3**). If victims of emotional maltreatment become parents, they are less likely to be able to provide the kind of stable and supportive relationships that their own children need. Without sufficient care and attention, these children are placed in an environment that puts them at an increased risk of child maltreatment, often leading to a continuation of the damaging cycle of emotional maltreatment.[26–28]

PREVALENCE

The lack of consensus as to a working definition of emotional maltreatment and the likelihood that it often goes unreported make it extremely difficult to accurately estimate its prevalence.[3] Researchers are limited in their means to extract and gather data on emotional maltreatment, most often asking study participants to self-report whether they were abused as children or if they have abused their own children. Conservative estimates have put the prevalence of emotional maltreatment to be in the range of 8% to 12% in the general population.[29,30]

Studies repeatedly show that emotional maltreatment is present in 75% to 90% of known cases of physical abuse or neglect,[6] but the fact that emotional maltreatment often underlies these more visually symptomatic forms of abuse can lead to it being overlooked during a child's initial evaluation. Trickett and colleagues[31] reviewed 303 children who were known to have been victims of some form of maltreatment. After

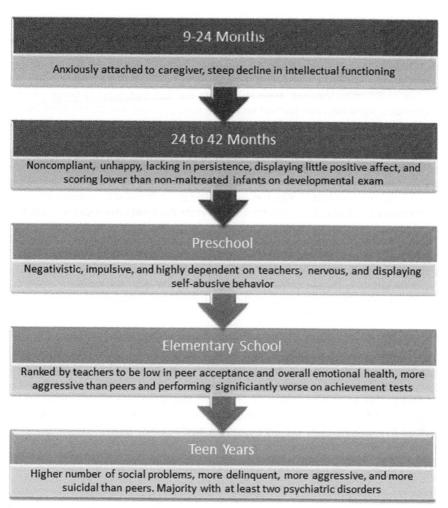

Fig. 2. Social and behavioral effects of emotional neglect. (*Data from* Erickson MF, Egeland B. Child neglect. In: Myers JE, Berliner L, Briere J, editors. The APSAC handbook on child maltreatment. 2nd edition. Thousand Oaks (CA): Sage Publications; 2002. p. 3–20.)

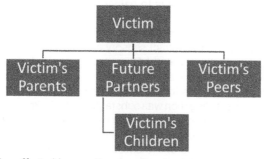

Fig. 3. Relationships affected by emotional maltreatment.

conducting in-person interviews and reviewing a summary of the child's involvement with the Department of Children and Family Services, including agency records, court reports, investigation documents on reports of maltreatment, and placement history, nearly half of the children were determined to have been victims of emotional maltreatment. Only 9% of these children had been identified as such at the time of their initial Children and Family Services' referral. Despite the fact that most of these children experienced more than one form of emotional maltreatment, most commonly terrorizing and spurning, it was often only the co-occurring physical abuse or neglect that was the focus of the Child Protective Services' investigation.

Another difficulty in estimating the prevalence of emotional maltreatment is that most definitions and studies that examine this form of maltreatment focus primarily on the child's relationship with his or her primary caregiver. As is the case with other forms of abuse or neglect, a child can be emotionally maltreated by anyone. Although the primary caregiver is the one who likely spends the most time with the child and, therefore, may have the greatest opportunity to inflict the abuse or neglect, often other people are in a position to emotionally maltreat the child. Studies that do not limit their definition to parent-child relationships find that children report being emotionally maltreated by a variety of perpetrators. These perpetrators are most often an older person who is important in the life of the child and can include relatives, teachers, coaches, babysitters, and other adults in a position of authority over the child.[29,32]

RISK FACTORS

The presence of multiple stressors puts an individual at increased likelihood to perpetrate emotional maltreatment. These risk factors include domestic violence, depression or other mental health concerns, alcohol or drug abuse, and learning disabilities.[33] Some of the specific parental attributes noted in cases of child emotional maltreatment include poor parenting skills, depression, suicide attempts or other psychological problems, low self-esteem, poor social skills, lack of empathy, social stress, and family dysfunction. The absence of another adult in the home, which prevents the caregiver from being able to spend time alone or away from the children, also puts children at an increased risk of emotional maltreatment.[34]

Domestic Violence

Domestic violence or intimate partner violence occurs more often among couples who have children than those who do not[35,36] and puts the child at an increased risk of emotional and physical maltreatment.[37] McDonald and colleagues[35] estimate that 15.5 million children (29.4%) are exposed to domestic violence in the United States each year, with 7 million children being exposed to what they classify as severe violence. Another study that used police reports to gather data, determined that children were present for 44% of the domestic violence incidents investigated by law enforcement. Of the children present for the domestic violence event, 81% were determined by the police officer to have experienced direct sensory exposure to the event with 4% being actually physically injured in the event.[36] A Canadian incidence study on child abuse and neglect determined that just less than half of the investigated emotional maltreatment cases involved exposure to some form of family violence, and in 63% of these cases, the emotional maltreatment allegation was substantiated by Child Protective Services.[38]

When the child's primary caregiver finds his or her own emotional needs being left unmet, as is often the case in an abusive environment, the caregiver may, in turn, find it difficult to meet the emotional needs of the child, often leading to a deterioration of the caregiver-child relationship.[39] Children who grow up in these environments can experience a wide range of behavioral problems including anxiety, depression, with-drawal, aggression, poor academic performance, and problems in their own dating re-lationships.[40,41] An analysis of existing data by Dube and colleagues[42] determined that children who were exposed to domestic violence were 6 times more likely to be emotion-ally abused, 4.8 times more likely to be physically abused, and 2.6 times more likely to be sexually abused than children who had no history of exposure to domestic violence.

Mental Health of Caregiver

In the United States, two-thirds of adults who meet criteria for psychiatric disorders across all diagnostic conditions are also parents.[43] Practitioners perceive one's ability to parent effectively to be adversely affected by mental health problems.[44] The stress of dealing with his or her own mental illnesses may limit the caregiver's ability to consistently and appropriately meet the emotional needs of the child. Maternal depression, in particular, may lead to increased feelings of irritability and hostility to-ward the child, more negative perceptions of infant behavior, and a weakened attach-ment relationship.[45–47]

IDENTIFICATION/INTERVENTION

Medical professionals are often in a unique position to identify younger children who may be at risk of emotional maltreatment, as these children often have limited contact with anyone outside of their home. Being alert for signs or symptoms of emotional maltreatment when any risk factors are identified and particularly when any other form of abuse is known or suspected can improve identification. Every interaction with the caregiver and child offers an opportunity to observe parenting techniques and evaluate the strengths/weaknesses of the caregiver-child relationship. How does the caregiver view the child? Does the caregiver find any redeeming qualities in the child, or is the child viewed as entirely responsible for any difficulties the care-giver may be experiencing? Negative facial expressions; threatening or violent actions or words; a rude, mocking, or hateful manner of speaking; and the use of overly nega-tive descriptors when talking of his or her child are often indicative of an unhealthy caregiver-child relationship. Medical professionals must familiarize themselves with specific examples of caregiver behaviors that may be indicative of an emotionally abusive or neglectful parenting style to aid in the identification of children who may be at an increased risk of emotional maltreatment (**Box 1**).

Box 1
Caregiver behaviors concerning for emotional maltreatment or neglect

Shows little or no sensitivity to child's needs

Emotionally or physically rejects child's attention

Exhibits frightening, threatening, or insulting behavior toward child

Refers to child as inherently bad or evil

Shows lack of concern/interest when talking about child

Responds to child inconsistently, often with emotional discharge

Data from Wolfe DA, McIsaac C. Distinguishing between poor/dysfunctional parenting and child emotional maltreatment. Child Abuse Negl 2011;35:802–13.

Observing the child's reactions to the caregiver's behavior can also offer clues to the hurtful nature of the interaction. The toddler brought to care for concerns of misbehavior (swears, will not sit in a chair for prolonged times, is a "terror") with a parent who is yelling at him, physically threatening, and swearing at him clearly warrants intervention. If the caregiver acts in an obviously harmful and destructive manner while being observed by others, his or her behaviors are likely to be even more threatening and damaging when occurring in the privacy of the caregiver's own home. Whenever caregiver behavior that is clearly damaging to the child is observed and raises a reasonable suspicion for abuse or neglect in the mind of the observer, a report must be made to Child Protective Services.

When indicated, clinicians are encouraged to make referrals to community programs or counseling services that provide assistance to families who may be going through stressful situations or when any of the aforementioned risk factors for emotional maltreatment are identified.[48,49] In many cases, the child's caregivers may have a great deal of unresolved conflicts in their own lives, and programs that work with these caregivers to help them address their own personal problems have led to improved outcomes for both the child and caregivers.[50] Programs that incorporate a multiagency, collaborative approach have had success in identifying victims of emotional maltreatment at a younger age and in helping to address the social, behavioral, and emotional symptoms these children often experience.[51]

In a study by Doyle, survivors of emotional maltreatment indicate that simply having someone in their life who gave "unconditional, positive regard, thought well of them, and made them feel important" was the single greatest contributing factor to their survival.[49] Medical professionals are often in a position to fill this role, especially for children who may have limited contact with anyone outside of their immediate family. By listening to children and taking their concerns and fears seriously, the medical professional can provide a positive influence and help the child explore and identify other possible positive role models and supports in their lives—a trusted teacher, relative, clergy, or coach. By making a report to Child Protective Services whenever any behavior is observed or suspected that is harming or damaging either emotionally or physically to a child, one can take the first step toward helping ensure the child and his or her family receive the services and assistance they need.

PREVENTION

Prevention techniques for emotional maltreatment are either universal (geared toward the entire population) or individualized to fit a specific set of people or circumstances. Universal intervention techniques attempt to create a change in the behavior and parenting techniques of the average parent across the entire population.[52] Programs designed to educate parents about proper parenting techniques and the negative effects of child maltreatment are found to reduce negative outcomes (even when significant risk factors for maltreatment are identified)[53] and decrease the incidence of reported and substantiated maltreatment cases by Child Protective Services.[54]

The variability of emotional maltreatment necessitates, at times, a more tailored approach at the individual or family level. This targeted approach focuses on the portions of the population identified as being at an increased risk of perpetrating emotional maltreatment. By narrowing the target population, these programs can address specific risk factors or poor parenting techniques. Families with known histories of abuse, domestic violence, mental health issues, financial difficulties, alcohol or drug misuse, or mothers with postnatal depression may benefit most from a more direct or targeted approach.[55]

SUMMARY

Emotional maltreatment often leads to lifelong cognitive, behavioral, and social consequences for children. Although it can affect any child of any age, children in the first few years of life seem to be at the greatest risk of suffering the most negative and damaging outcomes. Protecting and strengthening the child's relationship with his or her primary caregivers is of utmost importance when developing prevention/intervention strategies, as the child's wellness and outcome are often directly tied to that of his or her caregivers. Medical professionals can identify children at risk of emotional maltreatment by observing caregiver-child interactions, recognizing caregiver behaviors that may be indicative of an abusive or neglectful parenting style, and detecting risk factors for emotional maltreatment in the family's social history. Providing education and guidance concerning the impact of the caregiver-child interaction on the child's growth and development is a critical part of the intervention process and can encourage a shift of focus from the stress the family may be experiencing to the future health and development of the child. Future research must focus on developing prevention/intervention efforts that involve multiagency collaboration and incorporate community programs and social service providers that can provide resources and assistance to the many families that are either affected by or at risk of emotional maltreatment.

REFERENCES

1. Hart SN, Brassard MR, Binggeli NJ, et al. Psychological maltreatment. In: Myers JE, Berliner L, Briere J, et al, editors. The APSAC handbook on child maltreatment. 2nd edition. Thousand Oaks (CA): Sage Publications; 2002. p. 79–104.
2. Glaser D, Prior V. Predicting emotional abuse and neglect. In: Browne K, Hanks H, Stratton P, et al, editors. Early prediction and prevention of child abuse: a handbook. West Sussex (England): John Wiley & Sons, Ltd; 2002. p. 57–70.
3. Brassard MR, Hart S, Hardy DB. Psychological and emotional abuse of children. In: Ammerman RT, Hersen M, editors. Case studies in family violence. New York: Plenum Press; 1991. p. 255–70.
4. Binngeli NJ, Hart SN, Brassard MR. Definitions and meanings of psychological maltreatment. In: Conte JR, editor. Psychological maltreatment of children. Thousand Oaks (CA): Sage Publications Inc; 2001. p. 1–23.
5. Higgins DJ, McCabe MP. Multi-type maltreatment and the long-term adjustment of adults. Child Abuse Rev 2000;9:6–18.
6. Claussen AH, Crittenden PM. Physical and psychological maltreatment: relations among types of maltreatment. Child Abuse Negl 1991;15:5–18.
7. Rich CL, Gidycz CA, Warkentin JB, et al. Child and adolescent abuse and subsequent victimization: a prospective study. Child Abuse Negl 2005;29:1373–94.
8. Hart SN, Brassard MR. A major threat to children's mental health: psychological maltreatment. Am Psychol 1987;42:160–5.
9. Hart H, Rubia K. Neuroimaging of child abuse: a critical review. Front Hum Neurosci 2012;6:52.
10. Brassard MR, Donovan KL. Defining psychological maltreatment. In: Freerick MM, Knutson JF, Trickett PK, et al, editors. Child abuse and neglect: definitions, classifications, and a framework for research. Baltimore (MD): Brookes Publishing Co; 2006. p. 151–97.
11. Horwath J. Living with child neglect: the impact on children. In: Child neglect: identification and assessment. New York: Palgrave Macmillan; 2007. p. 41–68.

12. Perry BD. Childhood experience and the expression of genetic potential: what childhood neglect tells us about nature and nurture. Brain Mind 2002;3:79–100.

13. Stirling J, Amaya-Jackson L. Understanding the behavioral and emotional consequences of child abuse. Pediatrics 2008;122:667–73.

14. Shonkoff JP, Garner AS, Committee on Psychosocial Aspects of Child and Family Health, et al. The lifelong effects of early childhood adversity and toxic stress. Pediatrics 2012;129:e232–46.

15. Van der Kolk BA. The neurobiology of childhood trauma and abuse. Child Adolesc Psychiatr Clin N Am 2003;12:293–317.

16. Schore AN. Effects of a secure attachment relationship on right brain development, affect regulation, and infant mental health. Infant Ment Health J 2001;22:7–66.

17. De Bellis MD. The psychobiology of neglect. Child Maltreat 2005;10.150–72.

18. Stirling J. Neurobiology and the long-term effects of early abuse and neglect. In: Reece RM, Christian CW, editors. Child abuse: medical diagnosis & management. Elk Grove Village (IL): The American Academy of Pediatrics; 2009. p. 793–812.

19. De Bellis MD. Developmental traumatology: the psychobiological development of maltreated children and its implications for research, treatment, and policy. Dev Psychopathol 2001;13:539–64.

20. Briere JN, Elliott DM. Immediate and long-term impacts of child sexual abuse. Future Child 1994;4:54–69.

21. Tanaka M, Wekerle C, Schmuck ML, et al, MAP Research Team. The linkages among childhood maltreatment, adolescent mental health, and self-compassion in child welfare adolescents. Child Abuse Negl 2011;35:887–98.

22. Herringa RJ, Birn RM, Ruttle PL, et al. Childhood maltreatment is associated with altered fear circuitry and increased internalizing symptoms by late adolescence. Available at: http://www.pnas.org/content/early/2013/10/30/1310766110.short. Accessed November 11, 2013.

23. Nelson F, Mann T. Opportunities in public policy to support infant and early childhood mental health: the role of psychologists and policymakers. Am Psychol 2011;66:129–39.

24. Egeland B, Sroufe LA, Erickson M. The developmental consequence of different patterns of maltreatment. Child Abuse Negl 1983;7:459–69.

25. Erickson MF, Egeland B. Child neglect. In: Myers JE, Berliner L, Briere J, et al, editors. The APSAC handbook on child maltreatment. 2nd edition. Thousand Oaks (CA): Sage Publications; 2002. p. 3–20.

26. Braveman P, Barclay C. Health disparities beginning in childhood: a life-course perspective. Pediatrics 2009;124:S163–75.

27. Wickrama KA, Conger RD, Lorenz FO, et al. Family antecedents and consequences of trajectories of depressive symptoms from adolescence to young adulthood: a life course investigation. J Health Soc Behav 2008;49:468–83.

28. Kahn RS, Brandt D, Whitaker RC. Combined effects of mothers' and fathers' mental health symptoms on children's behavioral and emotional well-being. Arch Pediatr Adolesc Med 2004;158:721–9.

29. Finkelhor D, Ormrod R, Turner H, et al. The victimization of children and youth: a comprehensive, national survey. Child Maltreat 2005;10:5–25.

30. Scher CD, Forde DR, McQuaid JR, et al. Prevalence and demographic correlates of childhood maltreatment in an adult community sample. Child Abuse Negl 2004;28:167–80.

31. Trickett PK, Mennen FE, Kim K, et al. Emotional abuse in a sample of multiply maltreated, urban young adolescents: issues of definition and identification. Child Abuse Negl 2009;33:27–35.
32. Moran PM, Bifulco A, Ball C, et al. Exploring psychological abuse in childhood: I. Developing a new interview scale. Bull Menninger Clin 2002;66:213–40.
33. Cleaver H, Unell I, Aldgate J. How mental illness, learning disability, substance misuse and domestic violence affect parenting capacity. In: Children's needs – parenting capacity. Child abuse: parental mental illness, learning disability, substance misuse and domestic violence. 2nd edition. Norwich (United Kingdom): Crown Publications Inc; 2011. p. 49–84.
34. Garbarino J, Vondra J. Psychological maltreatment: issues and perspectives. In: Brassard MR, Germain R, Hart SN, editors. Psychological maltreatment of children and youth. New York: Pergamon Pres; 1987. p. 25–44.
35. McDonald R, Jouriles EN, Ramisetty-Mikler S, et al. Estimating the number of American children living in partner-violent families. J Fam Psychol 2006;20: 137–42.
36. Fantuzzo J, Boruch R, Beriama A, et al. Domestic violence and children: prevalence and risk in five major U.S. cities. J Am Acad Child Adolesc Psychiatry 1997;36:116–22.
37. Edleson JL. The overlap between child maltreatment and woman battering. Violence Against Women 1999;5:134–54.
38. Trocmé N, MacLaurin B, Fallon B, et al. Canadian incidence study of reported child abuse and neglect: final report. Ottawa (Ontario): Minister of Public Works and Government Services Canada; 2001.
39. Osofsky JD, Lieberman AF. A call for integrating a mental health perspective into systems of care for abused and neglected infants and young children. Am Psychol 2011;66:120–8.
40. McFarlane JM, Groff JY, O'Brien JA, et al. Behavior of children who are exposed and not exposed to intimate partner violence: an analysis of 330 black, white and hispanic children. Pediatrics 2003;112:e202–7.
41. Thackeray JD, Hibbard R, Dowd MD, Committee on Child Abuse and Neglect, Committee on Injury, Violence and Poison Prevention. Intimate partner violence: the role of the pediatrician. Pediatrics 2010;125:1094–100.
42. Dube SR, Anda RF, Felitti VJ, et al. Exposure to abuse, neglect, and household dysfunction among adults who witnessed intimate partner violence as children: implications for health and social services. Violence Vict 2002;17: 3–17.
43. Nicholson J, Biebel K, Katz-Leavy J, et al. The prevalence of parenthood in adults with mental illness: implications for state and federal policymakers, programs, and providers. In: Manderscheid RW, Henderson MJ, editors. Mental health, United States, 2002. Rockville (MD): Substance Abuse and Mental Health Services Administration; 2004. p. 120–37.
44. Dent RJ, McIntyre C. Health visitors, children and parental mental health problems. In: Reder P, McClure M, Jolley A, editors. Family matters: interfaces between child and adult mental health. Philadelphia: Taylor and Francis Inc; 2000. p. 185–96.
45. Lovejoy MC, Graczyk PA, O'Hare E, et al. Maternal depression and parenting behavior: a meta-analytic review. Clin Psychol Rev 2000;20:561–92.
46. Trapolini T, Ungerer JA, McMahon CA. Maternal depression: relations with maternal caregiving representations and emotional availability during the preschool years. Attach Hum Dev 2008;10:73–90.

47. Stanley C, Murray L, Stein A. The effect of postnatal depression on mother-infant interaction, infant response to the still-face perturbation, and performance on an instrumental learning task. Dev Psychopathol 2004;16:1–18.
48. Keen J, Alison LH. Drug misusing parents: key points for health professionals. Arch Dis Child 2001;85:296–9.
49. Doyle C. Emotional abuse of children: issues for intervention. Child Abuse Rev 1997;6:330–42.
50. Trowell J, Hodges S, Leighton-Laing J. Emotional abuse: the work of a family centre. Child Abuse Rev 1997;6:357–69.
51. Osofsky JD. Community outreach for children exposed to violence. Infant Ment Health J 2004;25:478–87.
52. Darlow J, McMillan AS. Safeguarding children from emotional maltreatment: what works. Philadelphia: Jessica Kingsley Publishers; 2010. p. 41–58.
53. Sanders MR, Ralph A, Sofronoff K, et al. Every family: a population approach to reducing behavioral and emotional problems in children making the transition to school. J Prim Prev 2008;29:197–222.
54. Printz RJ, Sanders MR, Shapiro CJ, et al. Population-based prevention of child maltreatment: the US triple p system population trial. Prev Sci 2009;10:1–12.
55. Straus MA, Hamby SL. Measuring physical and psychological maltreatment of children with the conflict tactics scales. In: Kaufman GK, Jasinski JL, editors. Out of the darkness: contemporary perspectives on family violence. Thousand Oaks (CA): Sage Publications Inc; 1997. p. 119–35.

Corporal Punishment

Adam J. Zolotor, MD, DrPH

KEYWORDS

- Corporal punishment • Spanking • Discipline • Behavior

KEY POINTS

- Corporal punishment is extremely common.
- Corporal punishment is associated with physical abuse in many studies.
- Anticipatory guidance around discipline should focus on building the skills to employ a variety of healthier techniques in an effective and consistent manner.
- Parents using escalating and ineffective discipline or those with psychosocial comorbidities will require additional resources.
- Systematic approaches to addressing discipline in the pediatric office setting can increase effectiveness and consistency.

INTRODUCTION

Corporal punishment (CP) includes use of any physical punishment against a child in response to perceived misbehavior. In the United States, this most often takes the form of spanking, but many other forms of CP are widely practiced in the United States and abroad. There can be a fine line between corporal punishment and physical abuse. In the United States, spanking and hitting with an object (such as a belt or switch) in the home are legal, if no significant injury occurs. For practical purposes, some child protective services agencies and consulting physicians use a 24 -hour rule; that is, if a mark from CP lasts greater than 24 hours, injury is said to have occurred, and the fine line between CP and physical abuse has been crossed.[1] CP should be considered in the context of discussions of child abuse for several reasons:

It is associated with numerous harms to the well-being of the child, including adverse developmental and behavioral harms.
It is closely associated with child physical abuse.
It is considered by many child rights advocates to be a form of physical abuse.

This article will consider the harms associated with CP, the clinical context for discussing CP, and the prevention of CP.

Department of Family Medicine, University of North Carolina at Chapel Hill, CB #7595, Chapel Hill, NC 27599-7595, USA
E-mail address: ajzolo@med.unc.edu

Pediatr Clin N Am 61 (2014) 971–978
http://dx.doi.org/10.1016/j.pcl.2014.06.003
0031-3955/14/$ – see front matter © 2014 Elsevier Inc. All rights reserved.

EXTENT OF CP

CP is widespread in the US. Population-based data on spanking is often difficult to compare based on differences in methodology and sampling. The most systematically comparable data on corporal punishment over time comes from the 1975 and 1985 National Family Violence Surveys and the 1995 Gallup survey on discipline.[2,3] A recent report compared the results from those studies over three decades to 2002 data from North and South Carolina to demonstrate a decline of 18% in spanking over nearly four decades. Analysis was restricted to children between ages three and 11 because spanking very young and older children is less common. Overall rates of spanking have declined 18% from 76.5% (1975—national sample) to 62% (2002–Carolinas) of children three to 11. Spanking peaks among three to 5 year olds, with a rate of 78.8% in 2002, down 4% from 82.2%in 1975. However, this still indicates that a large majority of preschool aged children are spanked. Hitting with an object is reported less often, with a rate of 33.2/% in 2002. This type of punishment peaks somewhat later, with nearly 50% of 7–9 year olds being hit in the past year.[4] It should be noted that this data comes from parent self-report. Therefore the decline might be a real decline in the use of spanking, but it also may reflect a decline in the social acceptability of spanking; increasingly, parents may be reluctant to disclose their use of CP. A more recent study of CP of children less than two demonstrated that 30% of children were spanked in the past year. Further, when analyzed by month of age, 50% of 17 month olds and 70% of 23 month olds were spanked in the last year.[5]

SEQUELAE OF SPANKING AND HITTING

Many experts and advocates recommend corporal punishment as an option for discipline or even a necessary part of good parenting.[6–8] It is clear that corporal punishment can be effectively used to alter immediate compliance, but this effect is short-lived.[9] However, it is also clear that corporal punishment has many unintended consequences. A systematic review of over 300 original articles on corporal punishment demonstrated that corporal punishment has adverse associations in childhood including: moral internalization (i.e. a belief by the child that she/he is bad), aggression, delinquent and antisocial behavior, decreased quality of parent-child relationship, and behavioral problems. In addition, corporal punishment during childhood is associated with long-term consequences later in adulthood: aggression, criminal and antisocial behavior, worse mental health, and abuse of one's own child and spouse.[9]

Spanking is associated with an increased risk of physical abuse. Previous research has shown that protective services substantiated abuse often results from escalated spanking[10] and is usually in response to perceived misbehavior.[11] Other studies have shown that abusive parents are 3–5 times more likely to spank than non-abusive parents.[12,13] If a child is spanked often, spanking will become less effective at modifying behavior. If spanking is ineffective, a parent may spank more, harder, or use an object.[10,14,15] A recent study reported that spanking frequency and intensity (use of an object) are associated with increasing probability of parents' reporting that they abused the child.[16]

Spanking very young children may have particularly important consequences. One longitudinal study of CP at age three found that, among girls, CP was associated with a lower IQ.[17] A subsequent study with a much larger sample and more effective control of confounding variables reported that spanking at 1 year of age was associated with aggressive behavior at 2 years of age and lower developmental scores at three compared to children who were not spanked.[18] A recent prospective cohort study reported that spanking at three was associated with increased aggressive behavior at five, further reinforcing that the groundwork for adverse developmental and behavioral consequences of spanking may be laid at a young age. Social learning theory supports these findings. Children that are spanked learn that hitting is the way to deal with anger or frustration leading to aggressive behavior in childhood and adulthood.[19]

Corporal punishment is also a human rights issue. Briefly stated, in most civil societies, it is illegal to strike an adult. Such use of force is considered a violation of human rights. The state of childhood should confer, if anything, special rights, not an abdication of those rights.[20]

CLINICAL ASSESSMENT

There are predominantly two reasons parents spank. Either they are angry/frustrated and/or they are trying to change behavior—usually by eliminating an undesirable behavior. The American Academy of Pediatrics recommends that pediatricians begin to assess discipline by 9 months of age.[21] By 8 months of infant age, 8% of parents report spanking, and 5% report spanking as early as at 3 months of age. Primary care providers should consider beginning such discussions by three to 4 months of age.[5]

Case 1: A mother brought her 4 year old to the doctor because he is having school problems. She states in the child's presence, "he is just bad, he won't listen, he is just like his dad." During the course of a 20 minute initial interview, she spanks or swats the child 15 times for touching things in the exam room and speaking out of turn. He barely notices.

Comments on case 1: It is clear that this mother is at her wits end. Spanking is ineffective and used so often that it is clearly extinct and she needs another option. The risk here is that she will spank harder to achieve a desired result. Much of the misbehavior could be eliminated and thus this need for negative reinforcement by engaging the child in a constructive activity (looking at a book). The pediatrician might model soothing and praising, re-directing the child, while asking the mom how she thinks the spanking is working and offering some other options. Motivational interviewing is a useful tool in helping families develop new discipline techniques. Motivational interviewing includes identifying a patient's self-interest in change, using their own words to express desire for change, planning for change, enhancing confidence by affirming small changes, and strengthening commitment to change.[22] This mother needs a lot more parenting help then you can provide in a typical office visit. She should be referred to a behavioral health professional or care manager if one works in your setting or a local parenting program. The pediatrician should also assess the mother for other psychosocial stressors, such as. depression, substance abuse, stressors, support, coping mechanism, and intimate partner violence.

It is valuable to assess the reason parents spank. See **Box 1** for suggested questions in assessing discipline.

There are many model programs and methods for addressing CP in a clinical setting. Clinicians and care managers can be trained to provide consistent evidence-based advice on child discipline (see Addressing Corporal Punishment).

One of the most challenging areas in assessing child discipline is to assess what the parent brings to the issue. Parents with mental health disorders, substance abuse disorders, those who are experiencing much stress, and those who were abused as a child or adult are at high risk for escalating CP and child abuse. Structured screening

---

Box 1
Assessment

- What do you do for discipline?
- What have you found to work? For how long?
- What does *John* do that makes it necessary to discipline him?
- How often do you spank *Jane*?
- Does spanking work? If "yes", "for how long?"
- What are you feeling when you spank *John*?
- How do you feel after you've hit or spanked John?
- Does *Jane* understand what you are trying to teach her?
- Do you sometimes spank with a belt, switch, or another object?
- Do you sometimes find it necessary to spank *John* harder or more often to teach him a lesson?
- What else have you tried to teach *Jane*? (see **Box 2**)

---

tools can be an efficient way to identify parents at risk for abuse. The Safe Environment for Every Kid program (see Addressing Corporal Punishment) uses this type of structured screening tool.[23]

Case 2: During a group well child visit you ask the mothers of 9 month olds "are you having any discipline issues? What is working for you?" Most mothers say they have started to say no but mostly avoid opportunities for misbehavior and re-direct. One mother says "I know you'll think it's awful, but I pop him when I have to" Another says (as if planted in the group) "what does he do that makes you have to pop him?" She replies "he messes with the remote control." To which another mom responds on cue, "maybe you could put it on top of the TV so he can't reach?"

Comments on case 2: These mothers have done your job. This advice may be more effective coming from her peers. They have instructed the mom on the avoidance technique. You might follow up with appropriate developmental expectations and setting priorities for teaching a 9 month old (e.g., no bite). You happen to know that this mom is also homeless and was a domestic violence victim during her pregnancy. If the CP issue was isolated, you might continue to provide advice and support. More resources such as a local parenting class might be useful as well as services for homeless families and intimate partner violence victims.

ADDRESSING CORPORAL PUNISHMENT
Approaches to Corporal Punishment

Parents can be taught alternative effective approaches for discipline. Ultimately, discipline is a means to teach children the important lessons of life. There are approaches other than corporal punishment that are more effective. Parents should be encouraged and taught to build a range of skills to successfully teach a child. Educational approaches foster change in knowledge, attitude, and behavior. However, the most effective approaches such as intensive home visiting are costly and often only available to serve high risk families. It is critical to provide parents with alternatives and resources in counseling regarding discipline. See **Box 2** for an approach to parents who choose to spank and **Box 3** for parent resources.

Box 2
Addressing corporal punishment

Empathize with the challenges of parenting

Tell parents that successful discipline requires a 'bag of tricks'

Explain extinction (when a technique stops working because of overuse)

Recommend against spanking when angry

Recommend avoiding spanking in young children (less than 2 years old)

Recommend avoiding use of a belt, switch, or other object

Give alternatives

- Time in (increase attention, praise and special time to promote desirable behavior)
- Time out (take a break from escalating misbehavior)
- Positive reinforcement (reward desirable behavior, can use a star, sticker, treat, or special activity). Can be used as a token economy in which a certain number of stars earns the child a reward of greater value.
- Negative reinforcement (An unpleasant consequence in immediate response to a misbehavior). Physical punishment is most often used this way, but other negative reinforcements include verbal reprimand (sharp 'no', expressing disappointment, taking away a privilege.)
- Passive inattention (ignore low level misbehaviors that are not a priority now for improving behavior, requires some understanding of normal development and prioritization)
- Avoidance (avoid the opportunity for misbehavior and thus the need for corrective action).

Provide resources

- Books
- Websites
- Local parenting classes

Some primary care providers and parenting educators will recommend to clients that they should never spank. This position may be useful in an advocacy role. However, since spanking is so normative in our society, the parent may tune out and the provider/educator may lose the opportunity to shift the parent to other techniques by expanding his or her tool box.

Box 3
Parenting resources

- *1–2–3 Magic: Effective Discipline for Children 2–12* by Thomas Phelan
- *The Pocket Parent* by Gail Reichlin and Caroline Winkler
- *How to Talk so Kids Will Listen and Listen so Kids Will Talk* by Adele Faber and Elaine Mazlish
- *Parenting with Love and Logic* by Foster Cline and Jim Fay
- *Discipline without Shouting or Spanking* by Jerry Wyckoff and Barbara Unell
- *The Discipline Book: How to Have a Better-Behaved Child from Birth to Age Ten* by Martha Sears and William Sears
- *Positive Discipline* by Jane Nelsen

In considering educational approaches to corporal punishment, it is useful to consider appropriate service delivery settings such as medical homes, schools, and community centers as well as developmentally appropriate timing for messages. As previously discussed, corporal punishment is common even in the first 6 months of life. There are two commonly used approaches toward universal education: primary care and mass media. Rigorous evaluations of stand-alone media campaigns to decrease CP are lacking. Media campaigns have been part of other evidence-based, community wide interventions such as Triple P (Positive Parenting Program). In this context, media campaigns may play a role in decreasing corporal punishment.[24]

Primary care medical visits are nearly universal in the US and most countries—in the first few years, and offer a good opportunity for education about discipline. A typical well child schedule in the US includes six visits through the first birthday. The American Academy of Pediatrics states unequivocally that children under two should not be spanked and that parents should be encouraged to develop and use alternative behavior management strategies for children of all ages.[21] Child health care professionals, public health programs, and child development programs should assist parents of very young children in developing a discipline skill set including positive and negative reinforcement without physical punishment as well as setting appropriate behavioral expectations for children. Well child visits are crowded with dozens of suggested topics for screening and anticipatory guidance, and primary care clinicians are limited by time and reimbursement to the number of topics they can address reasonably well.[25,26] However, primary care clinicians have been reported to be expert sources for parenting and safety advice.[27] One approach is the use of supplementary educational materials. One study randomized parents attending a primary care clinic to use an interactive DVD to view four behavior conflicts and parenting strategies out of 16 options versus usual care. Parents reported immediately after the intervention that they planned to spank less and that they felt the clinic visit had helped them to develop discipline strategies.[28] Other models that use primary care offices for parenting education have potential or demonstrated success in reducing corporal punishment but require relatively more resources.[23,29,30] The Safe Environment for Every Kid (SEEK) model offers brief training for primary care clinicians, structured screening, limited counseling, limited onsite social work support, and referral.[23,29] One additional approach that has involved primary care clinics is Triple P, in which some nurses were trained in Triple P approaches as part of county-wide interventions which have been shown to reduce corporal punishment.[24] Second to primary care, the next most common service for young children is daycare. Triple P has included daycare staff for training in parenting techniques as well. While many studies have evaluated daycare centers as places to disseminate parenting advice, CP rates related to parent education on this issue have not been studied.[24]

Parents who are at high risk of abusing their children due to risk factors such as young age, depression, substance abuse, partner violence, and poverty may need more intensive help than can be offered in a primary care setting. Such programs often focus on child rearing strategies in the context of children's health and development and parent wellness. Several programs have been found to reduce CP or improve positive discipline. Healthy Families America and Healthy Start have shown reductions in harsh punishment parenting.[31,32] The Nurse Family Partnership has shown more positive discipline. Incredible Years has reported less harsh discipline (verbal and physical), less CP, more positive discipline, and improved child behavior.[33] A particular therapeutic model, Parent Child Interaction Therapy, has been shown to improve positive parental responses to desirable behavior.[34]

SUMMARY

Primary care clinicians are trusted sources for parenting advice and have an opportunity to develop close relationships with families. Primary care is near universal in the United States and it is considered appropriate by most families to discuss discipline and psychosocial stressors. With limited intervention and resources, the primary care clinician can assess and offer assistance to all families. Practitioners should, however, be prepared to identify more serious discipline problems and co-morbidities (e.g. parental mental health and substance abuse disorders, child conduct disorders), and facilitate referrals to other services.

REFERENCES

1. Committee on Child Abuse and Neglect. When inflicted skin injuries constitute child abuse. Pediatrics 2002;110:644–5.
2. Straus MA, Donnelly DA. Beating the devil out of them: corporal punishment in American families and its effects on children. New Brunswick (NJ): Transaction Publishers; 2005.
3. Straus MA, Hamby SL, Finkelhor D, et al. Identification of child maltreatment with the Parent-Child Conflict Tactics Scales: development and psychometric data for a national sample of American parents. Child Abuse Negl 1998;22:249–70.
4. Zolotor AJ, Theodore AD, Runyan DK, et al. Corporal punishment and physical abuse: population-based trens for three-to-11-year-old children in the United States. Child Abuse Rev 2011;20:57–66.
5. Zolotor AJ, Robinson TW, Runyan DK, et al. The emergence of spanking among a representative sample of children under 2 years of age in North Carolina. Front Psychiatry 2011;2:36.
6. Baumrind D, Larzelere RE, Cowan PA. Ordinary physical punishment: is it harmful? Comment on Gershoff (2002). Psychol Bull 2002;128:580–9.
7. Focus on the Family. Discipline: wisdom for raising children in today's culture. New York: Colorado Springs; 2007.
8. Larzelere RE, Baumrind D, Polite K. Two emerging perspectives of parental spanking from two 1996 conferences. Arch Pediatr Adolesc Med 1998;152:303–5.
9. Gershoff ET. Corporal punishment by parents and associated child behaviors and experiences: a meta-analytic and theoretical review. Psychol Bull 2002;128:539–79.
10. Kadushin A, Martin JA. Child abuse: an interactional event. New York: Columbia University Press; 1981.
11. Gil DG. Violence against children. Cambridge (MA): Harvard University Press; 1973.
12. Oates RK, Davis AA, Ryan MG, et al. Risk factors associated with child abuse. Child Abuse Negl 1979;3:547–53.
13. Smyth SM. The battered child syndrome. London: Thomas Butterworth; 1975.
14. Kempe RS, Kempe CH. Child abuse. London: Fontana/Open Books; 1978.
15. Straus MA, Gelles RJ. Physical violence in American families: risk factors and adaptations to violence in 8145 families. New Brunswick (NJ): Transaction Publishers; 1999.
16. Zolotor AJ, Theodore AD, Chang JJ, et al. Speak softly–and forget the stick. Corporal punishment and child physical abuse. Am J Prev Med 2008;35:364–9.
17. Smith JR, Brooks-Gunn J. Correlates and consequences of harsh discipline for young children. Arch Pediatr Adolesc Med 1997;151:777–86.

18. Berlin LJ, Ispa JM, Fine MA, et al. Correlates and consequences of spanking and verbal punishment for low-income white, african american, and mexican american toddlers. Child Dev 2009;80:1403–20.

19. Taylor CA, Manganello JA, Lee SJ, et al. Mothers' spanking of 3-year-old children and subsequent risk of children's aggressive behavior. Pediatrics 2010;125: e1057–65.

20. Committee on the Rights of the Child. General comment number 1. The aims of education. UNICEF; 2001.

21. Stein MT, Perrin EL. Guidance for effective discipline. American Academy of Pediatrics. Committee on Psychosocial Aspects of Child and Family Health. Pediatrics 1998;101:723–8.

22. Center for Evidence Based Practices, Motivational Interviewing. Available at: http://www.centerforebp.case.edu/practices/mi. Accessed March 28, 2014.

23. Dubowitz H, Lane WG, Semiatin JN, et al. The safe environment for every kid model: impact on pediatric primary care professionals. Pediatrics 2011;127: e962–70.

24. Prinz RJ, Sanders MR, Shapiro CJ, et al. Population-based prevention of child maltreatment: the U.S. Triple p system population trial. Prev Sci 2009;10:1–12.

25. Norlin C, Crawford MA, Bell CT, et al. Delivery of well-child care: a look inside the door. Acad Pediatr 2010;11:18–26.

26. Rourke L, Leduc D, Constantin E, et al. Update on well-baby and well-child care from 0 to 5 years: what's new in the Rourke Baby Record? Can Fam Physician 2010;56:1285–90.

27. Zolotor AJ, Burchinal M, Skinner D, et al. Maternal psychological adjustment and knowledge of infant development as predictors of home safety practices in rural low-income communities. Pediatrics 2008;121:e1668–75.

28. Scholer SJ, Hudnut-Beumler J, Dietrich MS. A brief primary care intervention helps parents develop plans to discipline. Pediatrics 2010;125:e242–9.

29. Dubowitz H, Lane WG, Semiatin JN, et al. The SEEK model of pediatric primary care: can child maltreatment be prevented in a low-risk population? Acad Pediatr 2012;12:259–68.

30. Minkovitz CS, Hughart N, Strobino D, et al. A practice-based intervention to enhance quality of care in the first 3 years of life: the Healthy Steps for Young Children Program. JAMA 2003;290:3081–91.

31. Duggan A, Fuddy L, Burrell L, et al. Randomized trial of a statewide home visiting program to prevent child abuse: impact in reducing parental risk factors. Child Abuse Negl 2004;28:623–43.

32. DuMont K, Mitchell-Herzfeld S, Greene R, et al. Healthy Families New York (HFNY) randomized trial: effects on early child abuse and neglect. Child Abuse Negl 2008;32:295–315.

33. Letarte MJ, Normandeau S, Allard J. Effectiveness of a parent training program "Incredible Years" in a child protection service. Child Abuse Negl 2010;34: 253–61.

34. Thomas R, Zimmer-Gembeck MJ. Accumulating evidence for parent-child interaction therapy in the prevention of child maltreatment. Child Dev 2011;82: 177–92.

The Conversation
Interacting with Parents When Child Abuse Is Suspected

John Stirling, MD

KEYWORDS

- Child abuse • Forensic interview • Documentation

KEY POINTS

- The physician's role is medical, but medical concerns should always include the patient's safety and, thus, may include forensics.
- Open-ended questions, structured interviews, and active listening skills help provide accurate information.
- Questions should be phrased as simply as possible and pitched to the developmental level of the person being interviewed, whether adult or child.
- It can be hard for doctors to consider maltreatment by a caregiver in the differential, because to do so appears to sacrifice the partnership between parent and clinician.
- Preconceptions and prejudices interfere with accurate information gathering but are almost universal. Taking a history should begin with self-awareness.
- Clear, accurate documentation of history taking and medical decision making is essential to patient care and allows effective transfer of vital information to other agencies involved in guaranteeing the patient's safety.

INTRODUCTION

There is no such thing as a baby. If you set out to describe a baby, you will find you are describing a baby and someone.

—*Donald Winnicott, 1947*

The cooperative partnership of parent and physician in the interest of a child's health is one of the strengths and joys of pediatric medicine. Interactions with the child's caregivers, however, can become problematic when medical providers suspect a child may have been abused or neglected. When the doctor is forced to confront

Disclosure: None.
Center for Child Protection, Santa Clara Valley Medical Center, 751 South Bascom Avenue, San Jose, CA 95128, USA
E-mail address: JStirlings@aol.com

Pediatr Clin N Am 61 (2014) 979–995
http://dx.doi.org/10.1016/j.pcl.2014.06.008   **pediatric.theclinics.com**
0031-3955/14/$ – see front matter © 2014 Elsevier Inc. All rights reserved.

the possibility that the child patient may have come to harm through the actions or negligence of a trusted caregiver, trust in the family is shaken, and some difficult conversations lie ahead.

This article reviews some of the challenges and pitfalls in communicating with families when abuse is part of the differential diagnosis and offers some suggestions for improving communication with parents and children in these challenging clinical settings.

TAKING THE HISTORY FROM PARENTS AND CAREGIVERS WHEN ABUSE IS SUSPECTED

When the initial history appears to be at odds with an observed injury, the first step should be to review the history with the caregivers. Beginning with the history of the presenting complaint (injury), the physician needs to know when the child last appeared to be at his or her normal baseline and when after that the child first appeared to be injured. It is useful to ask, "How did you know?" in obtaining this information, distinguishing between what the historian witnessed versus what was told them or deduced logically. It is useful to inquire as to the presence of other witnesses to the event and recording their names if known. To the extent that it is possible, a reliable timeline should be constructed with the caregivers, from the time of the injury event to the child's arrival in the office or hospital.

It is useful to speak to multiple caregivers separately. This separation allows for a comparison of the histories provided and helps to minimize coercion by allowing shy or intimidated witnesses to speak freely.

A thorough review of systems and past medical history may prompt the family to recall other, earlier symptoms and can identify conditions that may prove pertinent to the diagnosis or to subsequent care. Finally, family and social history will help place the child's history in proper context, identifying sources of support and sometimes areas of vulnerability.

When informing the family of the decision to report the case to Children's Protective Services (CPS) or to law enforcement, it is important to be mindful of the effect of this decision on the family and to treat it as an important discussion. The decision to report should be disclosed respectfully but firmly, along with the reasons for the report. It may help to explain that medical providers are required by law to notify the authorities of any inadequately explained injury that occurs to a child. There is widespread confusion and misapprehension about the role and the workings of CPS, and this conversation is a good time to help the family understand what happens next, again, explaining that medical providers work with CPS and police agencies to gather information that may help in our diagnosis and treatment, for example, they can interview others outside of the hospital or visit the scene of the incident. This conversation is a good time to point out that the common goal of parents and professionals is to provide for the child's safety and to prevent future injury.

THE ART OF ASKING

Although knowing *what* to ask is obviously necessary, it is equally important to know *how* to ask the questions to best encourage the free exchange of accurate information.[1] The conversations that ensue after a suspicious injury, especially when there is suspicion of abuse, can be highly emotional for both parties, but the information gathered may be essential to making an accurate diagnosis. It can be helpful to plan the sequence of the interview in advance.

One Recommended Sequence for Conducting the Interview

1. *Introduce yourself*, and clarify your medical role in caring for the patient. Identify and acknowledge each person in the room, including each child. If possible, sit down and help put the others at ease.

2. *Establish rapport* by showing concern for the family's welfare and immediate needs. Take some time to gather an impression of their communication and coping skills and their emotional states. Useful questions on meeting a family for the first time might be, "What have you been told so far?" and "What do you know about the injuries?" Such questions begin a discussion of the injuries and establish the questioner in the appropriate role of a helpful expert. They also frame the discussion properly: as an attempt to provide the best possible health care for the child by obtaining all the available, accurate information.

3. *Gather information*, beginning with the chief complaint or presenting injury, using open-ended questions whenever possible and avoiding judgments (see later discussion). In obtaining information about the presenting complaint, the clinician should always remember that each caregiver usually will have a different perspective on the events, and attempts should be made to speak to each separately to facilitate free conversation and to assess concordance in their accounts.

4. *Learn about the patient*, including medical history; a review of systems; and educational, social, and family histories. Any information may prove valuable in evaluating possible abuse. Preexisting medical conditions may render a child more fragile and more susceptible to injury after accidental trauma. School or discipline problems may reflect a stressful environment. A social history may suggest other possible perpetrators of abuse or identify positive factors for recovery after trauma. To paraphrase Sir William Osler, it is as important to know which patient has been injured as it is to know which injury the patient has.

5. *Close with the family*. It is at this stage that the examiner may need to respectfully explain that maltreatment is being considered, and why. Discrepant histories and inexplicable injuries can be reviewed in the context of difficulty in making a medical diagnosis. Parents can be reminded that law requires that medical providers consult with CPS whenever an injury is medically inexplicable. The decision to report should be explained in the light of the legal mandate and the necessity of gathering more information than is available in the medical setting. True closure also implies giving the family time and opportunity to react to the decision and helping them process the information. If appropriate, explain the next steps anticipated in medical care and when you expect to see them again. Provide a means to contact the appropriate medical provider if more information becomes available.

First Principles of Interviewing

In proceeding through a sequence like the one above, it is helpful to remember a few basic principles.

LISTEN BEFORE TALKING

An oft-cited axiom in the medical profession is that "They don't care how much you know until they know how much you care." Parents of injured children can be expected to experience anxiety, often extreme, as well as uncertainty, fear, and, in some cases, guilt. They may well find it difficult to organize their own thoughts, let alone understand and answer questions, until they have had time to give voice to their concerns. Opening with a sympathetic query ("A workup like this can be pretty overwhelming. I'd like to help. What's going through your mind right now?") can serve to open the door while offering comfort to stressed parents.

This invitation to share, coupled with a demonstration of sympathy, serves an additional purpose: by opening a conversation, the physician has an opportunity to assess important characteristics of the caregiver. These include emotional state and emotional relationship with the child, facility with language, and cognitive ability, all characteristics that are relevant to the evaluation.

It is useful, as information is obtained, to pause and reflect on what has been said. Pausing to verbally summarize and allow the others to affirm what has been said allows the interviewer to demonstrate mutual understanding.

DON'T ANSWER YOUR OWN QUESTIONS

Interviewing necessitates asking questions, but not all questions are equally useful. Ideally, queries to caregivers will invite them to tell their historical narrative in their own words. Optimal questions that will elicit this narrative are termed *open-ended* questions, in that they do not limit the response options. Examples of open-ended questions include "What happened next?" or a request to "Tell me more about that." Research shows that beginning an interview with open-ended questions leads to more information.[2]

A more restrictive form, common in medical interviews, is the restrictive (yes-or-no) question. In a yes-or-no format, the question allows only 2 possible options. This form of questioning allows the interviewee to choose an answer but does not invite a narrative that could provide richer information. For example, a 6-year-old being interviewed about possible sexual abuse might be asked "Did he have his pants on or off?" and find herself unable to describe an assailant who left the trousers on, but unzipped. Similarly, "Has your husband ever hit you like this before?" will usually obtain less information than the similar "Have you and your husband been having problems?"

The most restrictive class of questions is known as *leading* questions, in which the interviewee is asked to endorse a proffered version of the events. Usually seen in legal cross-examination, it takes the form "X is true, isn't it?" Interviewers who feel sure of an answer often tend to fall back on this mode ("That must have hurt, huh?" or "She's had all her shots, hasn't she?"), often to save time, but leading questions pose considerable danger of introducing bias. This bias can result from the interviewer's closing the door to other possible scenarios and from suggestibility and a desire to please on the part of the interviewee.

It can be difficult, and sometimes impossible, to conduct an interview using only open-ended questions, and most interviewers will occasionally resort to more restrictive formats. In these instances, however, it is advisable to open the format as soon as possible for fear of restricting the quality of the information obtained. For instance, a directed question such as "Did she fall off the bed?" would be followed immediately by the more open "Tell me more about that."

WAIT FOR AN ANSWER

In daily conversation, a long pause can be an indication that the other party is losing interest or that something has been said that is somehow awkward. When this happens, most people have an understandable tendency to try and fill the gap, either by changing the topic or by suggesting what they feel to be a reasonable response from their conversational partner. Although pardonable in our usual interactions, such efforts can be counterproductive in clinical history taking.

People under stress often feel confused and disoriented, and there are few things more stressful than a child's injury, even a clearly accidental one. A parent may need time before responding to a question, either to gather thoughts into a coherent response, to search for memories, or to overcome a reluctance to address a particular topic (perhaps a reluctance born of fear or guilt). When an interviewer rushes in to fill the silence, the obligation to respond is diminished, and information may be lost.

RETAIN (BENIGN) NEUTRALITY

Conversation implies a give and take, and an interviewer is obligated to "give" something to the conversation if the interchange is to proceed naturally. Here again, however, it is important to avoid conveying a bias while encouraging information exchange. Encouragement should be positive but nonspecific ("Thank you for helping me understand" rather than "Thank you for telling me [a specific fact]") for fear of moving the interview in a predetermined direction.

At times, it is appropriate to express sympathy, but this must be done cautiously, taking one's cues from the other's facial expressions and tone. It may be wise to ask the subject "How did you feel about that?" before offering support. Premature expressions of sympathy or concern may appear judgmental. Expressing sympathy for pain or for presumed shame before finding out if the event really was perceived as painful or embarrassing can shut down an interview quickly. It is far easier to discuss an emotionally charged situation if one need not worry about the listener's reaction or about being judged.

TALKING TO CHILDREN: SPECIAL CONSIDERATIONS

When abuse is suspected, the child victim or witness can be a valuable source of information, but retrieving and interpreting that information can be difficult. A body of research shows that, although it is clearly possible to obtain reliable information from young children, to do so requires both good interview technique and a realistic awareness of the child's capabilities. All of the interviewing principles outlined above are used when talking to children, but there are some that are particularly important in addressing younger interviewees.

Setting the Stage

It is often preferable to speak privately to a child about stressful subjects. If the child can be separated from the parent without distress, the interviewer can

- Obtain another perspective on the history given by the adult caregiver
- Avoid prompting or coaching by a parent
- Minimize intimidation (intended or not) by the parent
- Remove a source of distraction from the scene. This is especially helpful when the caregiver suffers visible emotional reactions to the disclosures.

If separation is not an option, parents may be cautioned to remain quiet and can be positioned behind the child, out of direct line of sight.

Body language is particularly important in conversations with children. It is best for the interviewer to appear relaxed but interested and to come down closer to (or even below) the child's eye level. Anxious children, especially the younger ones, may feel intimidated by prolonged direct eye contact or by what they perceive to be a domineering posture. It is sometimes helpful to turn a bit, facing some 60° or 90° away from an anxious child, while maintaining voice contact and casting occasional direct glances to convey interest.

Know with Whom You Are Speaking

As every parent knows, childhood is a period of constant change and growth, as new verbal, cognitive, and social skills are acquired. Conversing effectively begins with estimating the individual child's unique skillset at that point. Just as with adults, 1 or 2 minutes spent developing rapport can serve several functions. A benign conversation can assure the child that the adult is in fact interested, and that the child does have permission to speak. It can allay anxiety and make the child feel more comfortable. At the same time, conversing about some recent event or activity can give the interviewer a good idea of the child's vocabulary, grasp of syntax, ability to link cause and effect, and to sequence events in a storyline. Skilled interviewers will pay attention to the use of pronouns and ability to understand the "W" questions of who, what, where, and when. A working understanding of the particular child's use of language will guide the length and complexity of the interviewer's own sentences.

This initial period of exploration is especially important when the suspected victim is cognitively or linguistically delayed or when the interview is not being done in the child's native language.

Keep It Simple

Adults are more experienced with complex sentence structure than are children who can easily get lost while trying to understand a complicated question. Suggestions for simplifying questions[3] include:

- Use simple terms and avoid jargon
- Use proper names instead of pronouns to avoid confusion
- Phrase questions positively ("Did you see ___?" instead of "Didn't you see ___?")
- Use one main idea per question, and start with that

Suggestibility?

It is widely believed that children are more suggestible than adults, but it would be a mistake to let this concern prevent a discussion with the child victim or witness. Care must, of course, be taken to avoid conveying an expectation of a particular answer, whether by body language or by the technique of asking.[4]

Researchers point out that children have a desire to please adults, and that they will sometimes attempt to guess the right answer to an adult's question. Interview protocols urge that the questioner remind the child early on that he or she does not necessarily know what happened, advising the child that "I don't know," if true, is a perfectly acceptable answer.

Regardless of the child's age, open-ended questions ("What happened after that?") retrieve more information than suggestive or restrictive yes-or-no questions. Nonetheless, on occasion, it may be necessary to ask more directed questions. Whenever this is necessary, it is important to open up the interview again, following up with less-directed and thus less-restrictive questions. A directed yes-or-no question, such as "Did he touch your private parts?" for example, can be followed up by "Show me where" or simply by "Tell me more about that."

Providing encouragement to a child during the interview can be effective, but should be done carefully. It is best to phrase encouragement generally ("Thank you for helping me understand what happened," for instance, conveys less bias than "Thank you for telling me that ____ hurt you"). Prompts that repeat parts of the child's spontaneous answer have been shown effective in drawing out further information ("You said the man hurt your ear. Tell me more about that.").[5]

Finally, it is necessary to remember that children are relatively inexperienced with language and may misunderstand a word. This misunderstanding may be compounded when they use that word in a response. "He put his pee-pee in my pee-pee," for instance, may refer to sexual abuse or perhaps to using the same toilet. Taking the time to verify one's understanding frequently during a conversation with a child may be well worth the effort.

Medical History Versus Evidence

Although information gathered in the medical interviews of child victims may often prove useful to investigators from CPS or law enforcement, the main objective of the medical interview is to assess the child's health and to plan a course of treatment where necessary, and questions should serve that purpose foremost. Both medical and community professionals may share an interest in descriptions of the events in question and of its perpetrator(s), but police officers and other forensic interviewers may pursue this information in greater detail in their efforts to investigate the crime scene and apprehend their suspect. Medical professionals will be more interested in ascertaining the patient's reactions to the event, to the symptoms experienced, to past medical history, and to understanding the family's experience.[6]

THREE PITFALLS

The right questions, a well-planned interview sequence, supportive body language, and skillful technique are valuable tools, but pitfalls remain before the information can be put to effective use. Here are 3 common failings.

#1: Failing to Keep Intentional Injury Part of the Differential Diagnosis

Although child maltreatment is a relatively common problem with serious consequences, many physicians still find it hard to place maltreatment on the differential diagnosis. To do so implies a sacrifice: when confronting the possibility that parents or caregivers are themselves responsible for harm to the child, physicians are asked to put aside the parent-physician partnership on which pediatric care is traditionally based. The physician may feel forced to choose between trusting the family and trusting her own diagnosis, and the diagnosis is often doubted first.

It is good practice to question one's diagnosis, but when carried to extremes this doubt can prove dangerous. Before seriously considering maltreatment, the reluctant physician may end up accepting very unlikely scenarios, fabricating ones they might prefer, or searching exhaustively for ever more implausible noninflicted conditions to explain the findings while ignoring the more likely, but more distasteful, alternative.

Failure to consider the possibility of inflicted trauma can prevent the practitioner from reporting what should be reasonable suspicions to CPS or law enforcement agencies, depriving the physician of valuable allies in the attempt to assure the child's safety. For a child victim, this failure can prove catastrophic.[7] For further discussion of child abuse reporting, see elsewhere in this issue.

#2: Overlooking Bias

It is essential that any professional enter an interview with a clear and unbiased mind, open to all possibilities. Unfortunately, biases can be subtle and difficult to uproot. To a significant extent, what a person perceives is dependent on a framework of life experiences, of lessons learned in roughly similar previous situations. These perceptual frames can be useful when the new event corresponds to a previous one, allowing one to apply in the present lessons learned previously. It can be dangerous, however, when the new event is, in fact, different in an important way. If an inappropriate frame is used, one can misperceive an important aspect of the new experience.

For example, a nonoffending parent whose framework does not include the possibility that a trusted spouse might be capable of injuring the child may fail to perceive clear evidence that he has, in fact, done so, and may contrive (to perceive) several excuses to maintain the frame. Similarly, a doctor who is unable to acknowledge that abuse might have happened may inadvertently make excuses or ignore certain pieces of information to preserve this more comfortable frame. The opposite may also prove true: an interviewer who is convinced of the historian's guilt may well, with no conscious intent to do so, see sinister shadings in what is said and may work harder to seek out data that confirm the interviewer's view.

Pediatricians are not immune to the effects of perceptual framing. A 1985 hospital study found that race, socioeconomic status, maternal employment, type of abuse, and mother's role in the abuse all played a part in the physicians' decision to report to CPS.[8] Seventeen years later, researchers found that minority toddlers with accidental fractures were more likely to be investigated for abuse than were their white counterparts, even after controlling for socioeconomic status.[9]

Psychologists have termed this *confirmation* (or *confirmatory*) *bias*, the tendency to seek out information preferentially that supports an established hypothesis while ignoring dispositive information. Confirmation bias is especially strong in emotionally charged settings.[10]

One can never be sure about avoiding bias, but it helps to take some time for introspection, to review potentially confounding variables before engaging the parents, and to remain alert to one's own reactions during the interview. Does the interviewer have a personal trauma history? Are there cultural or racial expectations, either positive or negative, to be avoided? Are there characteristics of the child, parents, or injuries that resonate with something in the interviewer's own history? It pays to take one's own temperature before and during the interview to assess perceived similarities and differences with the interviewee and to monitor one's reactions at all times.

Caregivers, regardless of whether they are responsible for a child's condition, may find it difficult to participate in what they see as an investigation of their fitness as parents. Although this attitude may be understandable, it can still be easy to interpret a confused and irritated parent as hostile or to label a bewildered one as uncooperative. It is even easier if the physician is a bit irritated and bewildered, too.

Scripts, protocols, and standardized forms have all been used to guide forensic interviewers in assessing putative victims.[11,12] These aids impose a certain order on the questioning and assure that all interviewers ask the same questions of each interviewee. A protocol such as the CalOES 2–900 form adopted by the state of California (Appendix 1)[13] can help make sure that an interviewer or examiner does not omit an important part of the evaluation, either out of an unsuspected bias or simply from fatigue, distraction, or a lapse in memory. Regardless of whether such aids are used, it is essential to stay aware that perceptual frames can introduce bias and to take measures to minimize this effect. These begin with self-awareness, and can involve use of protocols, team interviewing, and peer case review.

#3: Inadequate Documentation

Medical providers are constantly reminded of the importance of documentation, and nowhere is this more important than in the abuse workup. In addition to the usual concerns about immediate patient care, liability, and proper billing, thorough documentation is often of value to community investigators and eventually, sometimes years later, to judges and juries in civil and criminal courts. The most skillful interview will be of little use if its information cannot be recalled later. Don't trust to memory!

As an aid to subsequent recall, the questions asked and the answers should be documented as nearly verbatim as possible. The temptation to synopsize should be avoided; information will invariably be lost. "The child told me she had been touched on her buttocks" is useful, but when "When asked what happened after he shut the door..." precedes the statement, it is clear that the disclosure had not been suggested by the interviewer.

Photographic documentation of visible injuries should be done wherever possible and the images made part of the medical record. Effective documentation involves photographing from various distances (wide angle, middle, and close up) and use of an on-screen measuring device. Images should be reviewed to assure their accuracy.[14]

UNDERSTANDING THE MEDICAL PROVIDER'S ROLE

In evaluating a child for possible abuse, there can be understandable confusion of the medical and forensic roles, as medical information may have an important role in determining someone's guilt or innocence. Nonetheless, the physician's primary responsibilities must remain medical. In meeting and working with a family, it is important to stress that the medical providers and family caregivers share a common goal: the health and welfare and safety of the child.

Medical evidence, although undoubtedly important, is not the only evidence, and medical certainty, as evidenced by our concept of the differential diagnosis, should never be confused with legal certainty. It is the role of the physician to evaluate and treat the victim's injuries while working with other professionals to guarantee the child's future safety. Conducting these difficult conversations with the child and caregivers is the beginning of that process.

REFERENCES

1. Krahenbuhl S, Blades M. The effect of interviewing techniques on young children's responses to questions. Child Care Health Dev 2006;32(3):321–31.
2. Hershkowitz I, Horowitz D, Lamb ME, et al. Interviewing youthful suspects in alleged sex crimes: a descriptive analysis. Child Abuse Negl 2004;28(4):423–38.
3. Walker AG, Kennistion J. Handbook on questioning children: a linguistic perspective. Washington, DC: American Bar Association; 2013.
4. Ceci SJ, Bruck M. Children's suggestibility: characteristics and mechanisms. Adv Child Dev Behav 2006;34:247–81.
5. Lamb ME, Hershkowitz I, Orbach Y, et al. Tell me what happened: structured investigative interviews of child victims and witnesses. Chichester (United Kingdom): Wiley; 2008.
6. American Professional Society on the Abuse of Children. Practice guidelines: investigative interviewing in cases of suspected child abuse. Chicago: Author; 2002.
7. Jenny C, Hymel KP, Ritzen A, et al. Analysis of missed cases of abusive head trauma. JAMA 1999;281(7):621–6.
8. Hampton RL, Newberger EH. Child abuse incidence and reporting by hospitals: significance of severity, class, and race. Am J Public Health 1985;75(1):56–60.
9. Lane WG, Rubin DM, Monteith R, et al. Racial differences in the evaluation of pediatric fractures for physical abuse. JAMA 2002;288(13):1603–9.
10. Nickerson RS. Confirmation bias: a ubiquitous phenomenon in many guises. Rev Gen Psychol 1998;2(2):175–220.

11. Orbach Y, Hershkowitz I, Lamb ME, et al. Assessing the value of structured protocols for forensic interviews of alleged child abuse victims. Child Abuse Negl 2000;24(6):733–52.
12. Lamb ME, Orbach Y, Hershkowitz I, et al. A structured forensic interview protocol improves the quality and informativeness of investigative interviews with children: a review of research using the NICHD Investigative Interview Protocol. Child Abuse Negl 2007;31(11–12):1201–31.
13. Available at: www.CalEMA.ca.gov.
14. Ricci LR. Medical forensic photography of the sexually abused child. Child Abuse Negl 1988;12(3):305–10.

APPENDIX 1

State of California
Office of Emergency Services
(www.oes.ca.gov)

MEDICAL REPORT:
SUSPECTED CHILD PHYSICAL ABUSE AND NEGLECT
EXAMINATION

CAL OES 2-900

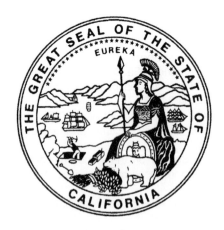

For copies of this form or assistance in completing the Cal OES 2-900, please contact
California Clinical Forensic Medical Training Center
(916) 930-3080 or
Contact Us @ www.ccfmtc.org

MEDICAL REPORT: SUSPECTED CHILD PHYSICAL ABUSE AND NEGLECT EXAMINATION
State of California
Office of Emergency Services
Cal OES 2-900

Confidential Document	**Patient Identification**

A. GENERAL INFORMATION   ☐ See Patient Label/Registration Face Sheet

1. Name of Medical Facility Where Exam Performed	Facility Address		2. Date of Exam	Time of Exam

3. Patient's Last Name	First Name	M.I.	Telephone	Cell Phone

4. Street Address	City	County	State	Zip Code

5. Age	Date of Birth	Gender ☐ Female ☐ Male	Ethnicity

6. Interpreter Used: ☐ No ☐ Yes   Language Used:_____

Name of Interpreter:_____   Telephone:_____
Affiliation of interpreter: ☐ Facility Interpreting Services
☐ Contracted Agency, specify:_____
☐ Family ☐ Friend ☐ Other, specify:_____

7. Name of Child's Caregiver ☐ Parent ☐ Legal Guardian ☐ Other, specify:_____	Gender ☐ Female ☐ Male	Telephone (w) (h) (c)
Street Address / City / County / State / Zip Code		

8. Name of Child's Caregiver ☐ Parent ☐ Legal Guardian ☐ Other, specify:_____	Gender ☐ Female ☐ Male	Telephone (w) (h) (c)
Street Address / City / County / State / Zip Code		

9. Name(s) of Siblings	Gender	Age	DOB	Name(s) of Siblings	Gender	Age	DOB
	M F				M F		
	M F				M F		

B. MANDATORY REPORTING FOR SUSPECTED CHILD ABUSE AND NEGLECT

Mandatory Child Abuse/Neglect Report made to both Law Enforcement and CPS Agencies (Pursuant to Penal Code §11166):

☐ Law Enforcement   ☐ Telephone Report ☐ Written Report Submitted   Name of Agency   Telephone   Date
Name of Person Taking Report:

☐ Child Protective Services ☐ Telephone Report ☐ Written Report Submitted   Name of Agency   Telephone   Date
Name of Person Taking Report:

C. RESPONDING PERSONNEL TO MEDICAL FACILITY

	Name	ID Number	Agency	☐ Unknown
Child Protective Services and/or Law Enforcement Officer				

D. PATIENT CONSENT AND AUTHORIZATION FOR EXAMINATION   (See instructions)

☐ Law Enforcement Authorized ☐ CPS Authorized ☐ Placed in protective custody ☐ Physician authority pursuant to state law ☐ Parent/Guardian consent

E. DISTRIBUTION OF Cal OES 2-900   (Check all that apply)

☐ Law Enforcement Agency (original) ☐ Hand Delivered ☐ Mailed ☐ Faxed	☐ Child Protective Services (copy) ☐ Hand Delivered ☐ Mailed ☐ Faxed
☐ Crime Laboratory (copy included with evidence)	☐ Medical Facility Records (copy)

F. PATIENT HISTORY

1. Name of Person(s) Providing History	Relationship to Patient

2. Child Accompanied to Facility By	Relationship to Patient

Patient Identification

3. History of Present Illness ☐ See dictation for additional information. ☐ N/A

If dictating, provide brief 2-3 sentence handwritten summary. Print or write legibly. Include date, time or timeframe, place of incident, and initial reporting party. Distinguish statements made by child in quotation marks from those statements made by other historians.

_____
_____
_____
_____
_____
_____
_____
_____
_____
_____
_____

G. PAST MEDICAL HISTORY

	Yes	No	Unknown	Describe
Birth History (if applicable)	☐	☐	☐	_____
Physical Abuse History	☐	☐	☐	_____
Sexual Abuse History	☐	☐	☐	_____
Neglect History	☐	☐	☐	_____
Emotional Abuse History	☐	☐	☐	_____
Domestic Violence Exposure	☐	☐	☐	_____
Alcohol/Drug Exposure	☐	☐	☐	Specify types of drugs if known, and collect urine toxicology up to 96 hours after ingestion:
☐ Prenatal ☐ Postnatal ☐ Alcohol ☐ Drug				_____
Hospitalization(s)	☐	☐	☐	_____
Surgery	☐	☐	☐	_____
Significant Illness/Injury	☐	☐	☐	_____
Any pertinent medical condition(s) that may affect the interpretation of findings?	☐	☐	☐	_____
Allergies	☐	☐	☐	_____
Medications	☐	☐	☐	_____
Immunizations Up To Date	☐	☐	☐	_____
Disabilities	☐	☐	☐	(Specify):_____
Growth & Development	☐	☐	☐	_____
☐ WNL ☐ ABN ☐ Unknown				

H. REVIEW OF SYSTEMS ☐ Negative except as noted below

_____
_____
_____
_____
_____
_____

☐ See dictation for additional information   ☐ N/A

I. NAME OF PERSON TAKING HISTORY (Print Name)	Signature	Telephone	Date

J. GENERAL PHYSICAL EXAMINATION

1. Temperature	Pulse	Respiration	Blood Pressure

2. Height (cm or in)	(%)	Weight (kg or lb)	(%)	Children under 2: (HC)	(%)

3. General physical appearance, demeanor, and level of physical discomfort/pain. Provide brief handwritten summary even if dictating. ☐ See dictation for additional information. ☐ N/A

Patient Identification

_____

_____

_____

_____

_____

4. Record results of physical examination.

	WNL	ABN	Not Examined	See Body Diagram	Describe Abnormal Findings. ☐ N/A ☐ See dictation for additional information
Skin					
Head					
Eyes					
Ears					
Nose					
Mouth/Pharynx					
Teeth					
Neck					
Lungs					
Chest					
Heart					
Abdomen					
Back					
Buttocks					
Extremities					
Neurological					
Genitalia					

5. If genital injuries are sustained, use copies of page(s) 6 and 7 (if applicable) from Cal OES 2-930 Forensic Medical Report: Acute (<72 hours) Child/Adolescent Sexual Abuse Examination Form or Cal OES 2-925 Forensic Medical Report: NonAcute (>72 hours) Child/Adolescent Sexual Abuse Examination to document findings and attach to this form.

J. GENERAL PHYSICAL EXAMINATION (continued)

6. Conduct physical examination and record findings using the diagrams.

Patient Identification

A | B

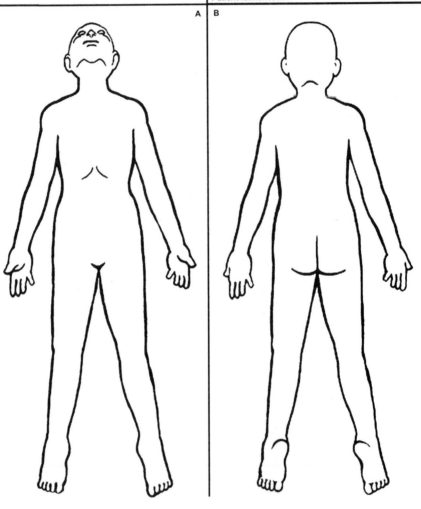

J. GENERAL PHYSICAL EXAMINATION (continued)

6. Conduct physical examination and record findings using the diagrams.

Patient Identification

C   D

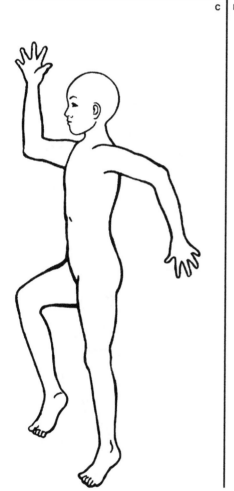
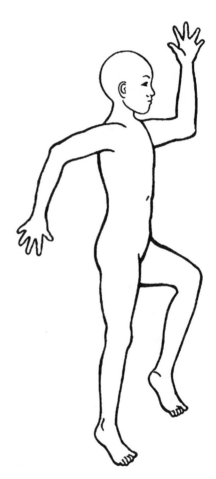

J. GENERAL PHYSICAL EXAMINATION (continued)

7. Examine the face, head, ears, hair, scalp, neck, and mouth for
   injury. Record findings using the diagrams.

Patient Identification

E
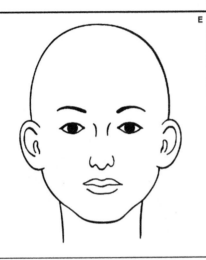

F
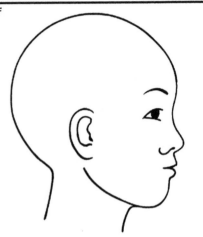

G
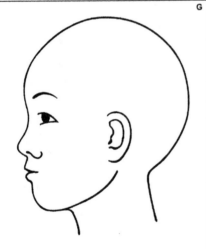

H
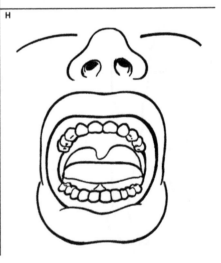

K. EVIDENCE COLLECTED AND SUBMITTED TO CRIME LAB

1. Clothing Collected ☐ No ☐ Yes ☐ N/A

Clothing Placed in Evidence Kit	Clothing Placed in Paper Bag

2. Foreign Materials Collected

	N/A	No	Yes	Collected by:
Swabs/suspected blood	☐	☐	☐	_____
Dried secretions	☐	☐	☐	_____
Fiber/loose hairs	☐	☐	☐	_____
Soil/debris/vegetation	☐	☐	☐	_____
Swabs/suspected saliva	☐	☐	☐	_____
Foreign body	☐	☐	☐	_____
Control swabs	☐	☐	☐	_____
Fingernail scrapings	☐	☐	☐	_____
Matted hair cuttings	☐	☐	☐	_____

Other types, describe:_____

L. TOXICOLOGY SAMPLES

	N/A	No	Yes	Time	Collected by:
Blood Alcohol / Toxicology	☐	☐	☐	___	_____
Urine Toxicology	☐	☐	☐	___	_____

M. REFERENCE SAMPLES

	N/A	No	Yes	Time	Collected by:
Blood (lavender top tube)	☐	☐	☐	___	_____
Blood card (optional)	☐	☐	☐	___	_____
Buccal swabs (optional)	☐	☐	☐	___	_____
Saliva swabs	☐	☐	☐	___	_____

N. DIAGNOSTIC STUDIES   ☐ Refer to dictation

1. Laboratory:

	WNL	ABN	N/A	Pending	Results
☐ CBC	☐	☐	☐	☐	_____
☐ Platelets	☐	☐	☐	☐	_____
☐ INR, PTT, PT	☐	☐	☐	☐	_____
☐ SGOT, SGPT	☐	☐	☐	☐	_____
☐ Urinalysis	☐	☐	☐	☐	_____
☐ Toxicology Screen	☐	☐	☐	☐	_____
☐ Other	☐	☐	☐	☐	_____

2. Diagnostic Imaging

	WNL	ABN	N/A	Preliminary Reading	Final Report
☐ Skeletal Survey	☐	☐	☐	☐	☐
☐ CT Scan	☐	☐	☐	☐	☐
☐ MRI	☐	☐	☐	☐	☐
☐ Other	☐	☐	☐	☐	☐

Describe:
_____
_____
_____

3. Exam Performed by Ophthalmologist:
☐ N/A ☐ No ☐ Yes ☐ Pending ☐ See Medical Record for Report
Name of Ophthalmologist:_____
Photographs Taken By:_____

O. PHOTO DOCUMENTATION

☐ No ☐ Yes ☐ N/A ☐ Film Retained
☐ Film Released to:_____
Photographs taken by:_____

35mm	Digital	Instant	Other
☐	☐	☐	☐ _____

Recommend follow-up photographs be taken in 1-2 days
☐ No ☐ Yes ☐ N/A

Patient Identification

P. REQUIRED SUMMARY AND INTERPRETATION OF HISTORY, EXAMINATION, AND DIAGNOSTIC STUDIES

Describe:
☐ Neglect
☐ Physical abuse
☐ Evaluation suspicious for physical abuse. Further information needed.
☐ Indeterminate cause
☐ Evaluation indicates non-abusive cause of medical findings.

_____
_____
_____
_____
_____
_____
_____
_____
_____
_____
_____
_____
_____

☐ See Additional Dictation   Dictation Reference Number:

Q. DISTRIBUTION OF EVIDENCE

	Released To
Clothing (items not placed in evidence kit) ☐ N/A	
Evidence Kit ☐ N/A	
Reference samples ☐ N/A	
Toxicology samples ☐ N/A	

R. PERSONNEL INVOLVED

Examination Performed By: (Print)	Signature of Examiner	
License No.	Telephone	Date

Examination Assisted By: (Print)	Signature	
License No.	Telephone	Date

Specimen labeled and sealed by:	Signature	
License No.	Telephone	Date

S. PATIENT DISPOSITION

☐ Admitted ☐ Home ☐ Protective Custody
☐ Follow Up Exam Needed (specify reason):_____

Cognitive Errors
Thinking Clearly When It Could Be Child Maltreatment

Antoinette L. Laskey, MD, MPH

KEYWORDS

- Cognitive errors • Child maltreatment • Confirmation bias • Anchoring
- Implicit biases

KEY POINTS

- Cognitive errors occur in every profession. Dozens of cognitive errors have been demonstrated to happen in medicine, many leading to poor patient outcomes.
- The diagnosis of child maltreatment can be susceptible to cognitive errors because of conditions of high stress, limited or questionable quality of data, and the subtlety of some diagnoses.
- Errors may be avoided through deliberate efforts to consider alternative diagnoses, avoiding premature closure, seeking objective input without social cues, and multidisciplinary collaboration.

Medical decision making is an exercise in process management: health care providers must gather data from multiple data sources, sometimes simultaneously, interpret signs and symptoms, sometimes without adequate history to fully understand the information provided, and direct patient management including further diagnostics and treatment, often without complete data. Most of the time the process seems to work adequately, that is, the patient is appropriately diagnosed and treated. Yet there continue to be studies that demonstrate failures in diagnosis and treatment related to factors that seem to be unrelated to the medical condition and more related to the patient's specific demographic characteristics.[1–4]

It is important that the diagnosis of child maltreatment be made accurately. Failure to correctly diagnose an abused child as abused (a false negative) could result in that child being returned to a potentially dangerous environment. Conversely, the overdiagnosis of child abuse (a false positive) could result in a child being removed from an environment wherein no one has caused harm to the child. The potential for errors

Disclosures: None.
Department of Pediatrics, Primary Children's Hospital, University of Utah School of Medicine, 675 East 500 South, Suite 300, Salt Lake City, UT 84102, USA
E-mail address: Antoinette.laskey@hsc.utah.edu

Pediatr Clin N Am 61 (2014) 997–1005
http://dx.doi.org/10.1016/j.pcl.2014.06.012
0031-3955/14/$ – see front matter © 2014 Elsevier Inc. All rights reserved.

in decision making related to child abuse extend far beyond the health care arena and include law enforcement, social welfare systems, prosecutorial decisions, and judge or jury decisions. Understanding the potential pitfalls in decision making is especially important for process improvement. Social psychologists have spent considerable effort in understanding how humans think, but only relatively recently have physicians looked to the literature to understand what clinicians can do better.

Humans have evolved to process an astonishing amount of information, often dealing with large simultaneous sensory inputs assaulting all of their senses. How is it that we are able to take in information, filter out what is not immediately relevant, and arrive at a reasonable conclusion? Are there shortcuts we can use to improve our processing speed without sacrificing the quality of the decision making? Perhaps most importantly, is it possible to avoid cognitive errors that we make and are compounded when community professionals from other disciplines, such as law enforcement and child protection services, are involved in a decision process?

COGNITIVE PROCESSES: AN OVERVIEW

Humans routinely make decisions in an overwhelming, complex environment. There are also limited cognitive resources available at any given moment to process all of the information available. Given the inability to completely process all of the data, humans have adapted by using cognitive shortcuts, which can be both hardwired and derived. One easy-to-appreciate example of a hardwired shortcut is that of recognizing potential danger. It does not take a prior experience with a potential threat, such as an obviously hostile animal, to realize that care must be taken.

Derived shortcuts also are common occurrences that increase over the course of a lifetime. Driving represents a classic example of a derived shortcut. Memories of learning to drive often will conjure the stress associated with the myriad of data bombarding the novice driver. It is only after years of practice that the process becomes nearly fully automated. What was once a difficult, stressful, and complex effort changes into a background process that frees the mind to handle other tasks. However, this automation can be an impediment to rapid responses to the unexpected. Deviations from the norm will take longer to recognize and process when one is not fully engaged in the task at hand.

Just as driving or tying one's shoes, or doing any number of complex learned tasks becomes less of an elaborate mental juggling act, so too does one's ability to complete tasks associated with the work. In the early years of a person's career, every part of the job requires thought and deliberation. As one gains experience and feedback on process and decision making, the process becomes more refined and automated. However, just as automation improves efficiency in tasks such as driving, it can also decrease the ability of an individual to recognize and respond to deviations from the norm.

Decision theory is the study of identifying what is known, what is unknown, and the other factors involved in arriving at an optimal (and therefore correct) decision. Social psychologists use multiple techniques to understand the processes involved in decisions. Decisions are very often reliant on heuristics, which are the shortcuts used to aid in decision making sometimes referred to as rules of thumb; new, incoming data are constantly incorporated and compared with previously gathered information. If they match previously acquired data, a shortcut in the thought process may be used to arrive at the answer. Heuristics can certainly be helpful in improving efficiency, but also may lead one astray if they compound biases in the thought process.

Biases may be either explicit or implicit. An implicit bias is one that an individual holds without being aware. Implicit biases can be difficult for an individual to acknowledge or control, given that they are happening without any real understanding or conscious effort. It has been clearly demonstrated that even people who profess to be egalitarian in their beliefs, and act outwardly in egalitarian ways, hold implicit biases that can influence decision making.[5] It is especially important to draw a distinction between implicit and explicit biases. Explicit biases are very much part of a person's conscious awareness and can be considered less socially desirable. Examples of explicit biases include overt racism, sexism, or ageism.

Much is now known about how humans process complex information. Research has shown that it is possible to improve thinking and reduce errors in judgment. Multiple studies have demonstrated that cognitive errors may lead to incorrect medical diagnoses. It is therefore important that professionals engaged in these high-stakes decisions, such as the diagnosis of child abuse, make efforts to understand how and when these errors might occur and how best to mitigate their effects.

COGNITIVE ERRORS AND CHILD MALTREATMENT

There are many common assumptions made by professionals that might not apply when the case involves child abuse. First, health care professionals assume that parents will be open and honest when seeking medical care for their child. However, if the perpetrator is a parent, he or she may not share the relevant information leading up to the symptoms that brought the child to medical attention, or worse, this person may lie and obfuscate. Second, there is a generally held belief that health care professionals use science and logic alone to reach a correct diagnosis, yet there is evidence to the contrary that "the art of medicine" is actually antithetical to science in some cases.[6] There are situations wherein a better, more scientifically sound approach to medical care is available to clinicians who resist implementation of the new protocol because they "know what is best."[7] Third, primary care providers often feel they know their patients' families and can judge who is at risk and who is not. Finally, primary care providers often feel that they would be able to detect problems in parent-child relationships by how a child interacts with their parent (eg, the child seems well bonded to the mother so there is no reason to think the mother could be abusing him).[8,9] None of these factors is meant as an indictment of a profession or group of individuals; rather, it is an acknowledgment of the complexities of the human thought process in light of difficult decisions.

The problems inherent in the human thought process are abundant. Many cases of potential child maltreatment are subtle and there are few "a-ha" moments that bring absolute clarity. Sometimes, despite best efforts, professionals are not fully engaged in the work of the day and rely more readily on derived shortcuts without realizing this is occurring. Often, parents and caregivers do not know what information is relevant or most important to share when talking to medical personnel or investigators, causing them to offer information that could be construed as misinformation or attempts at deception. Moreover, in other circumstances parents or caregivers may lie deliberately.

A closer look at common cognitive errors can help illustrate how they can confound arrival at an optimal answer. An in-depth exploration of all possible cognitive errors is beyond the scope of this article (**Table 1**).

Implicit Stereotypes

Stereotypes have a negative connotation, suggesting willful discrimination. Implicit stereotypes, however, are those that are typically not in the conscious awareness of the holder. Stereotypes are derived shortcuts that allow rapid categorization of people

Table 1
Common errors and possible solutions

Type of Cognitive Error	"Symptoms"	Possible Solution
Implicit stereotypes	Relying on generalizations to describe a family or caregiver. Examples: "bad parent," "nice family"	Using another colleague to staff the case because he or she will not have the same initial impression of the family
Anchoring	Difficulty considering alternative diagnoses even if all the information does not fit as one would expect	Devil's advocate (either a colleague or simply proposing countertheories to one's self), intentionally proposing alternative diagnoses to see if the working diagnosis is still the best fit
Triage cueing	Sending a patient to a specialist based on a very specific symptom or finding (which could be an anchor)	Multidisciplinary approach to diagnosis allows multiple viewpoints given identical case details, prevents "thinking in your box"

and naturally develop over a lifetime of exposures to information from the environment. When asked to conjure a mental image of an elderly person or a nurse or a homeless person, it is likely that this is not a difficult task. Clearly the image called to mind does not accurately represent all who are in that category, being a mental shortcut, but it does serve a purpose. Likewise, if a medical provider interacts with a family in a clinical setting, it is not difficult to understand that a subconscious categorization occurs, putting them into a "good" or "bad" family category without objective data to support this segregation. Some data that are used to categorize people are present immediately on first contact: the style of clothes or body art, the age, the speech patterns, and the color of the skin all are seen, processed, and sorted without conscious effort. Just as stereotypes are heuristics that allow us to categorize people easily, if not necessarily accurately, biases also exist and are frequently implicit. Social psychologists have demonstrated repeatedly that in-group preferences, that is, preferring those who are like as opposed to those who are different, are more natural than out-group preferences. For this reason, it is more natural to give the benefit of doubt to those who are similar to the observer and hold those who are not to a different standard.

In perhaps the most powerful demonstration of implicit biases, the Implicit Association Test developed by Nosek and Banaji (Available at https://Implicit.Harvard.edu) has been used to demonstrate people's natural tendency to easily categorize consistent pairings while having more difficulty categorizing inconsistent pairings. In the classic example, the time lag in a rapid categorization test is measured when a subject is required to associate a negative word with a white person's face or a positive word with a black person's face. It has been shown to be demonstrably slower than when the pairing is a positive word and a white face or a negative word and a black face. Because the positive or negative association is implicit, people are often surprised to learn their results and frequently express frustration because they perceive themselves to be egalitarian.

The relevance of stereotypes and implicit biases is found throughout the child maltreatment literature. Hampton and Newberger[10] found that hospitals were more likely to report a family to child protective services (CPS) if the patient was black, the parents were young, or the family was poor. In a study of patients presenting to the emergency department, Jenny and colleagues[11] found that abusive head trauma was missed nearly one-third of the time on initial presentation to medical care, and cases were more commonly missed if the patient was white or from an intact family. In another study of children admitted to an urban academic medical center with skeletal injuries, children with skeletal injuries who were from minority or low-income families were more likely than white or insured children (a proxy for socioeconomic status) to be evaluated for abuse and to be reported for abuse.[4] In an attempt to create an experimental model for the influence of race and socioeconomic status on the diagnosis of child abuse, Laskey and colleagues[12] used a methodology adapted from the psychology literature, and showed a difference in the frequency of the diagnosis of abuse among low-income white children in comparison with other categories. In this study, practicing primary care pediatricians were asked to rate the likelihood that an injury of ambiguous etiology (ie, it could potentially have been either accidental or inflicted) was abusive. The results demonstrated that socioeconomic status had more of an effect on the diagnosis of abuse than did race, despite identical clinical histories.[12]

In the law review literature, stereotypes have been shown to influence behavior and memories in investigators, prosecutors, and juries. The concept of misremembering, that is, creating a new memory from pieces of information that are reassembled into a new memory, has been shown to occur in stereotypical ways. In one study, a story of a crime is presented and the race of the characters is changed. The results showed that people tended to forget mitigating factors for black characters, and hostile actions were more likely to be attributed to them, even if they were not the aggressors in the story. Similarly, hostile actions by white characters were often forgotten. Of note, research subjects were often very confident in their memories, even when those memories were wrong.[13]

It should be apparent, therefore, that implicit stereotypes and implicit biases play an important role in how information is processed, particularly when a quick decision is required or a decision that relies on less than optimal information is necessary. How might this affect the accuracy of determinations when it comes to child maltreatment? Implicit beliefs may lead one to accept a story at face value because the alternative (eg, the diagnosis of child abuse) does not fit an implicit belief. If presented with a "nice" family and a child with injuries possibly related to child abuse, it might be an easier path to follow to consider alternative diagnoses. It is not uncommon that a bleeding condition, metabolic or genetic bone disease, nutritional deficiency, previously unrecognized congenital anomaly, or an accident is more aggressively pursued as the potential cause rather than to consider the unfortunately more common explanation of abuse. This is not to say that these conditions should be dismissed from the differential diagnosis, but neither should abuse be ignored in the evaluation. Alternatively, an ascertainment bias (also known as self-fulfilling prophecy), that is, looking for something only where it is expected to be found, may occur. If one only believes that "bad parents" (defined in whatever subconscious way that a health care provider believes) abuse their children, people who fit such a model of bad parenthood will be much more likely to be evaluated for abuse than those who do not. Of course cases are more likely to be found where one looks, leading to a circular fulfillment of the bias.

Anchoring

Anchoring is a problem of premature closure. When first presented with information, both explicit information and implicit data that are perceived but are not explicitly presented, the human tendency is to begin an immediate sorting and processing of the data. Data about a patient and family are available for this on first contact with the chart. Names often are markers of social position and frequently have racial or ethnic clues.[14] Race is commonly assigned by appearance and not by a parent's report. A clinical interaction begins with questions by a provider and answers from a caregiver or parent. From the outset, the clinician is building and testing hypotheses to explain the chief complaint and the associated findings. Sometimes these initial impressions form an anchor from which it is challenging to change course. Once the basic categorizations are made, further information is processed in that context. Anchors can be descriptors (eg, "difficult parent," hypochondriac), or a working diagnosis or historical piece of data (eg, fever several days ago but not currently, illness in household).

Just as stereotypes can lead to ascertainment bias, anchors may result in a confirmation bias. Humans like to be correct and will often work to find support for a theory. Examples abound of people's willingness to disregard information that is contradictory to a held belief and then embracing supporting information, even if it is dubious. Confirmation biases are especially problematic in accurate decision making because once a hypothesis has been generated, the tendency is to abandon opposite hypothesis testing. This action can result in the inability to accurately process new historical information or new test results.

When doctors perform testing, the analysis of the new data is often in the context of whether it fits with the working theory. Although it is often said that something is being "ruled out," research has shown that what is happening more often is a "rule in." As one builds a mental case for a given condition, information that does not support the theory is more difficult to "see," or be incorporated into the overall picture. It is not unusual that the information is not even truly processed at the same level as the supporting data. It is the avoidance of cognitive dissonance that leads to a cycle of seeking confirmation of one's theories and finding support in data that are obtained, even if there may be more than one way to interpret the new information.[15]

Triage Cueing

The adage "to the hammer, the world is a nail" is an apt description of triage cueing. When a patient is referred to a specialist, a specific question is often posed that the specialist would be ideally suited to answer. However, this begs the question of whether the information used to arrive at the referral to the specialist was correct or whether any cognitive errors may have occurred along the way. If a physician is evaluating an infant with bruising, referral to a hematologist will result in an evaluation of whether the patient has a bleeding disorder. If such a workup fails to demonstrate abnormality, the question has been answered and the case is returned to the hands of the primary care physician (PCP). But was the question answered? Whose responsibility is it to pursue the cause of the bruising? This closing of the loop sometimes does not occur.

It is the natural inclination of a specialist to answer the question that is asked, not answer the unasked question. Triage cueing, that is, the referral based on an assumption of diagnosis, could result in missing the ultimate diagnosis if the referral was to the wrong specialist. In child abuse pediatrics, the nature of the evaluation is inherently multidisciplinary. When a PCP consults with a child abuse pediatrician, the effects of triage cueing can be mitigated by having it be the responsibility of the child abuse pediatrician to engage other specialists while sharing the broad base of information gathered in the course of the medical evaluation.

A corollary to triage cueing is diagnosis momentum. In cases of caregiver-fabricated illness (previously known as Munchausen syndrome by proxy and medical child abuse), patients often have exhaustive problem lists with many diagnoses. When a parent seeks care with a new clinician, and provides what appears to be a detailed medical history and even supporting documentation for the child's diagnoses, it is easy to start with these data and move forward with the evaluation and management. The problem lies in the complexity of the case and the disinclination to "start from the beginning." Diagnosis momentum uses the preassigned diagnosis as a given fact. Unfortunately, the disorder inherent in caregiver-fabricated illness relies on this flaw in thinking. It is not uncommon to discover on thorough review of the medical documentation that many of the diagnoses carried by these patients are in fact conditions that were in a differential diagnosis and then ruled out. Similar to anchoring bias, labels are sticky and will build over time, placing these children at extreme risk of morbidity and mortality.[16]

COUNTERING ERRORS IN THINKING

It is not possible to avoid all errors in a process that has so many unknowns. The goal of safe, effective medical care should be the minimization of errors wherever those errors may arise. Psychologists have shown that there are processes that can be used to improve decision making. The following are some easy-to-apply strategies to improve decision making.

1. An important countermeasure is the use of the devil's advocate who, either as an individual working on a case or as a member of a broader team of professionals, can pose the question, "what are the alternative explanations for the information currently available?" When this question is asked as a member of a diverse team, it is possible to consider alternative hypotheses and propose tests and theories while minimizing the effects of a confirmation bias.
2. Avoid subjective or emotive descriptors. Many biases are compounded inadvertently by the way people naturally communicate. Descriptors are important to building a mental image. In medicine, handoffs between professionals, such as occur during shift changes or between teams in the hospital setting or even between professions when a case is passed from the medical team to CPS are frequently filled with descriptors. These details influence the receiver of the information by coloring how new incoming information is processed. If a parent is framed in a negative light, the new provider will interact with that parent from the anchor of this negative information. If a diagnosis is suggested as the working hypothesis, it will form an anchor against which new incoming data will be compared. Clearly it is important to relay information gathered to promote effective communication about a patient. The key to minimizing the cognitive errors in the system is to consider how that information is relayed. Data presented in handoffs should be evaluated to determine if it is necessary to the care of the patient, objective or subjective, and known versus hypothesized.
3. Seek objective input from colleagues on challenging cases. Another strategy that can be used with socially charged situations, such as when a particular situation is triggering a visceral reaction (eg, "this is a good family" or "this person is really frightening"), is to present purely objective data to a colleague. Although clearly a diagnosis cannot be made in a vacuum of information, by stripping away some of the social cues that might trigger an implicit bias, the diagnostic process can be improved. The history, medical presentation, physical examination findings, and test results can be objectively interpreted by someone who has not had his or her implicit biases activated. It is important when using this approach to present the data as cleanly as possible without any extraneous commentary to avoid swaying the interpretation.

4. Multidisciplinary thinking. Child abuse pediatricians often work as part of a larger multidisciplinary and interdisciplinary team. A key strategy to avoiding errors such as anchoring or triage cueing is to think broadly, the "think outside of the box" approach. Because the diagnosis of child abuse is a difficult one to make with serious consequences for a wrong diagnosis in either direction, it is especially important to use the collective wisdom of a team. Because each provider on the medical team will interpret the information through the lens of his or her specialty, open discussion of supporting information in addition to refuting information will improve the quality of the diagnosis, avoiding a singular focus.

SUMMARY

The diagnosis of child abuse is one that no provider wants to make, including those in primary care. It is known that cognitive errors happen, but they are not inevitable and steps can be taken to minimize them. It is through introspection that process improvement can be achieved. Diagnosis and medical management can be optimized through collaboration, discussion, and effective teamwork. Mistakes can lead to a better understanding of how humans think. As James Joyce said, "mistakes are the portals of discovery."

REFERENCES

1. Loring M, Powell B. Gender, race, and DSM-III: a study of the objectivity of psychiatric diagnostic behavior. J Health Soc Behav 1988;29(1):1–22.
2. McKinlay JB, Potter DA, Feldman HA. Non-medical influences on medical decision-making. Soc Sci Med 1996;42(5):769–76.
3. Feldman HA, McKinlay JB, Potter DA, et al. Nonmedical influences on medical decision making: an experimental technique using videotapes, factorial design, and survey sampling. Health Serv Res 1997;32(3):343–66.
4. Lane WG, Rubin DM, Monteith R, et al. Racial differences in the evaluation of pediatric fractures for physical abuse. JAMA 2002;288(13):1603–9.
5. Nosek BA, Greenwald AG, Banaji MR. The implicit association test at age 7: a methodological and conceptual review. Social psychology and the unconscious: the automaticity of higher mental processes. East Sussex (UK): Psychology Press; 2007. p. 265–92.
6. Suarez-Almazor ME, Russell AS. The art versus the science of medicine. Are clinical practice guidelines the answer? Ann Rheum Dis 1998;57(2):67–9.
7. Bohmer R, Edmondson A, Feldman L. Intermountain healthcare. Harvard Business Review School 2002. Case 603, 066.
8. Flaherty EG, Sege RD, Griffith J, et al. From suspicion of physical child abuse to reporting: primary care clinician decision-making. Pediatrics 2008;122(3):611–9.
9. Sege R, Flaherty E, Jones R, et al. To report or not to report: examination of the initial primary care management of suspicious childhood injuries. Acad Pediatr 2011;11(6):460–6.
10. Hampton RL, Newberger EH. Child abuse incidence and reporting by hospitals: significance of severity, class, and race. Am J Public Health 1985;75(1):56–60.
11. Jenny C, Hymel KP, Ritzen A, et al. Analysis of missed cases of abusive head trauma. JAMA 1999;281(7):621–6.
12. Laskey AL, Stump TE, Perkins SM, et al. Influence of race and socioeconomic status on the diagnosis of child abuse: a randomized study. J Pediatr 2012; 160(6):1003–8.e1001.

13. Levinson JD. Forgotten racial equality: implicit bias, decision-making and misre-membering. Bepress Legal Series 2006:1630.
14. Bertrand M. Are Emily and Greg more employable than Lakisha and Jamal? A field experiment on labor market discrimination. National Bureau of Economic Research; 2003. (Working Page 9873).
15. Croskerry P. Achieving quality in clinical decision making: cognitive strategies and detection of bias. Acad Emerg Med 2002;9(11):1184–204.
16. Flaherty EG, MacMillan HL, Christian CW, et al. Caregiver-fabricated illness in a child: a manifestation of child maltreatment. Pediatrics 2013;132(3):590–7.

Cultural Considerations and Child Maltreatment

In Search of Universal Principles

Gauri Kolhatkar, MD, MPH[a],*, Carol Berkowitz, MD[b]

KEYWORDS

- Culture • Cultural competence • Child maltreatment • Corporal punishment
- Physical discipline • Child abuse and neglect • Universal child rights

KEY POINTS

- Culturally competent services, sensitive to diverse health beliefs and practices and to cultural and linguistic needs, are essential in achieving parity in care and facilitating positive health outcomes for children and families across all cultures.
- Cultural competence requires individuals and organizations to (1) appreciate diversity, (2) assess their own cultural perspectives and biases, (3) bridge cross-cultural differences, (4) acquire and disseminate knowledge regarding culture, and (5) continually address the changing needs of the culturally diverse population they serve.
- Owing to worldwide variability in resources and cultural/social norms, policies of child protection and definitions of child maltreatment vary.
- The use of culturally respectful models in the determination of child maltreatment does not mandate universal tolerance of all cultural practices.
- The United Nations Convention on the Rights of the Child (UN CRC) establishes universal principles for approaching child maltreatment and child protection.
- The application of the UN CRC requires an understanding of what is happening locally, including how a cultural group is situated within its social and political milieu, in addition to relevant laws and policies.

[T]he action most worth watching is not at the center of things but where the edges meet....shorelines, weather fronts, international borders. There are interesting frictions and incongruities in these places, and often, if you stand at the point of tangency, you can see both sides better than if you were in the middle of either one. This is especially true...when the apposition is cultural.
—Anne Fadiman, The Spirit Catches You and You Fall Down[1]

Disclosure of Relationships: The authors have no relationships to disclose.
[a] Child Abuse Pediatrics, Harbor-UCLA Medical Center, 1000 West Carson Street, Box 437, Torrance, CA 90509, USA; [b] Department of Pediatrics, Harbor-UCLA Medical Center, David Geffen School of Medicine at UCLA, 1000 West Carson Street, Box 437, Torrance, CA 90509, USA
* Corresponding author.
E-mail address: gkolhatkar@labiomed.org

Globalization, technology, media, and human migration patterns have all contributed to creating a landscape of cultural diversity that is being increasingly recognized within health care delivery models.[2] Groups have belief-systems that shape how they perceive health and illness, and whether and where they choose to seek out health care. Anne Fadiman's pivotal documentation of the 1980s clash between a Hmong refugee family and their daughter's health care providers in a Northern California community hospital highlighted what is now a well-recognized theme within the health care system. Importantly with regard to maltreated children, culture can affect their perception and disclosure of trauma, expression of symptoms, treatment-seeking behaviors, and attitudes toward treatment and recovery.[3,4] Especially challenging is the question of how health professionals resolve the tension between respecting cultural norms or child-rearing practices and the importance of determining what constitutes harm and child maltreatment.[4] Addressing this complex question necessitates an understanding of the culture of the child and the family, and also of the health care provider. In addition, consideration must be given to the social and cultural norms and policies of the society within which the circumstances are being evaluated. Moreover, there exists a universal standard of child rights that must be upheld to protect children of all cultures from harm and maltreatment.

BACKGROUND: CULTURE AND CULTURAL COMPETENCY
Defining Culture

Culture is a set of "beliefs, attitudes, values and standards of behavior" that are passed down generationally, and are so entrenched within a cultural group that they are obvious and need not be overtly stated or challenged and defended.[3] Key elements of culture are depicted in **Fig. 1**.[3] Culture is "not monolithic and static but variable and dynamic," and is modified by time and continual interactions within its larger environment.[5] Some of these dynamic processes are listed in **Table 1**.[6]

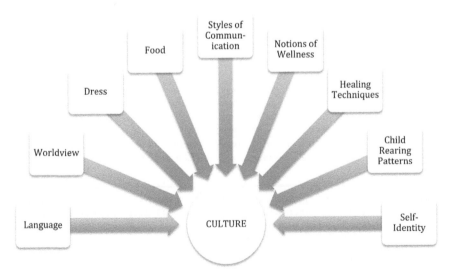

Fig. 1. Components of culture. (*Adapted from* Abney VD. Cultural competency in the field of child maltreatment. In: Myers JE, Berliner L, Briere J, et al, editors. The APSAC handbook on child maltreatment. Thousand Oaks: Sage Publications; 2002.)

Table 1 Dynamic cultural processes	
Enculturation	Process whereby a person is socialized into his or her own cultural group and learns its specific beliefs (eg, what a child undergoes as he or she is raised within one cultural group)
Intergenerational tensions	Process whereby 2 generations within one culture challenge each other's beliefs
Acculturation	Process whereby an individual responds to his or her nonprimary culture, and vice versa
Migration	Process of movement of an individual or a group to a separate or new geographic area (eg, immigrants seeking new opportunity; refugees fleeing persecution; Native Americans placed on reservations)

Adapted from Raman S, Hodes D. Cultural issues in child maltreatment. J Paediatr Child Health 2011;48:30–7.

Cultural Competence

An appreciation and understanding of cultural diversity is an essential component of clinical care. "Cultural competence refers to the process by which individuals and systems respond respectfully and effectively to people of all cultures, languages, classes, races, ethnic backgrounds, religions, and other diversity factors in a manner that recognizes, affirms, and values the worth of individuals, families, and communities and protects and preserves the dignity of each."[7] Cultural competence is vital to reducing disparities and to achieving parity in delivery of services and care across a diverse population.[8] Extensive guidelines have been published, giving providers and organizations a standard set of skills for culturally competent care.[6,9–13] The Joint Commission has summarized 5 basic elements required of individuals and organizations, which are helpful for health care providers who seek to provide care that is deemed culturally competent (**Table 2**).[6,12–14]

Achieving cultural competence is not a linear process with a definitive end point of full competency. Rather it is an iterative, dynamic process whereby providers continually appraise their own cultural belief systems and practices in addition to the needs of the populations they serve.[3,15] Some examples of providers' cultural limitations in assessing child maltreatment are listed in **Box 1**.[16] Recognizing these limitations, and those of one's beliefs, is referred to as "cultural humility," and is vital to exercising a culturally respectful approach to child maltreatment.[9]

CULTURE'S INFLUENCES

A foundational understanding of the influence that culture has on child-rearing practices, manifestations of symptoms of abuse, and health behaviors is essential to establishing a culturally competent practice of care.

Cultural Influences on Child Rearing

Cultures define "proper" and "improper" practices for parents. By understanding the diversity of culturally dictated factors influencing parenting and behaviors, health care providers are able to maintain cultural awareness and respect.[17]

Factors influencing parenting practices and parental intent

Multiple factors and values influence how parents view and treat their children. Certain characteristics of children influence their risk of abuse within different cultures. For

Table 2
Components of provider and organizational cultural competence

Component	Examples
Appreciate and value diversity	Recognize and respect that communities are their own cultural experts
Undergo continual self-assessment	Understand the impact of one's personal cultural identity on how one practices health care Aware of stereotypes Aware that patients are influenced by their culture but are not defined by them
Manage the dynamics of difference	Identify patients' preferred language and provide trained language/communication assistance services Consider involvement of a patient's family/cultural community in health-related discussions
Acquire and institutionalize cultural knowledge	Support ongoing sharing of cultural knowledge Support effective communication among staff to address diverse patient needs
Adapt to cultural diversity/community needs	Use population-level demographic data to determine community needs Collect feedback from patients, families, and the community

Adapted from Refs.[6,12,13]

instance, the sex of a child may predispose or protect that child from abuse.[18–20] An example is the strength of belief in male-child preference in regions of South Asia, which may influence the regional prevalence of female infanticide. Moreover, disabilities or health conditions in children may affect their value or burden.[18,19] A child's perceived economic utility or ability to preserve familial heritage may provide protection against maltreatment.[21] In addition, unique consideration should be given to the vulnerability of lesbian/gay/bisexual/transgendered/questioning youth, given the wide range of cultural beliefs regarding sexual orientation.[20] Cultural factors relating to the caregiver or family unit also affect the likelihood of maltreatment: these include family size and structure, sex roles, resources affecting stress and isolation, mental illness,

Box 1
Limitations in cultural awareness of service providers assessing child maltreatment

Stereotyping

Fear of appearing racist

Inadequate training

Denial of abuse in ethnic minorities

Communication difficulties (for example, the lack of use of interpreters, when indicated)

Overidentifying with caregivers

Fear of labeling a practice as maltreatment

Lack of child-centered approach

Cultural biases about disability and mental illness

Adapted from Polnay J, Polnay L, Lynch M, et al, editors. Child protection reader. 2007. Available at: http://www.rcpch.ac.uk/child-health/standards-care/child-protection/publications/child-protection-publications. Accessed November 13, 2013.

and history of abuse.[18–26] Furthermore, economic stress and intergenerational poverty significantly affect cultural beliefs and practices.[6]

Collier and colleagues,[27] in their study of Palauan teachers' perception of child maltreatment, expose the gray area of parental intent. Parental behaviors were less often perceived as abusive if their intent was for discipline, which included such practices as children being beaten for not doing their homework. In addition, the practice of Palauan parents tying their toddlers by the leg to a post to keep them safe while they farmed was the scenario that was least likely to be viewed as abusive and reportable; this highlights the interface of local cultural values, practical considerations of daily responsibilities, and parental intent.[27] Given that the intent was to protect, would providers with a Western cultural background also view this practice as acceptable? Although the practice is not deemed to be physically harmful within Palauan culture, the questions of the child's subjective well-being and of whether the child may still incur psychological trauma as part of the practice are difficult to fully ascertain, especially using a Western framework.

Culture and parental discipline

Among the most contentious and perhaps the most germane topic within child maltreatment for primary care providers is that of parental discipline.[6] "Child physical maltreatment most often results not from sadism or desire to harm, but from intent to punish or teach."[28] In particular, corporal punishment and its perception as either abusive or acceptable are varied across cultures and dynamics over time. Corporal punishment has historically been seen as acceptable, with most parents in the United States 2 decades ago reporting that they spanked their children, and with more than half of the medical providers in a survey supporting spanking in certain circumstances.[29] In the United States, laws banning corporal punishment of children in schools and in the home vary by state. In their multi-country (6 countries, 19 communities) survey of parental discipline as part of the World Studies of Abuse in the Family Environment (WorldSAFE) project, Runyan and colleagues[30] determined that a median of 16% of children in all countries surveyed experienced harsh or potentially abusive discipline in the prior year.[31]

New studies and greater understanding of the impact of parental violence against children, and the increased recognition of children as bearers of rights, have led to a shift from regarding physical punishment as an effective and acceptable parenting practice to a risk factor for maltreatment.[28] The American Academy of Pediatrics (AAP) Policy on Effective Discipline provides evidence that spanking can escalate: spanking increases the chance of physical injury to young children, may lead to more agitated or aggressive behaviors in children over the long term, and also may lead caregivers to perpetuate the use of physical punishment.[29] Children who are spanked experience poorer behavioral and cognitive longitudinal outcomes.[32] In recent years, the judicial systems evaluating corporal punishment cases in India, Israel, Italy, Fiji, Kenya, Namibia, Nepal, South Africa, and Zambia have ruled in favor of the rights of children.[28] Nevertheless, only 2% of the world's children, according to a UNICEF report, are protected from corporal punishment in the home.[33] Thus, there is still a global acceptance across many cultures of physical discipline.[34–37] Child rights advocates seeking legal protection of children from corporal punishment focus their efforts on changing cultural norms by motivating caregivers and educating the general public about the evidence-based negative health outcomes of this practice.

Cultural Influences on Health Behaviors

Fadiman's account of the Hmong family's clash with their daughter's Western health care providers illustrates innumerable manifestations of culture-related discordance of patients and clinicians.[1] Specifically, cultural beliefs and practices can affect adherence to health care recommendations, health-seeking behaviors, and acceptance of medical treatment.[38] For example, Fadiman describes how the Western medical ascription of seizures as a treatable medical problem stood in direct contrast to the Hmong belief that these seizures are a cherished unique and spiritual connection.[1] If a cultural group does not accept the premise behind the need for a medical intervention, nonadherence to care or delay in seeking care is expected. Alternative cultural practices may be administered in addition to or in lieu of allopathic medical care.

Clinicians should acquire knowledge of traditional remedies that may result in findings that raise concern for maltreatment. In particular, many cultural healing practices result in patterned skin markings. Moxibustion, the application of a heated object to the skin at therapeutic points, is used in many cultures. For example, the Vietnamese practice of coining involves application of a hot coin to the skin.[39] Cupping, the application of alcohol to the rim of a cup that is then heated and applied to the skin, may result in circular skin burns of varying severity.[39] *Maquas*, deep burns to the skin near diseased organs, are seen in Arabic cultures. In addition, garlic is used in many cultures for healing in various manners and, if applied to the skin for prolonged periods of time, results in bullae or burn-like lesions.[39] These findings may be misdiagnosed as abusive injuries by a clinician who has not considered these other potential practices. Such findings may present an opportunity for clinicians to illustrate alternative healing practices that may not cause physical injury.[39]

Cultural and religious beliefs that caregivers cite to overtly refuse medical care pose a unique challenge for clinicians who must decide if refusal of treatment constitutes maltreatment. Circumstances can range from vaccine refusal to blood-transfusion refusal to prayer over a convulsing child. The central issue is the determination of whether the child's health care needs are being met.[38] In the United States, a review of child deaths caused by lack of medical care for religious exemptions over a 20-year period determined that nearly all deaths were preventable.[40] Therefore, the AAP takes opposition to religious exemptions to medical care, stating that this disrupts society's ability to equally protect every child and ensuring the fulfillment of their basic needs.[41,42] Although this opinion is not universally upheld within regional United States legal systems, the US Supreme Court has ruled that the "right to practice religion freely does not include the liberty to expose the community or child to communicable diseases, or the latter to ill health or death."[43]

Cultural Influences on Manifestations of Abuse

When a child is maltreated within a family, cultural norms will dictate whether and how an individual or a family will disclose abuse, how they will seek help, and how they will respond to treatment and prevention initiatives. Disclosures of abuse can be discouraged by several factors that are weighted heavily in certain cultures: these include shame; taboos and modesty; sexual scripts; virginity; women's status; honor, respect, and patriarchy; and religious beliefs.[9] Some of these belief systems may limit open discussion about sexual matters, thereby limiting opportunity for disclosure, particularly of sexual abuse. Arab culture's emphasis on collectivism and the benefit of the family over the individual, filial piety, hierarchical parent-child roles, and family honor and loyalty, in addition to a cultural stigma of mental health problems, may affect a victim and his or her family's response to abuse.[44] In addition, disclosure can be impeded by "reporting costs," which are the consequences of a disclosure to an official source, such as loss of privacy, family support, or finances.[9] The concepts of historical trauma, whereby there is societal transmission of trauma to subsequent generations, and of unresolved or disenfranchised grief, whereby such grief cannot be publicly acknowledged or mourned or supported, may also influence disclosure and help-seeking behaviors.[45] Furthermore, the "model minority stereotype," as experienced by South Asians within American culture, may cause them to internalize an excessively idealized identity and, therefore, not disclose circumstances that may dishonor that model minority myth.[46] These examples illustrate the cultural variability in the disclosure of abuse.

In addition to disclosure, symptoms of abuse, for example, depression and suicidality or externalized symptoms such as anger or sexualized behavior, are variable depending on ethnic background.[4] A survey of Taiwanese schoolchildren showed that children identified as victims of physical abuse had fewer symptoms of subclinical posttraumatic stress disorder in comparison with victims studied in Western cultures.[47] This difference could be attributed, for example, to the fact that physical discipline by family elders is accepted in Chinese societies and that Chinese children therefore accept this as punishment for unwanted behaviors.[47] African American sexually abused girls have been noted to demonstrate more symptoms of trauma-related avoidance or withdrawal than their Hispanic counterparts. Although the effects of each ethnic group's level of acculturation cannot be measured, this increase in symptoms of avoidance and withdrawal can be potentially attributable to a history of disenfranchisement of African Americans within the child protective system in comparison with other ethnicities.[48] Thus, practitioners must be aware of the ethnic and cultural variability that may exist in the presentation of symptoms following abuse.

GLOBAL VARIABILITY

Significant variability exists in how child maltreatment is determined worldwide, in how children are protected from child maltreatment, and in how the acts of child maltreatment are handled. This variability is a reflection of diversity of not only cultural beliefs and practices but also of the nature and magnitude of resources available.

Global Variability in the Determination of Child Abuse

Variability in perceptions of parental and cultural practices affects what is perceived to be maltreatment across countries. The variability in such perceptions can occur even among world authorities in child maltreatment. The 2012 International Society on the Prevention of Child Abuse and Neglect (ISPCAN) World Perspectives survey of child maltreatment experts in 69 countries found that a majority defined physical abuse by parents or caregivers using specific examples, and sexual abuse (namely incest, sexual touching, or pornography) as child abuse.[35] However, other behaviors, such as physical discipline, child labor, and child abandonment were not agreed upon in the ISPCAN study, which points to the variability that exists globally.[35] There was further variability when low-income countries were compared with middle- and high-income countries.[35]

Variability in Child Protection Policies and Their Implementation

The variability in the determination of child maltreatment is both a function of and a result of each society's child protection system and response to child maltreatment. The challenges of defining child maltreatment cross-culturally must be placed within the context of the applicable laws. Ninety percent of the countries in the ISPCAN study reported having some form of official policy against child maltreatment, with most of these having actual laws on mandated reporting for child abuse and neglect.[35] Mandated reporting and laws help protect victims from what is otherwise managed informally within families.[9] Within the United States, although there is a federal law defining child abuse and neglect, mandated reporting laws still vary by state.[49]

Not unexpectedly, there is significant worldwide variability in the implementation of laws and policies, as far as the prosecution for maltreatment and the provision of child protection services for victims and their families is concerned.[35] The barriers to implementation of effective child protection practice include social norms. Perspectives on family, privacy, and support of physical punishment are a few of such named limitations.[35] However, the global variability is also due to limitations in governmental and community resources and the overall state of poverty in various regions.[35] Thus, the global variability in laws and policies regarding child maltreatment and their implementation is not exclusively reflective of a variation in cultural beliefs regarding child maltreatment, but of a greater problem relating to limitations in resources and systems to protect children.

UNIVERSAL PRINCIPLES IN CHILD MALTREATMENT
A Child Rights Approach

A culturally respectful approach does not necessitate universal tolerance of all cultural practices. Abney cautions that relativism* may predispose to the acceptance of a cultural practice without regard to its negative impact.[3] Acts accepted within certain cultures may still be deemed abusive if judged by a validated, accepted, cross-cultural universal standard.[15] Methodological challenges do exist in conducting culturally informed research, such as limitations inherent in defining cultural groups by race and ethnicity[3,5,50] and limitations in the application of research findings originating from Western countries.[31] However, extensive research documenting the negative health effects of adverse childhood experiences enforces the need to use evidence-based standards of child maltreatment that apply cross-culturally.[51]

When cultural practices are detrimental to a child, health care and service providers face the challenge of reconciling a culturally competent approach with the universal moral principles regarding child rights and protection. The Second United Nations Educational, Scientific, and Cultural Organization (UNESCO) World Report on Cultural Diversity states that the acknowledgment of cultural diversity and the establishment of child rights are not in opposition nor mutually exclusive. It posits, "human rights emanate from the very fabric of cultures, as recognized by the nations that have become signatories to human-rights instruments....Cultural diversity and intercultural dialogue are key levers for strengthening the consensus on the universal foundation of human rights."[2] That is, there exist universal, cross-cultural moral principles.[18]

The 1999 World Health Organization Consultation on Child Abuse drafted the following definition, based on the United Nation Convention on the Rights of the Child (UN CRC): "child abuse or maltreatment constitutes all forms of physical and/or emotional ill-treatment, sexual abuse, neglect or negligent treatment or commercial or other exploitation, resulting in actual or potential harm to the child's health, survival, development or dignity in the context of a relationship of responsibility, trust or power."[20] Article 24 within the UN CRC highlights that "parties shall take all effective and appropriate measures to abolish traditional practices prejudicial to the health of children."[6] This statement of intent forms a standard framework of universal child rights to protect children from harmful practices.

---

* The concept of relativism is discussed extensively in anthropological literature. It evolved as a response to historically ethnocentric practices. A relativist perspective "holds that judgment criteria are relative and vary with each individual and his or her environment," implying there are challenges and biases in the practice of one culture studying the practices of another.[15]

A STEPWISE APPROACH FOR THE PRIMARY CARE PROVIDER

Armed with this basic understanding of universal child rights and cultural diversity, how may a clinician serving a diverse population assess child well-being and determine child maltreatment? Structured approaches exist and involve evaluation of cultural, legal, and ethical considerations.

Establishing a Culturally Competent Practice

In the clinical setting, providers and organizations should address the basic elements of cultural competence as delineated in **Table 2**. The clinician should assess the degree of patient acculturation into their surroundings to determine which communication, education, and treatment strategies are most appropriate. For example, language barriers or limitations in understanding of cultural practices in a patient's new environment may need to be addressed. This process also facilitates determining how to approach communicating with the family; less acculturated families may initially benefit from education, provided by the health care practitioner, community agencies, or more experienced members of a family's cultural group, on the range of acceptable and legal parenting practices.[11] This approach includes how to speak with families in a culturally respectful manner (**Table 3**), and educating families on the harmful consequences and laws regarding certain practices.[52] In the case of parental nonadherence to medical care attributed to cultural beliefs, clinicians should acknowledge the role of those beliefs within that family's cultural identity.[6] A culturally competent provider and institution should seek the assistance of community agencies and cultural organizations that may facilitate these interactions with patients and families.

Characterizing Caregivers' Acts and Determining Harm to the Child

Because there is a range of parenting practices across the world, determining which parental acts of omission or commission are categorized as harmful requires a structured approach.[20] A culturally responsive approach exists in the assessment of maltreatment, whereby differences in child rearing between and within cultures are acknowledged.[6] However, this does not suggest universal tolerance of all practices. A clinician encountering an unfamiliar and potentially harmful parenting practice should consult the literature and/or an expert in the field, including the specialty of child maltreatment, so that a well-informed assessment may be made.[11]

Table 3
Culturally respectful approach to speaking with families about a harmful cultural practice

Components	Considerations
1. "Optimize the environment"	Privacy; need for interpreter
2. "Use appropriate and value neutral terminology"	Use of open-ended questions
3. "Ensure a professional and sympathetic response"	Maintaining respect for the patient
4. "Recognize that the law creates a barrier to open communication"	Awareness that the law may limit disclosure. Fostering a safe and comfortable environment for the family to communicate with the health care team

Adapted from Simpson J, Robinson K, Creighton SM, et al. Female genital mutilation: the role of health professionals in prevention, assessment, and management. BMJ 2012;344:37–41.

The clinician must assess the degree of harm to the child as a result of a caregiver act. In addition to noting caregiver acts of commission or omission, providers should approach understanding child maltreatment from a child-centric perspective. Are the basic needs of a child (adequate food, supervision, and protection; clothing; health care; education; a stable home; and the emotional needs for love and nurturance) being met? Dubowitz and Black,[38] in discussing medical neglect, identify 3 factors that health care providers should address when evaluating parenting practices,[38] the first of which is the assessment of actual or potential harm. Although most legal and clinical spheres require actual harm to have occurred to make a determination of maltreatment, potential harm may also be considered if there is a high likelihood of harm and/or if the potential nature of that harm is deemed severe. In the example of concern for medical neglect, clinicians should ascertain if preferable alternative treatments exist and, if so, whether these were integrated into the child's care. If effective or curative medical therapy is available and not sought out because of alternative cultural beliefs or practices, the concern arises that harm is being done.[38] A second element is the severity of the harm, including consideration of future sequelae. The third is the frequency of an act of commission or omission of maltreatment.[38] Thus, practitioners must consider the physical and emotional harm done to the child in addition to cultural aspects of parental intent.[6]

Raman and Hodes[6] classify caregiver acts into categories ranging from beneficial to harmful, and match them with an associated professional response (**Table 4**).[53] This simple framework acknowledges that understanding and respecting traditional practices must not prevent the identification of those that are harmful.[53] Although some of the examples they cite in their publication as harmful are still debated in cultural and legal spheres, this overall framework is helpful to the clinician who is categorizing the potential effects of parental acts.[6]

Understanding Applicable Laws and Moral Principles

It is important that applicable child protection policies and laws are considered. Laws and policies vary greatly, even regionally within countries such as the United States,

Table 4
Continuum of cultural practices in child rearing

Practice	Examples	Professional Response
Beneficial	Breastfeeding Infant massage Showing respect	Promote
Neutral	Toilet training at 1 y Gentle squeezing of nasal bridge for hiccups	Respect
Potentially harmful	Bed sharing (if other risk factors present, such as smoking, drug misuse, or overweight parents) Taping a coin over an umbilical hernia Prolonged application of garlic to the skin	Educate
Harmful	Chili in vagina Female genital mutilation Honor killings Forced marriage Extreme neglect	Prevent

Adapted from Raman S, Hodes D. Cultural issues in child maltreatment. J Paediatr Child Health 2011;48:30–7; with permission.

with regard to definitions of child abuse and to when a child maltreatment report must be made.[49] Determination of which laws are applicable is not always a straightforward process. However, in addition to local child maltreatment experts, publicly available legal guides online such as the US Department of Health and Human Services Administration for Children and Families Child Welfare Information Gateway (www.childwelfare.gov), may provide information on regional laws and practices.

Clinicians can be challenged by the tension between maintaining cultural respect while respecting applicable laws, exemplified in the discourse among United States health care providers surrounding female genital mutilation.[54,55] Nevertheless, adherence to relevant laws surrounding mandated reporting must be respected if child maltreatment is suspected.[49] Failure to report suspicion of maltreatment by a mandated reporter is a criminal offense in most United States jurisdictions punishable by prison and/or a fine. Conversely, mandated reporters in the United States are provided immunity from criminal and civil liability for reporting.[49]

Although the law may help a health care practitioner recognize child maltreatment in a given scenario, it does not provide a framework for how to respond in every case. Ultimately, when faced with these nuanced scenarios that can occur at the intersection of culture and child maltreatment, providers should rely on the universal guiding principles of child rights as designated in the UN CRC and their mandated reporting laws.

CULTURE AND PROTECTIVE FACTORS AGAINST CHILD MALTREATMENT

There are important aspects of culture that benefit the well-being of children and mitigate child maltreatment. Certain factors modulated by culture have also been shown to positively affect disclosure, victim treatment and outcomes, and child abuse prevention. Some of these include a strong cultural focus on the mother-child relationship, strong social sanctions against abuse, open discussions of sexuality, and formal and informal resources that protect children.[56] As providers establish appropriate cultural respect and understanding of cultural practices, they must recognize diverse positive and protective factors against maltreatment. Addressing and supporting such factors within the parent-child dyad, within their families, or within their cultural communities can help a provider establish rapport and enhance the aspects of a culture that benefit the health and wellness of children. For example, providers can

---

Box 2
Protective factors against child maltreatment

1. Nurturing and attachment (between the child and parent/caregiver)

2. Parenting skills and parental knowledge of child development

3. Parental resilience

4. Social connections (with community)

5. Concrete support for families (by their communities)

6. Social and emotional competence in children

Adapted from United States Department of Health and Human Services. Child Welfare Information Gateway. Making meaningful connections: 2014 prevention resource guide. Chapter 2: working with families using the protective factors. Washington, DC; 2014. p. 12–23. Available at: https://childwelfare.gov/preventing/preventionmonth/resource-guide/. Accessed April 1, 2014.

identify specific cultural practices that parents may use to nurture and form attachments with their children, such as infant massage, which is used in some cultures. Providing anticipatory guidance about child development to enhance parenting skills, and encouraging caregivers to use their informal systems of support that may be culturally specific are simple yet powerful strategies in the clinical setting.[38] A clinician attuned to specific cultural practices that are beneficial to a child may enhance these by positively motivating parents during their clinical encounters.[57] **Box 2** lists protective factors that may be identified within all cultural communities and can be emphasized in the health care setting to enhance child well-being.[58]

SUMMARY

With the privilege of being pediatric providers in a modern and multicultural society comes the responsibility to respect cross-cultural differences while maintaining a moral standard of safety and health for children.[53] There is growing evidence that in countries where there has been an increase in the recognition of and societal response to child maltreatment, there have been decreasing trends in prevalence.[31] This evidence is of fundamental importance to the discussion of culture and child maltreatment. While health care providers acknowledge, understand, and respect how culture affects all aspects of child maltreatment and child protection at the individual, caregiver, family/community, and societal levels, they must also hold at their core the integrity of the principles of universal rights for children. To this end, all countries must continue to strive to increase resources in child protection and welfare. In 2011, the United Nations Committee on the Rights of the Child added a formal comment to the CRC, emphasizing that a "child rights–based approach" must be underscored in child care and in child protection, focusing on the global health of the child, including their "psychological, social, moral and spiritual health, well-being and development."[59] In this spirit, health care providers must strive toward prevention, namely primary prevention, including efforts at addressing education and resources in addition to supporting the protective aspects of cultures, as the modality with which to mitigate child maltreatment and promote child wellness across all cultures.[31,56]

REFERENCES

1. Fadiman A. Preface. In: The spirit catches you and you fall down. New York: Farrar, Straus & Giroux; 1997. p. vii–ix.
2. United Nations Educational, Cultural and Scientific Organization. Investing in cultural diversity and intercultural dialogue. UNESCO World Report, 2nd edition: executive summary. 2009. Available at: http://www.unesco.org/new/en/culture/resources/report/the-unesco-world-report-on-cultural-diversity/. Accessed December 22, 2013.
3. Abney VD. Cultural competency in the field of child maltreatment. In: Myers JE, Berliner L, Briere J, et al, editors. The APSAC handbook on child maltreatment. Thousand Oaks (CA): Sage Publications; 2002. p. 477–86.
4. Cohen JA, Deblinger E, Mannarino AP, et al. The importance of culture in treating abused and neglected children: an empirical review. Child Maltreat 2001;6: 148–57.
5. Korbin JE. Culture and child maltreatment: cultural competence and beyond. Child Abuse Negl 2002;26:637–44.
6. Raman S, Hodes D. Cultural issues in child maltreatment. J Paediatr Child Health 2011;48(1):30–7.

7. National Association of Social Workers (NASW). NASW standards for cultural competence in social work practice. 2003. Available at: www.naswdc.org/practice/standards/NASWculturalstandards.pdf. Accessed November 13, 2013.
8. Office of Minority Health. What is cultural competency? U.S. Department of Health and Human Services; 2013. Available at: http://minorityhealth.hhs.gov/templates/browse.aspx?lvl=2&lvlID=11. Accessed March 17, 2014.
9. Fontes LA, Plummer C. Cultural issues in disclosures of child sexual abuse. J Child Sex Abus 2010;19:491–518.
10. Betancourt JR, Green AR, Carrillo JE. Cultural competence in health care: emerging frameworks and practical approaches: field report. The commonwealth fund; 2002. Accessed at: http://www.commonwealthfund.org/Publications/Fund-Reports/2002/Oct/Cultural-Competence-in-Health-Care-Emerging-Frameworks-and-Practical-Approaches.aspx. Accessed January 17, 2014.
11. Terao SY, Borrego J, Urquiza AJ. A reporting and response model for culture and child maltreatment. Child Maltreat 2001;6:158–68.
12. The Joint Commission. Advancing effective communication, cultural competence, and patient- and family-centered care: a roadmap for hospitals. Oakbrook Terrace (IL): The Joint Commission; 2010. Available at: http://www.jointcommission.org/assets/1/6/ARoadmapforHospitalsfinalversion727.pdf. Accessed March 24, 2014.
13. Office of Minority Health. National standards for culturally and linguistically appropriate services (CLAS) in health and health care. U.S. Department of Health and Human Services; 2010. Available at: https://www.thinkculturalhealth.hhs.gov/CLAS/clas_standard1.asp. Accessed March 17, 2014.
14. Commonwealth of Australia. Cultural competency in health: a guide for policy, partnerships and participation. Government of Australia National Health and Medical Research Council; 2005. Available at: http://www.nhmrc.gov.au/guidelines/publications/hp19-hp26. Accessed November 13, 2013.
15. Renteln AD. Relativism and the search for human rights. Am Anthropol 1988;90:56–72.
16. Polnay J, Polnay L, Lynch M, et al, editors. Child protection reader. Commonwealth of Australia: Royal College of Paediatrics and Child Health; 2007. p. 32–3. Available at: http://www.rcpch.ac.uk/child-health/standards-care/child-protection/publications/child-protection-publications. Accessed November 13, 2013.
17. Reisig JA, Miller MK. How the social construction of "child abuse" affects immigrant parents: policy changes that protect children and families. International Journal of Social Inquiry 2009;2:17–37.
18. Korbin JE. Chapter 2: culture and child maltreatment. In: Helfer ME, Kempe RS, Krugman RD, editors. The battered child. 5th edition. Chicago: University of Chicago Press; 1997. p. 29–48.
19. Finkelhor D, Korbin J. Child abuse as an international issue. Child Abuse Negl 1988;12:3–23.
20. Krug EG, Dahlberg LL, Mercy JA, et al, editors. World report on violence and health. Geneva (Switzerland): World Health Organization; 2002. p. 195. Available at: http://www.who.int/violence_injury_prevention/violence/world_report/en/. Accessed January 17, 2014.
21. Ferrari AM. The impact of culture upon child rearing practices and definitions of maltreatment. Child Abuse Negl 2002;26:793–813.
22. Drake B, Jolley JM, Lanier P, et al. Racial bias in child protection? A comparison of competing explanations using national data. Pediatrics 2011;127:471–8.

23. Webb E, Maddocks A, Bongilli J. Effectively protecting black and minority ethnic children from harm: overcoming barriers to the child protection process. Child Abuse Rev 2002;11:394–410.

24. Euser EM, van Ijzendoorn MH, Prinzie P, et al. Elevated child maltreatment rates in immigrant families and the role of socioeconomic differences. Child Maltreat 2010;16:63–73.

25. Coohey C. The relationship between familism and child maltreatment in Latino and Anglo Families. Child Maltreat 2001;6:130–42.

26. LeVine RA, Dixon S, LeVine S, et al. Part I: African infancy: frameworks for understanding. In: Child care and culture. Cambridge (MA): Cambridge University Press; 1994. p. 1–56.

27. Collier AF, McCluro FH, Collier J, et al. Culture-specific views of child maltreatment and parenting styles in a Pacific-Island community. Child Abuse Negl 1999;23:229–44.

28. Durrant JE. Physical punishment, culture, and rights: current issues for professionals. J Dev Behav Pediatr 2008;29:55–66.

29. Committee on Psychosocial Aspects of Child and Family Health. Guidance for effective discipline. Pediatrics 1998;101:723–8.

30. Runyan DK, Shankar V, Hassan F, et al. International variations in harsh child discipline. Pediatrics 2010;126:e701–11.

31. Runyan DK. Child maltreatment: a global perspective. In: Berman S, Palfrey JS, Butta Z, et al, editors. Global child health advocacy: on the front lines. 1st edition. American Academy of Pediatrics; 2013. p. 297–302.

32. MacKenzie MJ, Nicklas E, Waldfogel J, et al. Spanking and child development across the first decade of life. Pediatrics 2013;132:e1118–25.

33. Pinheiro PS, editor. Chapter 1. An end to violence against children. World report on violence against children. Geneva (Switzerland): United Nations Secretary General; 2006. p. 11. Available at: http://www.unicef.org/violencestudy/reports.html. Accessed January 17, 2014.

34. Runyan DK, Zolotor AJ. International issues in child maltreatment. In: Jenny C, editor. Child abuse & neglect: diagnosis, treatment and evidence. St Louis (MO): Elsevier; 2011. p. 620–7.

35. Dubowitz H. Executive summary. In: Dubowitz H, editor. World perspectives on child abuse. 10th edition. Aurora (IL): International Society for Prevention of Child Abuse and Neglect; 2013. p. 1–6.

36. Gracia E, Herrero J. Beliefs in the necessity of corporal punishment of children and public perceptions of child physical abuse as a social problem. Child Abuse Negl 2008;32:1058–62.

37. Maiter S, Alaggia R, Trocmé N. Perceptions of child maltreatment by parents from the Indian subcontinent: challenging myths about culturally based abusive parenting practices. Child Maltreat 2004;9:309–24.

38. Dubowitz H, Black MM. Child abuse: medical diagnosis management. 3rd edition. China: American Academy of Pediatrics; 2008. p. 428–63.

39. Knox BP, Starling SL. Abusive burns. In: Jenny C, editor. Child abuse & neglect: diagnosis, treatment and evidence. St Louis (MO): Elsevier; 2011. p. 222–38.

40. Asser SM, Swan R. Child fatalities from religion-motivated medical neglect. Pediatrics 1998;101:625–9.

41. Committee on Bioethics. Conflicts between religious or spiritual beliefs and pediatric care: informed refusal, exemptions, and public funding. Pediatrics 2013;132:962–5.

42. Committee on Bioethics. Religious objections to medical care. Pediatrics 1997; 99:279–81.
43. Legal Information Institute. Prince v. Massachusetts. Cornell University Law School; 1992. Available at: http://www.law.cornell.edu/supremecourt/text/321/ 158. Accessed May 12, 2014.
44. Haboush KL, Alyan H. "Who can you tell?" Features of Arab culture that influence conceptualization and treatment of childhood sexual abuse. J Child Sex Abus 2013;22:499–518.
45. DeBruyn L, Chino M, Serna P, et al. Child maltreatment in American Indian and Alaska native communities: integrating culture, history, and public health for intervention and prevention. Child Maltreat 2001;6:89–102.
46. Kanukollu SN, Mahalingam R. The idealized cultural identities model on help-seeking and child sexual abuse: a conceptual model for contextualizing perceptions and experiences of South Asian Americans. J Child Sex Abus 2011;20: 218–43.
47. Chou CY, Su YJ, Wu HM, et al. Child physical abuse and the related PTSD in Taiwan: the role of Chinese cultural background and victims' subjective reactions. Child Abuse Negl 2011;35:58–68.
48. Clear PJ, Vincent JP, Harris GE. Ethnic differences in symptom presentation of sexually abused girls. J Child Sex Abus 2006;15:79–98.
49. United States Department of Health and Human Services. Child welfare information gateway. Available at: https://www.childwelfare.gov/systemwide/laws_ policies/state/. Accessed January 17, 2014.
50. Putnam-Hornstein E, Needell B, King B, et al. Racial and ethnic disparities: a population-based examination of risk factors for involvement with child protective services. Child Abuse Negl 2013;37:33–46.
51. Felitti VJ, Anda RF, Nordenberg D, et al. Relationship of childhood abuse and household dysfunction to many of the leading causes of death in adults. The Adverse Childhood Experiences (ACE) Study. Am J Prev Med 1998;14: 245–58.
52. Simpson J, Robinson K, Creighton SM, et al. Female genital mutilation: the role of health professionals in prevention, assessment, and management. BMJ 2012; 344:37–41.
53. Koramoa J, Lynch MA, Kinnair D. A continuum of child-rearing: responding to traditional practices. Child Abuse Rev 2002;11:415–21.
54. Committee on Bioethics. Ritual genital cutting of female minors. Pediatrics 2010; 125:1088–93.
55. Palfrey J. AAP response to eLetters regarding the "policy statement – ritual genital cutting of female minors". American Academy of Pediatrics; 2010. Available at: http://pediatrics.aappublications.org/content/125/5/1088.abstract/ reply#pediatrics_el_50189. Accessed January 17, 2014.
56. Fontes LA. Chapter 1: multicultural orientation to child maltreatment work. In: Child abuse and culture. New York: The Guilford Press; 2005. p. 1–29.
57. Schwartz RP. Performing preventive services: a bright futures handbook. 2012. p. 175–7. Available at: http://www2.aap.org/oralhealth/docs/AppendixF_MI.pdf. Accessed February 13, 2014.
58. United States Department of Health and Human Services. Child Welfare Information Gateway. Making meaningful connections: 2014 prevention resource guide. Chapter 2: Working with families using the protective factors. Washington, DC; 2014. p. 12–23. Available at: https://childwelfare.gov/preventing/ preventionmonth/resource-guide/. Accessed April 1, 2014.

59. Bennett S, Hart S, Wernham M. The UN convention on the rights of the child general comment 13: towards enlightenment and progress for global child protection. In: Dubowitz H, editor. World perspectives on child abuse. 10th edition. Aurora (IL): International Society for Prevention of Child Abuse and Neglect; 2013. p. 124–7.

Has This Child Been Abused?

Exploring Uncertainty in the Diagnosis of Maltreatment

Rebecca L. Moles, MD*, Andrea G. Asnes, MD, MSW

KEYWORDS

- Child abuse • Physical abuse • Sexual abuse • Uncertainty • Bias
- Child protective services

KEY POINTS

- In cases of suspected child abuse, a clear understanding of the sources for potential uncertainty and a stepwise approach to managing uncertainty are of vital importance.
- Uncertainty in an evaluation for suspected physical abuse may stem from a question of whether a child's presentation is secondary to injury or the result of a medical problem, about whether the cause of an injury is accidental or abusive, and about the timing of the injury.
- An evaluation for suspected sexual abuse can be confounded by uncertainties about the veracity and meaning of a child's disclosure of abuse and the significance of any examination findings.
- In the setting of uncertainty, a consideration of family risk factors and potential strengths may aid the clinician in making a final determination and recommendations for the child's safety.

INTRODUCTION

The practice of medicine has often been described as an art. Using the term "art" implies that medicine is somehow fluid, moldable, and influenced by the artist's skill level, experiences, emotions, and tools. Medical schools teach raw skills, such as history taking and note writing, in addition to the pathophysiology of disease processes. The art in medical practice lies in the application of these skills and knowledge to a particular patient. Medicine may be viewed as art within which both the physician

Disclosures: None.
Department of Pediatrics, Yale School of Medicine, PO Box 208064, New Haven, CT 06510, USA
* Corresponding author.
E-mail address: Rebecca.Moles@yale.edu

Pediatr Clin N Am 61 (2014) 1023–1036
http://dx.doi.org/10.1016/j.pcl.2014.06.009
0031-3955/14/$ – see front matter © 2014 Elsevier Inc. All rights reserved.

pediatric.theclinics.com

and the patient are the artists, working together toward the masterpiece of diagnosis and treatment. In very young or very old patients, the caretakers often become the artists on behalf of the patients.

A necessary and fundamental component of the practice of the art of medicine is uncertainty.[1] Uncertainty is what drives research and new discoveries. If there were no uncertainty in diagnosis and treatment, there would be no need for a second opinion, and no need for clinical trials, case-control studies, or meta-analyses of data. Uncertainty, at its most basic level, is beneficial in medicine. At the level of an individual case, however, uncertainty is challenging, frustrating, and frightening, at times for both the patient and the physician. To admit uncertainty in a diagnosis or treatment plan may lead to a concern for malpractice by the treating physician.[2]

Child abuse cases have unique complexities. A diagnosis of child abuse affects those with whom a child lives, may result in a parent's incarceration, or may force a day-care provider to close her business. Incorrectly diagnosing child abuse as an accident may cause a child to be returned to an unsafe home and suffer additional injuries or death. Studies demonstrating lack of agreement on case etiology among child abuse pediatricians (CAPs) highlight the regular role uncertainty plays for a clinician faced with potential child abuse.[3,4] Primary care medical providers may feel particularly uncertain about all aspects of a child abuse case, from when and if to report to child protective services (CPS), to what to say to parents about reporting, to what medical testing to order, to how to follow a child in the primary care office once CPS has become involved.

The purposes of this article are to define and discuss uncertainty in the case of physical and sexual abuse, and to suggest an approach to cases to assist with managing uncertainty while still providing valuable information to the medical and CPS systems to promote the health and safety of children.

DEFINING UNCERTAINTY

Medical providers frequently must make important decisions in the care of a patient in uncertain situations. There are countless patient care situations in which uncertainty plays a potent role. Beresford[5] suggested that uncertainty falls into 3 main categories: (1) technical uncertainty, whereby inadequate scientific knowledge exists to predict disease processes or outcomes; (2) personal uncertainty, such as when the medical provider is unaware of the patient's wishes or when personal connection to the patient may affect judgment; and (3) conceptual uncertainty, which occurs when a provider must choose between 2 or more options that are incomparable, such as determining which of 2 complex and seriously ill patients receives an urgent imaging appointment or when trying to predict outcomes of the same procedure in 2 vastly different patients. This article discusses each of these in the context of an evaluation of a child suspected of being a victim of physical abuse.

Technical Uncertainty

In cases of suspected child abuse, technical uncertainty plays a role in both the expertise of the individual medical provider and the body of knowledge that makes up the evidence base supporting or refuting a diagnosis of abuse. In cases of suspected physical abuse, a common question facing the clinician is whether the injury the child has sustained is adequately explained by the history provided by the caregiver. Primary care clinicians may be uncertain about how to answer this question because of a lack of training about and experience with injury mechanics in children of varying developmental abilities. CAPs may be faced with a lack of definitive, evidenced-based data toward which to turn. Both primary care providers and CAPs are likely to be challenged by incomplete information from caregivers about the circumstances of a child's injury. In addition, primary care clinicians, who may be inexperienced in working with CPS, may be both uncertain about whether a child's presentation meets the threshold for a CPS report and unused to providing information to CPS investigators. These uncertainties may cause primary care physicians to overreport or underreport concerns, and to inadvertently undermine the work of CPS.[6]

Personal Uncertainty

Personal uncertainty, as defined as being unaware of the patient's wishes or how personal involvement or connection to the patient may affect clinical decisions, is a nearly universal component of child abuse work. In cases of suspected child abuse, the parent or other caregiver of a child is, by definition, under suspicion for being the perpetrator of the abuse. The primary care provider may find that abuse does not enter the differential diagnosis of an explanation for an injury, owing to the provider's previously established trust in the family. Similarly, the child abuse pediatrician or similar provider must guard against the possibility of the family or parents' wishes interfering with objective assessment of the data. The facts pointing to abuse as the diagnosis can be blurred by the clinician's emotional desire to please the family by pursuing some other cause for the presenting illness or injuries.

The role of personal connection is stronger and, potentially, more hazardous for the primary care physician. The provider may find it difficult or impossible to consider that a parent the provider trusts and with whom the provider has an established relationship may have harmed the child.

Conceptual Uncertainty

The last type of uncertainty in Beresford's model is conceptual uncertainty, whereby the challenge lies in applying abstract information to a concrete scenario. One of the many skills taught in medical school is how to critically review the medical literature, asking questions such as "how can I apply this information to my particular patient?"[7] Each case of child abuse is unique, and the art of medicine lies in applying a vast amount of experiential and literature-based knowledge to a particular patient. There is likely no case report in which the patient is identical to the one the clinician is evaluating. The provider must synthesize elements of experience, descriptive studies, clinical trials, and meta-analyses into the care of a particular patient, and specifically incorporate such data into a determination of whether the child was or was not abused. The determination of child abuse often relies on the opinions of other medical specialists in addition to investigative data from CPS and law enforcement. Each of these specialists has his or her set of technical, personal, and conceptual uncertainties. The degree of uncertainty in an individual case evaluation is the sum of that found in the clinician plus the uncertainties in each of the subspecialists and investigators who render opinions used by the clinician. The additive nature of uncertainty results in multiple opportunities for a correct diagnosis to be missed or clouded.

In the primary care setting, 2 possible sources of conceptual uncertainty may be present. First, the experiential base of the provider, that is, the number of child abuse evaluations managed by the specific provider, may be quite low. Second, familiarity with and depth of understanding of the literature are likely much lower than that of the child abuse expert with subspecialty training. The primary care provider may be more swayed by outlier cases in his or her past; for example, the child removed from a family for bruising found to have a bleeding disorder, or the subtle finding in an infant who was not followed up which became significant once the child died of abuse. In addition, primary care providers may be faced with children in their practice for whom a report to CPS has been made, but not substantiated. Limited but memorable past experience with potential abuse may leave the provider uncertain about what to watch for, when to be alarmed, and when and if another report to CPS is warranted.

Uncertainty Beyond the Medical Diagnosis

An additional complication in child abuse work is the level of certainty in the diagnosis required by each member of the multidisciplinary team responsible for the care and safety of the child. CPS must first determine the likelihood that abuse has occurred. Once this decision is made, CPS must derive and institute a safety plan for the abused child. Certainty about the timing of an injury can assist CPS is determining a perpetrator and in forming comprehensive safety plans. Strictly speaking, CPS need not be certain that the child was abused. If, however, CPS determines that a care plan that involves temporary or permanent placement of a child outside of the home is indicated, CPS must demonstrate that a "preponderance of the evidence" exists to show that abuse of the child is more likely than not likely.

Law enforcement and prosecution rely on the burden of proof of "beyond a reasonable doubt" and "within a reasonable degree of medical certainty." To convict a caregiver of causing an abusive injury, the medical and investigative proof that the child was abused and that the person being charged is the perpetrator must be beyond a reasonable doubt. Child abuse cases often do rise to the certainty level at which CPS can intervene to protect a child, but a caregiver may not be criminally charged or face trial.

The classifications or subsets of uncertainty outlined can provide scaffolding around which to conceptualize uncertainty in child abuse cases. Understanding where uncertainty is likely to appear, added to the clinician's personal recognition of the areas of uncertainty likely to be present during an evaluation, may assist the clinician in minimizing both doubt and the emotional burden that uncertainty brings to a case.

Reporting to Child Protective Services

The primary care provider faced with a child who may have been maltreated has one key question to answer: does the presentation warrant a report to CPS? Local statutes for mandated reporting share common language that should simplify decision making in this setting. Legally, mandated reporters must contact CPS immediately when they suspect that a child has been maltreated. Certainty is not required, and a delay may result in further injury or even death of a child. Despite the clarity of the law in this setting, however, providers have been shown to fail to report in the context of clear concern.[6]

APPROACH TO UNCERTAINTY IN PHYSICAL ABUSE CASES

A framework within which to consider uncertainty in physical abuse can be useful in the setting of decision making, and is provided in **Fig. 1**. Although each case is unique, this figure proposes a standardized thought process that may aid the clinician faced with a child suspected of being a victim of physical abuse. The depth of the case review may differ between a primary care provider and a child abuse consultant, but the process is similar.

Timing of Injury

Providers can diagnose an injury as having been caused by abuse, but the timing of the abuse is uncertain. In this setting, the question faced by medical providers "was

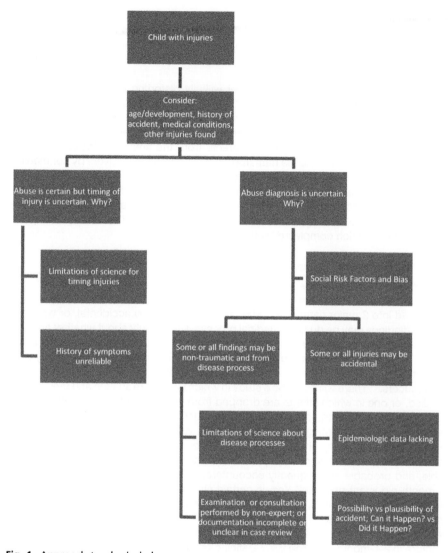

Fig. 1. Approach to physical abuse cases.

this child abused?" has been answered affirmatively. The natural secondary question to address is, then, "when was the child abused?", which is the frequently the same as asking, "by whom was the child abused?" In some cases, a child's injuries can be determined to have certainly been caused by abuse, but determining when the injuries were inflicted, and by whom, often cannot be determined based on medical science. Why is timing so difficult to determine? One reason is that medical science is not as specific as investigators wish it to be. Bleeding on a computed tomography scan of the brain can be classified as "acute," a term that covers hours to a few days. The child may have been in the care of several caregivers over the "acute" time period.[8-10] In child abuse cases, the child often cannot provide a history because the child is nonverbal or minimally verbal, or too ill or scared to provide the details. Clinicians are reliant on the caregivers of the child to provide the history of symptoms that inform the determination of timing of the injury. The caregivers providing the history are often the same caregivers who are under suspicion for inflicting the injury. Details that may be important in determining the timing of the injury may be omitted by the caregiver in an effort to deflect blame.

Even when a child's caregivers are not willfully distorting the history, accurately timing an injury may be very challenging. Some children are raised in such chaotic environments that obtaining a history of onset and progression of medical symptoms may be impossible even with truthful caregivers. In some cases, law enforcement or CPS workers may have removed the parents from the hospital. Medical providers are often then reliant on histories gathered from the parents/caregivers by nonmedical investigative staff without the benefit of a direct history. Additional complexity is added when a CAP or other clinician is reviewing the records of a child seen at another institution for the purpose of giving a second opinion for a medical or legal reason. The reviewing physician is then limited to the information provided and to the adequacy of the documentation completed by the treating physicians.

Uncertain Diagnosis of Abuse

Uncertainty arising from the possibility of accidental injury

When the diagnosis of abuse is itself uncertain, the reasons for uncertainty can be separated into 2 major categories: when the injuries may be accidental, or when the injuries/findings may be due to a medical process. Uncertainty about whether an injury is accidental is more likely when the suspected victim is ambulatory or there is a history of a fall or other trauma provided by the parent. The medical literature may offer validation for unusual histories, such as a femur fracture sustained by infants using Exersaucers.[11] There will never be a study in which infants are shaken and their injuries studied, or one in which infants are dropped from the height of an adult and their injuries quantified and categorized. Clinicians must rely on a combination of professional experience, existing epidemiologic data, and details of the specific case at hand when determining whether an offered history is possible to explain the mechanism, severity, and timing of the injury. In child abuse work the terms possible, plausible, and probable are frequently encountered. Is an accidental femur fracture in a 4-month-old infant possible? Yes, in certain circumstances, such as in a fall with an adult, or in a baby device, or during a car accident. Is an accidental femur fracture in a 4-month-old plausible? Perhaps, if the history of the accident is clear and the injury mechanism described is of sufficient force to cause a fracture. Is an accidental femur fracture in a 4-month-old probable? Defining probable as "most likely," the answer is no, when considering all femur fractures in 4-month-olds.[12–14]

Uncertainty arising from the possibility of a medical condition

The cause of an injury or finding also may be uncertain when some or all of the findings may be due to, or are complicated by, a medical condition. An example of this scenario is a child with bruising. Bruising may be from normal childhood play or may signify a bleeding disorder in a child. Bruising may also be the first, and perhaps only, sign of physical abuse. Delaying an abuse evaluation or failure to ensure the safety of a child while the child awaits an evaluation by a hematologist may return the child to an unsafe situation and may allow additional injury, or death, to occur from abuse.[15] The concepts of possible, plausible, and probable apply in cases where a medical diagnosis is suggested as an alternative diagnosis to abuse. It is possible that an infant with a bruise on the ear has a previously unrecognized bleeding disorder, but it is neither probable nor plausible. Even when a comorbid medical diagnosis is present, such as in a premature infant with multiple bruises, the presence of the co-morbid condition does not preclude a diagnosis of abuse. Parents, lawyers, or clinicians may identify alternative but unlikely medical explanations for injuries attributable to abuse, such as a metabolic disease leading to multiple fractures. Although medical causes should certainly actively be pursued and managed, a search for an esoteric, extraordinarily rare disease cannot and should not interfere with the timely diagnosis of abuse, with protection of the child when such a diagnosis is warranted.

APPROACH TO UNCERTAINTY IN SEXUAL ABUSE CASES

Key differences between physical and sexual abuse cases require a separate approach (**Fig. 2**). Concerns of sexual abuse generally arise when a child makes statements about abuse or sexual acts, has concerning behaviors, or has physical examination or laboratory findings concerning for abuse. Although children's disclosures of sexual abuse can be clear and specific, often they are subtle or even incomplete. Uncertainty in this setting is often compounded by the fact that physical findings to

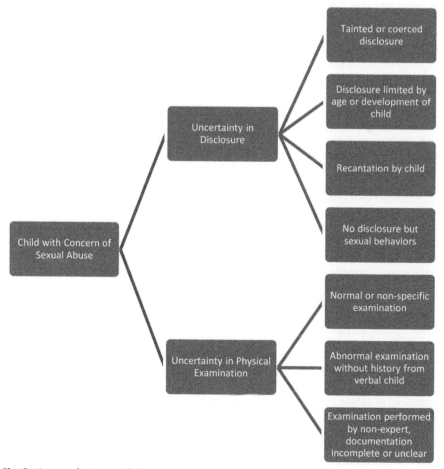

Fig. 2. Approach to sexual abuse cases.

support a disclosure in sexually abused children are rare.[16] An incomplete or subtle disclosure can occur when a child makes a statement about abuse to an adult or to another child but then does not repeat the disclosure during the course of a forensic evaluation. Very young children may make one statement to an adult, then change aspects of that statement during the forensic interview, or make vague statements that are developmentally appropriate but that introduce uncertainty into the evaluation. Particular concern for a coerced disclosure can arise when children in disputed custody arrangements allege abuse.

The Children's Advocacy Center (CAC)[17] movement, with its focus on skilled, child-friendly interviews, may assist in determining true sexual abuse from innocent touching or coaching by a parent. CAC-style interviews are not available in all geographic areas, however, and even if such services are available, well-meaning daycare, school, family, or investigative personnel may inappropriately question a child before a CAC interview is scheduled. Regardless of the interview setting, some children may be too young, frightened, or developmentally unable to provide the details and context to determine if abuse has occurred.

Concern that a child may be a victim of sexual abuse also may arise from the actions of the child rather than by voiced reports from a child. There is a wide variation of sexual behaviors that are considered "normal," and these behaviors vary by age and developmental stage of the child.[18] Increased sexual content of social media leading to high visibility of sexual images and references for children may influence the nature of "normal" play behaviors and shift them to more sexualized behaviors. A certain diagnosis of sexual abuse is often not possible if based solely on the presence of sexualized behaviors in a child.

Examination

The examination of the genitalia itself may be the cause of uncertainty. Many, if not most, general pediatric providers have not received specific training in the full spectrum of normal anatomic variations, particularly with respect to the female genital examination and anal examination for both sexes.[19] When providers of varying experience in recognizing normal findings examine the same child, significant disagreement and resultant uncertainty can ensue.[19,20]

Even for CAPs well versed in the spectrum of normal physical findings, sources of uncertainty persist. For example, examination findings previously reported in the medical literature as diagnostic for penetrating injury are now considered normal or nonspecific.[21–27] Another challenge arises when a verbal child displays examination findings considered diagnostic for penetrating genital trauma but persistently denies abuse.

THE IMPACT OF UNCERTAINTY ON SAFETY
Safety Determination

Primary care and pediatric providers, when faced with a suspicion of abuse, must report to CPS. This action can be challenging when the provider is not absolutely sure that abuse has taken place, but reporting statutes are designed to cause providers to involve CPS when a reasonable suspicion of abuse is present. From the standpoint of safety, in the setting of a reasonable suspicion making a report is always optimal. Failing to report when a concern is present not only may compromise the safety of a child, but also may result in adverse consequences, such as a fine or even criminal prosecution, for the provider who does not act to protect a child at risk.

For CAPs who have expertise in evaluating cases of suspected abuse, certainty in assessment is always the goal. At the close of a medical assessment, uncertainty about the diagnosis of abuse in a particular child will sometimes persist. Whereas medical uncertainty may be fully acceptable in some realms, such as when a child presents with a febrile illness and a rash that cannot be identified but fully resolves, this is not the case with suspected abuse. With injuries that may be due to abuse or the possibility of sexual abuse, the possibility of simply accepting uncertainty does not exist, not just because of the possibility that an incorrect diagnosis may lead to additional harm or death to a child, but because the conclusions in child abuse pediatrics drive CPS and law enforcement decision making.

Even when the diagnosis of abuse is uncertain, medical providers can and do play an important role as partners with CPS and law enforcement. Although the medical evaluation may be complete, CPS must still decide what comes next for the child. CPS officials can benefit from a deeper understanding of why the medical case is uncertain and what medical and social follow-up the medical provider suggests. If provided with a simplified opinion that abuse is just as likely as nonabuse, without a dialogue about the nuances of the particular case, CPS involvement may range from closing the investigation, putting limited services in place, or even taking custody of a child. Input from the clinician is invaluable for the CPS workers charged with making safety determinations.

Although the conclusion of uncertainty is never the goal of the medical provider, it may be seen as preferable to an incorrect conclusion. The implications of an incorrect diagnosis when abuse is suspected are many and potentially devastating, and have the potential to affect children, families, and communities as well as to negatively affect the clinician's professional and personal status. When abuse is mistaken for an accidental or medical diagnosis, a child may be hurt or sexually assaulted again, or killed. When abuse is wrongly diagnosed and an alternative explanation for a child's presentation exists, the child may be removed from his or her family, with profoundly negative implications for the child and the caregivers. Mistakes may engender both community distrust of CPS and increased risk-adverse behaviors by CPS that can lead to overly punitive and restrictive disposition planning for children and families. Being wrong can lead to allegations of medical malpractice in addition to deep and abiding feelings of guilt and self-doubt. An approach to management of uncertainty in these challenging cases is outlined in **Table 1**.

The stakes are undoubtedly high in the setting of decision making in abuse determinations. While clinicians remain uncertain, health care providers must be willing to partner with CPS by offering additional information, such as about identifying and managing risk, which will help CPS to arrange dispositions for children.

Table 1
Risk factors for physical abuse in social realms

Child	Parent	Family	Community
Unwanted	Mother <19 y at child's birth	Family violence	Poverty
Disabled (including behavioral, learning, emotional disability)	Substance abuse	Family isolation	Unemployment
Multiple	Mental illness	Single parent	Community violence
Preterm	Developmental delay Abuse in childhood	Many children <5 y Household flux	Residential flux

Data from Refs.[36–41]

Safety Planning in Physical Abuse

In cases of possible physical abuse, the starting point is usually an injury. An example of this scenario occurs when a possible, plausible explanation for an injury exists, but the injury is severe and the mechanism of injury was unwitnessed. Consider a 2-month-old infant with a buckle femur fracture such as could occur in the setting of a direct impact onto a bended knee. A sole caregiver reports having dropped the infant with a fall onto the leg. The mechanism is possible, but the event was unwitnessed and the 2-month-old infant did not sustain the fracture under her own power. A complete workup for occult injury is unrevealing, and therefore reassuring, but not sufficient to fully dispel a concern for abuse. A crucial step is a careful scene investigation with a request for the caregiver to reenact the injury mechanism. Sometimes, such as when the details of the scene are grossly different to what was reported to the evaluating medical provider, such a request is sufficient to result in doubt in the veracity of the caregiver's offered history. If the scene evaluation and reenactment are reassuring, a careful review of evidence-based risk factors may be helpful. It may be useful to consider these risk factors as they pertain to the child herself, the caregiver, the family, and the community in which the family resides (**Table 2**).

The presence of risk factors does not and should not result in a conclusion of abuse. Rather, their presence should inform decision making and planning in the setting of uncertainty. In the case of the 2-month-old infant, a history of significant family violence in the past should result in amplification of the services offered to the family and careful surveillance. On the other hand, careful attention must be paid to avoiding bias in decision making. Living in a socially disadvantaged neighborhood should not confer guilt on caregivers. Some risk factors, such as substance abuse and domestic violence, have emerged in recent study to be more potent predictors of abuse risk for children, and are therefore better drivers of CPS safety planning (Duffy JY, Hughes M, Asnes AG, et al. Child maltreatment and risk patterns among participants in a child abuse prevention program. Submitted for publication).

When additional risk factors are identified in the setting of a possible diagnosis of physical abuse, several steps should be undertaken.

1. Provision of services to address risk factors is fundamental. These services may include drug/alcohol testing and treatment, mental health assessment and treatment, or interventions to address family violence.
2. Prolonged family assessment may be helpful. CPS may extend its investigation over time to monitor a family. Such longitudinal assessment can lead to valuable information about a family's strengths and additional vulnerabilities, assess the effectiveness of interventions, and adapt the interventions to fit the developing needs of the child. A prolonged case with a family also can allow the child or children to "age out" of infancy and toddlerhood, ages at which children may be the most vulnerable to abuse.[28]
3. Primary care providers also can be instrumental in offering ongoing surveillance to families for whom a concern for physical abuse has been raised. Infants are frequently evaluated in the primary care setting with multiple opportunities to monitor for additional signs of injury (such as bruising or oral injury) that would confirm abuse. When an infant has been evaluated for a possible abusive injury, but no clear diagnosis has been made and some degree of concern remains, the primary care provider's knowledge about the concern can be invaluable. CAPs and CPS workers should make and maintain contact with primary care providers in the setting of an injury that has raised concern.

Table 2
Types of uncertainty and suggestions for management

Type of Abuse	Type of Uncertainty	Sources of Uncertainty	Management of Uncertainty

Physical	Technical	Unclear diagnosis of abuse
		  Possible accident
		  Possible medical condition
		  Uncertain timing of injury
			Use local CAP or experienced clinician
			Scene investigation information (with CPS and/or law enforcement)

	Personal	Caregiver characteristics that influence level of concern (eg, parents sought care appropriately, intact family, educated parents)	Be aware of potential biases in suspicion and reporting Allow objective findings (such as fracture in a nonambulatory child) to guide action, not family appearance
	Conceptual	Clinician's inexperience with possible abuse Differing opinions of subspecialty clinicians on likelihood of abuse	AAP guidelines on evaluation of physically abused child Use local CAP or experienced clinician Case conference with multiple subspecialists to address differences

Sexual	Technical	Unclear diagnosis of abuse
		  Subtle, incomplete, or coerced verbal disclosure of abuse
		  Inconclusive physical examination
			Use CAP or experienced clinician
			Local CAC
			myCasereview[a] or other case review platforms

	Personal	Discomfort with normal examination in the setting of significant disclosure of abuse	Report suspected abuse to proper local CPS and/or law enforcement Recall that a normal examination does not rule out abuse
	Conceptual	Clinician's inexperience with possible abuse	AAP guidelines on evaluation of suspected sexual abuse Use CAP or experienced clinician Local CAC myCasereview[a] or other case review platforms

Abbreviations: AAP, American Academy of Pediatrics; CAC, Children's Advocacy Center; CAP, child abuse pediatrician; CPS, child protective services.
[a] Midwest Regional Children's Advocacy Center's myCasereview.[35]
Data from Refs.[17,32–35]

Safety Planning in Sexual Abuse

CPS is unlikely to be able to adequately assure the safety of a child in whom a concern of sexual abuse has been raised but a clear diagnosis is unobtainable. This scenario is one of the more challenging that primary care providers confront. When worries for a child's immediate safety persist after a forensic evaluation that has not resulted in a CPS intervention, such as removal of a child from the home or removal of the alleged perpetrator from the child's environment, clinicians must provide ongoing surveillance. An approach similar to the list of risk factors for physical abuse also applies to sexual abuse. Mental health, domestic violence, and substance abuse issues in the family should be addressed. Parents with a history of sexual abuse themselves require mental health support. A prolonged family assessment with ongoing involvement from a skilled social worker will offer ongoing monitoring and ensure that recommendations are followed through. Education of the family about behaviors seen in sexually abused children (such as earlier engagement in sexual activity), and about steps to limit exposure of children to sexualized media content, are vital.[29] Of perhaps utmost importance is ensuring that the children and family follow through with evidence-based treatments for sexual abuse. Even when the diagnosis is uncertain but concern for sexual abuse remains, evidence-based treatments, such as trauma-focused cognitive-behavioral therapy and the child and family traumatic stress intervention, can reduce the development of posttraumatic symptoms and, as a result, other negative consequences that can follow sexual abuse.[30,31] As with physical abuse, the primary care provider's role is key in the maintenance of the child's safety and identification of additional concerns. Primary care providers should be vigilant about passive and active risky behaviors, such as early sexual debut and self-injurious behaviors. Armed with the knowledge of a previous, yet perhaps unsubstantiated concern of sexual abuse, the primary care provider is better equipped to assess common pediatric problems such as bedwetting, vaginal discharge or itching, or gender identity concerns.

SUMMARY

Uncertainty is an inevitable factor in medical practice. Uncertainty in the diagnosis and management of suspected child abuse is, and will be, a potent source of challenge to providers who care for children. Recognition of the likely sources of uncertainty coupled with the approaches offered will give providers tools to minimize the negative outcomes that can stem from uncertainty in this setting.

REFERENCES

1. Ghosh AK. Understanding medical uncertainty: a primer for physicians. J Assoc Physicians India 2004;52:739–42.
2. Ghosh AK. Dealing with medical uncertainty: a physician's perspective. Minn Med 2004;87(10):48–51.
3. Laskey AL, Sheridan MJ, Hymel KP. Physicians' initial forensic impressions of hypothetical cases of pediatric traumatic brain injury. Child Abuse Negl 2007;31(4): 329–42.
4. Lindberg DM, Lindsell CJ, Shapiro RA. Variability in expert assessments of child physical abuse likelihood. Pediatrics 2008;121(4):e945–53.
5. Beresford EB. Uncertainty and the shaping of medical decisions. Hastings Cent Rep 1991;21(4):6–11.
6. Flaherty EG, Sege RD, Griffith J, et al. From suspicion of physical child abuse to reporting: primary care clinician decision-making. Pediatrics 2008;122(3):611–9.
7. Guyatt GH, Rennie D. Users' guides to the medical literature. JAMA 1993; 270(17):2096–7.
8. Biron DL, Shelton D. Functional time limit and onset of symptoms in infant abusive head trauma. J Paediatr Child Health 2007;43(1–2):60–5.
9. Adamsbaum C, Grabar S, Mejean N, et al. Abusive head trauma: judicial admissions highlight violent and repetitive shaking. Pediatrics 2010;126(3):546–55.
10. Starling SP, Patel S, Burke BL, et al. Analysis of perpetrator admissions to inflicted traumatic brain injury in children. Arch Pediatr Adolesc Med 2004;158(5):454–8.
11. Grant P, Mata MB, Tidwell M. Femur fracture in infants: a possible accidental etiology. Pediatrics 2001;108(4):1009–11.

12. Flaherty EG, Perez-Rossello JM, Levine MA, et al. Evaluating children with frac tures for child physical abuse. Pediatrics 2014;133(2):e477–89.

13. Leventhal JM, Thomas SA, Rosenfield NS, et al. Fractures in young children. Distinguishing child abuse from unintentional injuries. Am J Dis Child 1993;147(1): 87–92.

14. Thomas SA, Rosenfield NS, Leventhal JM, et al. Long-bone fractures in young children: distinguishing accidental injuries from child abuse. Pediatrics 1991; 88(3):471–6.

15. Sheets LK, Leach ME, Koszewski IJ, et al. Sentinel injuries in infants evaluated for child physical abuse. Pediatrics 2013;131(4):701–7.

16. Adams JA, Harper K, Knudson S, et al. Examination findings in legally confirmed child sexual abuse: it's normal to be normal. Pediatrics 1994;94(3):310–7.

17. National Children's Alliance. Available at: http://www.nationalchildrensalliance.org/. Accessed July 16, 2014.

18. Friedrich WN, Fisher JL, Dittner CA, et al. Child sexual behavior inventory: normative, psychiatric, and sexual abuse comparisons. Child Maltreat 2001;6(1):37–49.

19. Ladson S, Johnson CF, Doty RE. Do physicians recognize sexual abuse? Am J Dis Child 1987;141(4):411–5.

20. Adams JA, Wells R. Normal versus abnormal genital findings in children: how well do examiners agree? Child Abuse Negl 1993;17(5):663–75.

21. McCann J. Use of the colposcope in childhood sexual abuse examinations. Pediatr Clin North Am 1990;37(4):863–80.

22. McCann J, Voris J. Perianal injuries resulting from sexual abuse: a longitudinal study. Pediatrics 1993;91(2):390–7.

23. McCann J, Voris J, Simon M. Labial adhesions and posterior fourchette injuries in childhood sexual abuse. Am J Dis Child 1988;142(6):659–63.

24. McCann J, Voris J, Simon M. Genital injuries resulting from sexual abuse: a longitudinal study. Pediatrics 1992;89(2):307–17.

25. Adams JA. Evolution of a classification scale: medical evaluation of suspected child sexual abuse. Child Maltreat 2001;6(1):31–6.

26. Adams JA, Knudson S. Genital findings in adolescent girls referred for suspected sexual abuse. Arch Pediatr Adolesc Med 1996;150(8):850–7.

27. Adams JA. Medical evaluation of suspected child sexual abuse: 2011 update. J Child Sex Abus 2011;20(5):588–605.

28. U.S. Department of Health and Human Services Administration for Children and Families, Children's Bureau. Child maltreatment 2012. 2013. Available at: http://www.acf.hhs.gov/programs/cb/research-data-technology/statistics-research/child-maltreatment.

29. Putnam FW. Ten-year research update review: child sexual abuse. J Am Acad Child Adolesc Psychiatry 2003;42(3):269–78.

30. Berkowitz SJ, Stover CS, Marans SR. The child and family traumatic stress intervention: secondary prevention for youth at risk of developing PTSD. J Child Psychol Psychiatry 2011;52(6):676–85.

31. Mannarino AP, Cohen JA, Deblinger E, et al. Trauma-focused cognitive-behavioral therapy for children: sustained impact of treatment 6 and 12 months later. Child Maltreat 2012;17(3):231–41.

32. Kellogg ND. Evaluation of suspected child physical abuse. Pediatrics 2007; 119(6):1232–41.

33. Jenny C, Crawford-Jakubiak JE, Committee on Child Abuse and Neglect, American Academy of Pediatrics. The evaluation of children in the primary care setting when sexual abuse is suspected. Pediatrics 2013;132(2):e558–67.

34. Fortin K, Jenny C. Sexual abuse. Pediatr Rev 2012;33(1):19–32.
35. Midwest Regional Children's Advocacy Center's myCasereview (formally THICM). Available at: www.mrcac.org/medical-academy/. Accessed July 16, 2014.
36. Appleyard K, Berlin LJ. Supporting healthy relationships between young children and their parents: lessons from attachment theory and research. Durham (NC): Center for Child and Family Policy, Duke University; 2007.
37. Coulton CJ, Crampton DS, Irwin M, et al. How neighborhoods influence child maltreatment: a review of the literature and alternative pathways. Child Abuse Negl 2007;31(11–12):1117–42.
38. Ertem IO, Leventhal JM, Dobbs S. Intergenerational continuity of child physical abuse: how good is the evidence? Lancet 2000;356(9232):814–9.
39. Govindshenoy M, Spencer N. Abuse of the disabled child: a systematic review of population-based studies. Child Care Health Dev 2007;33(5).552–8.
40. Rumm PD, Cummings P, Krauss MR, et al. Identified spouse abuse as a risk factor for child abuse. Child Abuse Negl 2000;24(11):1375–81.
41. Stier DM, Leventhal JM, Berg AT, et al. Are children born to young mothers at increased risk of maltreatment? Pediatrics 1993;91(3):642–8.

Working with Child Protective Services and Law Enforcement: What to Expect

Nancy D. Kellogg, MD

KEYWORDS

- Child protective services • Law enforcement • Reporting child abuse • HIPAA
- Testifying

KEY POINTS

- Lack of recent education in child abuse and a lack of knowledge about reporting laws and practices impede reporting tendencies among physicians.
- Primary practice characteristics, such as limited time to adequately evaluate a child for abuse, lack of quick accessibility to a child abuse specialist, desire to preserve a professional relationship with the family, and negative prior experiences with reporting affect the clinician's ability to diagnose and report child abuse.
- Reporting child abuse entails both an emotional and cognitive response in the reporter.
- Improved communication with child protective and law enforcement investigators, child abuse specialists, and other resources enhances the clinician's confidence in reporting suspected abuse.
- Suggested approaches to improving the clinician's ability to detect, report, manage, and collaborate with investigators include seeking opportunities to update knowledge, implementing a screening tool, establishing contact with child abuse resources in the community, and communicating effectively and promptly with child abuse investigators.

INTRODUCTION

The process whereby a clinician decides that child abuse is a diagnostic possibility is often marked with doubt and fear. Abusive parents can present convincing lies, and children with suspicious injuries can have unusual accidents. Personal thresholds for reporting suspected child abuse vary considerably with bias, training, subspecialty, and situational factors. In addition, clinicians may mistrust or misunderstand the roles and responsibilities of the investigators and legal professionals involved after a report is made. The goals of this article are to improve understanding of the community responses to a report of child abuse, and to enhance the ability of the clinician to

Disclosure: None.
Center for Miracles, 315 North San Saba, Suite 201, San Antonio, TX 78207, USA
E-mail address: KELLOGGN@uthscsa.edu

Pediatr Clin N Am 61 (2014) 1037–1047
http://dx.doi.org/10.1016/j.pcl.2014.06.013
0031-3955/14/$ – see front matter © 2014 Elsevier Inc. All rights reserved.

work effectively with Child Protective Services (CPS), law enforcement, and legal professionals to ensure child safety and family integrity, when appropriate.

WHAT HAPPENS WHEN YOU REPORT CHILD ABUSE
Reporting Laws

In all states of the United States, health care providers are mandated by law to report suspected child abuse or neglect to designated child protection and/or local law enforcement agencies.[1] Although terminology varies, laws generally require a report when the clinician suspects abuse or has reason to believe that a child has been abused or neglected. Proof that abuse has occurred is generally not required to make a report of child abuse. However, in some states the standard for reporting does require the professional to believe that the child's mental or physical health has been adversely affected by maltreatment. In this latter circumstance, the physician is required to assess harm for those injuries resulting from abuse or neglect.

When Does Sexual Contact Equate to Sexual Abuse?

In general, any sexual contact involving children younger than 17 years and adults should be reported to CPS and/or law enforcement. Sexual contact involving children and family members or individuals residing in the child's home are usually investigated by CPS in addition to law enforcement. Sexual contact between minors and nonrelated adults, and nonconsensual sexual contact involving minors are reported to law enforcement. Clinicians should also report parents who are aware that abuse is occurring but fail to protect the child.

State laws vary with regard to mandatory or discretionary reporting of sexual activity between 2 consenting minor children.[2] Some states mandate reporting for any child below a designated "age of consent," whereas other states mandate reporting when the sexual activity is deemed physically or emotionally abusive or harmful. Penal code definitions for "sexual assault of a minor" typically use age-based criteria that differ from reporting mandates.

State laws protect the confidentiality of reporters; child protection and law enforcement professionals may not release the name of the reporter to the family or individuals involved in the investigation. However, physician reporters are often asked to provide records, affidavits, and testimony during or following the investigation, so the reporter is often known or revealed to the family. Many clinicians prefer to inform the family that they are reporting to child protection or law enforcement "so we can make sure everything is being done to keep your child safe."

Clinicians are protected from liability as long as they make a report of suspected abuse "in good faith"[3]; in some states, there is a presumption of good faith unless it is disproved.[4] Many state statutes specifically deny immunity for any reporter who knowingly makes a false or malicious report, and may impose either civil or criminal penalties for false reporting. Similarly, there are penalties for failing to report suspected abuse or neglect; punishments range from fines to imprisonment.

Child Protective Services Responses

CPS is responsible for determining whether the child is safe, and for implementing measures or "safety plans" to ensure the child remains safe during the investigation. When an individual makes a report to a child protection agency, the report may be either closed without investigation or assigned to investigation. Reports to investigation are assigned a priority ranking that determines the time within which the child protection worker must initiate the investigation. In general, reports involving younger children or serious injuries are prioritized. The results of the investigation are provided to the reporter in most states.[5] Physicians may be contacted by a child protection worker for additional information whether or not the physician is the reporter. The Health Insurance Portability and Accountability Act (HIPAA) permits disclosure of information without authorization of a legal guardian for situations relating to the investigation of abuse or neglect.[6] Although the physician should inform the parent or legal guardian when such disclosures are made, HIPAA also permits the physician to withhold the child's information from the parent if there is a possibility that the parent is the abuser or is protective of a suspected abuser.[6] The physician should confer with the child protection investigator if there is uncertainty about whether release of information to the parent could jeopardize the child's safety.

A timely report to CPS not only protects children, but can also initiate services to strengthen families. In some states, the court can mandate that family members participate in services while the child is kept safe with another relative. In general, CPS is required to make reasonable efforts to prevent removal of the child from the family if the child's safety can be assured while services are being offered. Services for families are expected to be strength-based, family-centered, trauma-informed, and respectful of culture, customs, beliefs, and needs.

When children cannot remain safely with their families, CPS provides out-of-home placements and, in some cases, adoption services. Foster children often have emotional or behavioral problems, chronic disabilities, developmental delays, and poor academic performance.[7] However, foster care also offers the opportunity to address unmet medical, dental, and mental health needs, and to provide a medical home. After initial health screening, children in foster care should receive comprehensive medical, dental, developmental, and mental health evaluations, with ongoing primary care monitoring of their health status.[7]

Law Enforcement Responses

Most states permit the physician to report to either child protection or law enforcement agencies when abuse is suspected. Referrals made to one agency often result in a joint investigation with the other agency. In general, child protection agencies investigate allegations of abuse or neglect involving a family member or occurring in a registered day care, whereas law enforcement investigates possible crimes involving both family member and non–family member suspects. A physician should call law enforcement if immediate safety measures are needed (**Box 1**).

Legal Responses

After a report of child abuse is made the physician may be required to testify, most commonly in either a child protection hearing or criminal trial, or both. After receiving

---

Box 1
Examples of when to call law enforcement emergently when there is a suspicion of abuse or neglect

- Parent is belligerent or violent
- Parent is threatening to leave when child needs further medical assessment or treatment
- Concern that parent will not comply with recommendations to take child to hospital immediately for further testing or admission
- To request a visit to the home to check on the child's welfare after the child has been dismissed from clinic (and child protective services is not yet involved)

a subpoena, the physician should place himself on standby (a phone number or contact person should be listed on the subpoena) and speak to the attorney issuing the subpoena. Physicians may request to be called to testify just prior to when testimony is needed (taking account of travel time). Although courts do not have to honor this request, it is reasonable to ask for consideration of patients who will have to be rescheduled because of physician testimony. The attorney requesting testimony should confer with the physician before testimony to review the medical findings and anticipated questions (**Box 2**). Sometimes telephone or videoconference testimony is allowed for certain legal proceedings.

PROBLEMS PHYSICIANS FACE WHEN CHILD ABUSE IS SUSPECTED

Physicians confront several questions in considering the decision to report suspected abuse and neglect:

- Is this really abuse?
- Are these parents capable of abusing their child?
- Would physician intervention with the parents be more effective than the child protection responses?
- Would referring the child and family to a social worker be better than making a report to a child protection agency?
- Will CPS really do anything?
- Will CPS take unnecessary drastic measures, jeopardizing the family rather than helping them?
- Will reporting affect the clinician's relationship with the family? If the family is lost from the clinician's practice, is the ability to monitor and protect the child in the future also lost?
- How much time will it take to make a report?
- How much time will be needed to prepare and provide testimony relating to the medical assessment of this child's injury or condition?

The importance of each question varies considerably among health care providers, depending on practice characteristics, education and knowledge in child abuse, past experiences with CPS, and personal experiences and opinions.

What Is the Threshold for Reporting?

State laws for reporting rely primarily on the individual's judgment that the child may have suffered abuse or neglect. A physician does not have to make a definitive diagnosis of child abuse to report.[5]

Box 2
General questions during testimony

- Name, educational background
- How clinician became involved with caring for the child
- What were the clinical findings: history, examination, ancillary testing
- What was the diagnosis
- What were the differential diagnoses, and how were they excluded
- What was done after the diagnosis was made (report, admit to the hospital, ordered a skeletal survey, and so forth)

In making a decision to report, physicians may consider where an injury falls on the continuum between abuse and accident or medical condition (**Fig. 1**).[8] Similarly, physicians may consider a continuum between neglect and accidental or medical causes when evaluating the need to report a child with failure to thrive. Sometimes it may not be clear where an injury falls on the continuum between abuse and neglect, but generally all injuries along this continuum are reported; for example, a 15-month-old with scald burns from a large pot with hot water that was placed on the kitchen floor and left unattended may have sustained the burns through inflicted or accidental causes, but both raise significant concerns for child safety.

The distinction between reasonable corporal punishment and physical abuse is challenging for many clinicians. The American Academy of Pediatrics has suggested: "child abuse should be considered as the most likely explanation for inflicted skin injuries if they are nonaccidental and there is any injury beyond temporary reddening of the skin."[9] However, physicians who are tolerant of corporal punishment are less likely to report.[10] In general, the younger the child, the lower the threshold should be for reporting.

Obstacles to Reporting Suspected Abuse

Even when abuse is suspected, 28% to 43% of pediatricians do not report to child protection or law enforcement.[11,12] Some physicians require a higher level of certainty before reporting,[13,14] or consider that there should be repeated incidents of abuse before a report is made.[14] Whereas most practitioners agree that child abuse is an important problem, fewer consider it important within their practice.[12] Other obstacles to reporting include:

- Inadequate opportunity in an office practice to adequately assess and report suspected abuse, owing to limited office visit time[15]
- Lack of concrete evidence for some types of child maltreatment such as psychological abuse or physical neglect[14]
- Lack of trust/understanding of what child protection agencies do[13,16]
- Not wanting to lose or jeopardize a relationship with the family[16]
- Having resources (such as social work) and knowledge to give the family the help they need[13]
- Fear of the consequences, including personal safety, lawsuits, and threat to the child's safety, of repercussions from reporting or inadequate child protection response[11]
- Inconvenience and discomfort related to testifying/being in court[15]

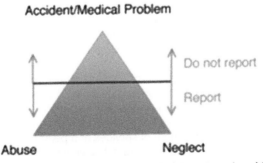

Fig. 1. Leventhal's triangle. (*From* Asnes AG, Leventhal JM. Managing child abuse: general principles. Pediatr Rev 2010;31:50; with permission from American Academy of Pediatrics, 2014.)

Impact of Education on Reporting

In one study of primary care providers,[13] those who received recent (within 5 years) formal education in child abuse following their residency were 10 times more likely to report child abuse than were providers without such training. Although child abuse has been a subspecialty of pediatrics since 2006, not all pediatric residencies require didactic and/or clinical training in child abuse. In addition, pediatricians may rely primarily on visible and explicit signs of injury, and may lack awareness of psychosocial factors that contribute to the diagnosis of child abuse.[14] Pediatricians who are less likely to report suspected child abuse or neglect are also more likely to indicate that they lack knowledge of reporting laws and processes.[11]

Impact of Prior Experience with Reporting

Most pediatricians tend to agree that CPS workers respond quickly, and are professional and thorough,[13,16] but only half indicate that they were more willing to report after their experiences with CPS.[13] About two-thirds considered they were not kept informed after the report was made,[13,16] and most thought that neither the child nor the family, nor the pediatrician's relationship with the family, benefited from the report.[13] In some cases, physicians felt less confident in diagnosing and reporting suspected abuse because CPS determined that no abuse had occurred when they reported previously.[15] Reporting suspected abuse tends to be an emotionally charged, memorable event for the practitioner, just as learning that signs of abuse were missed in a patient found later to be a victim of abuse.[15]

CHALLENGES TO WORKING WITH COMMUNITY RESOURCES
Lack of Understanding Regarding What CPS Does

During investigation, CPS workers consider several factors and sources of information in determining whether abuse has occurred, including:

- Additional information about the incident from witnesses and collaterals (this may include information requested by the physician)
- Previous CPS referrals (of which the reporter is frequently unaware)
- Criminal history of parents and in-home caretakers
- Drug-testing results for parents and in-home caretakers
- Past medical and mental health records for the parents and children
- History of family violence

This additional information may lead CPS to take custody of a child even when the reporter may consider the injury or condition to be minor. Alternatively, CPS may rule out abuse by family members in a child with egregious inflicted injury because a non–family member or day-care provider is determined to be the perpetrator. Reports of abuse that potentially involve a day-care provider are typically investigated by a unit separate from CPS.

A CPS investigator may refer a family for ongoing services during and following the investigation. These services may be offered even when abuse is not substantiated. Family-based or family preservation unit workers monitor family compliance with the services provided. The types of services offered to families vary considerably from state to state, as does the length of services and period of monitoring. Services provided may include parenting classes, mental health assessment and services, domestic violence intervention, case management, protective day-care arrangements, and counseling for children and families. Sometimes, in formulating a safety plan for children during the investigation, CPS may require the parent to seek necessary medical or mental health care for themselves or their children. In conferring with CPS investigators, pediatricians should clearly state recommendations with regard to compliance with medications, medical follow-up appointments, and referrals to other professionals. In some cases, CPS may make these recommendations a required part of the safety plan for the family.

Lack of Understanding What CPS and Law Enforcement Need from the Physician

In working with child protection and law enforcement professionals, the physician has the opportunity to ensure that the medical findings and implications for abuse or neglect are clearly understood. In one study,[17] more than 40% of physicians who evaluated or reported suspected child abuse did not document their opinion on the likelihood of abuse or neglect, or why they suspected abuse. Information that is generally helpful to child protection and law enforcement professionals is summarized in **Box 3**.

Lack of Understanding of How to Utilize a Child Abuse Specialist

Physicians find it helpful to have colleagues and child abuse experts available to discuss decisions about reporting abuse.[15] Because a decision to report child abuse is typically made during or immediately following a patient's visit, clinicians need quick access to resources that help them make this decision and manage the child's immediate needs for safety.

SUGGESTED APPROACHES TO WORKING WITH COMMUNITY RESOURCES
Seek Opportunities to Update Knowledge

Educational offerings in child maltreatment can improve detection, willingness to report, and knowledge about reporting laws and processes. The American Academy of Pediatrics (AAP) Section on Child Abuse sponsors several educational opportunities, including presentations at AAP conferences. In one focus group study[15] of

---

Box 3
Common questions that investigators have about medical findings

Suspected abuse

- What are the specific concerns for abuse? (unexplained injury, inadequately explained injury, pattern of injury, child states he/she was abused, and so forth)

- What characteristics of the injury are concerning? (pattern, location, severity, size, and so forth)

- Is this a serious injury? (required medical treatment, risks of further complications, impairs function temporarily or permanently, risk of death, and so forth)

- Will this child need medical follow-up for this injury?

Suspected neglect

- What are the specific concerns for neglect? (failure to follow important medical advice or treatment, evidence of inadequate provision of basic needs, inadequate growth, injury resulted from inadequate supervision, and so forth)

- What examination or laboratory tests support a concern for neglect? (growth charts, signs of malnutrition, sequelae of noncompliance with medical treatment, low drug levels, delay in seeking medical care for condition)

- Is this serious? (severity of growth failure, repetitive pattern of ignoring medical advice, risks of not taking medication, and so forth)

- Will this child need medical follow-up for this condition?

Box 4
What to do when you suspect child abuse or neglect

I. If you *suspect* child abuse or neglect:
- Report to child protective services (CPS) by
  i. Phone [hotline number] OR
  ii. Online report: http://www.childhelpusa.org
- Report to law enforcement if:
  i. You suspect a non–family member is the abuser, or
  ii. You feel rapid intervention may be needed (severe abuse, threatening parents, fear of parent flight with child)
  iii. Note that a law enforcement report should be made to the agency with jurisdiction over the location *where the abuse likely occurred—not necessarily where the child lives*
- Make the report as quickly as possible
- When you make a report (either to CPS or law enforcement), be sure to record the case report ID number in the medical record
- Consider whether other tests are needed
- Consider whether hospitalization is needed:
  i. To treat serious injuries, especially in younger children and infants
  ii. To facilitate the abuse evaluation
  iii. To keep the child in a safe location pending further evaluation by CPS or law enforcement
- Carefully and completely document all/any interactions with the child or parent, preferably in quotations

II. Interactions with the parent
- Stress your role to act in the child's best interest to ensure that the child is safe
- If the abuser is unknown, but may be the parent, or the parent appears to be protecting an abuser, then you are not required to release verbal or written information to the parent if it may place the child in danger. This is an exception to the rules of the Health Insurance Portability and Accountability Act (HIPAA)

III. Information release to CPS or law enforcement
- You can and should promptly release all information pertinent to the child's injuries promptly to CPS or law enforcement, when they request it. This is also an exception to the HIPAA rules

IV. When to call the child abuse specialist
- Child abuse clinic day and nighttime phone numbers
  i. You suspect any kind of abuse or neglect and want guidance on the next steps
  ii. You have a question about which diagnostic tests might need to be done and whether a child might need to go to the emergency room for further assessment
  iii. Other questions the child abuse specialist might be able to help with:
    1. "Does the history reasonably explain the injury(ies) in this child?"
    2. "Is this appropriate or abusive punishment?"
    3. "What does this positive drug screen in a mother/child mean?"
    4. "What other nonabusive causes are possible?"

V. When to call/refer to hospital emergency department and/or Sexual Assault Nurse Examiner (SANE) program

- [phone number]—7 days a week, 24 hours a day; ask for the emergency physician or forensic nurse examiner on duty
  i. Sexual abuse may have occurred within the past 96 hours
  ii. The child is a suspected victim of sexual abuse or assault and has symptoms of anogenital bleeding or pain

primary care physicians, office-detailing was suggested as an effective educational format. In addition, addressing fear as a mitigating factor for reporting behavior should be incorporated in educational approaches.[11] A field experience with CPS may improve understanding of CPS processes, communication, and compliance with reporting laws.[13]

Consider Using a Screening Tool

In one study[18] of emergency department nurses in 7 hospitals, the child abuse detection rate increased 5-fold after 20 months of using a 6-question screening tool. Other approaches include use of an algorithm,[19] chart check lists,[20,21] and self-instructional kits[22]; however, these approaches have been tested primarily in emergency department settings rather than office settings. Use of a pocket guide (**Box 4**) with succinct reminders of reporting processes and community resources may be useful in primary care practices.

Identify a Child Abuse Expert or Resource

The presence of child abuse specialists does not undermine the role of the general practitioner in the detection, diagnosis, and management of child abuse.[23] Similarly to situations that require a referral from a general practitioner to a pediatric cardiologist, child abuse pediatricians may be consulted for a variety of reasons:

- The clinical presentation is atypical but concerning for abuse
- Assistance is needed in selecting the most appropriate diagnostic tests
- Injuries are complex or critical, and an expert is needed to provide uniform information for investigators
- Collegial input is needed before a decision to report to CPS or referral to a child abuse specialist can be made
- Assistance is needed in finding the appropriate facility or specialist to further assess the possibility of abuse

As of 2014, there are 264 board certified child abuse pediatricians in the United States. The AAP has mapped the locations of several of these specialists (http://www2.aap.org/sections/childabuseneglect/MedicalDiagnostic.cfm). Other experts in child abuse can usually be identified within medical schools or by contacting a regional Children's Advocacy Center.

Cooperate, Collaborate, and Communicate with Investigators

Physicians are generally dissatisfied with the feedback they receive, or the lack thereof, from CPS following a report of suspected abuse.[13,15] Physicians can, however, contact CPS workers or supervisors to provide updates and to request clarification on what information can be released to the family, particularly if there is a concern that the parent may be an abuser or protective of an abuser.[6] In many states, workers have "gone mobile" and are more readily reached through the cell phones they carry during field work. CPS and law enforcement may request medical records; records requested for the purposes of a child abuse investigation may be released without parent authorization or consent.[6] Processing requests for records in a timely fashion will facilitate the investigation and enhance communication.

Face-to-face contact often facilitates collaborative work. Physicians may invite CPS supervisors to the office to meet the pediatric staff and to provide an overview of reporting laws and CPS processes. CPS can also assist in identifying the community resources that provide services to children and families at risk for abuse and neglect.

SUMMARY

Making the decision to report suspected child abuse is a stressful event. Lack of knowledge about indicators of abuse, reporting laws and processes, and investigator roles and responsibilities impede recognition and reporting of abuse. Threats of testimony, lawsuits, family anguish, and diagnostic uncertainty compete with concerns about missing true cases of abuse, with deleterious consequences for the child. Updating knowledge in child maltreatment and reporting procedures, using standard approaches to screen for abuse, and establishing collaborative relationships with investigators, colleagues, and child abuse experts in the local community optimizes the physician's role in the recognition and management of child maltreatment.

REFERENCES

1. US Department of Health and Human Services, Administration for Children and Families Child Welfare Information Gateway. Mandatory reporters of child abuse and neglect: summary of state laws. 2010. Available at: http://www.childwelfare. gov/systemwide/laws_policies/statutes/manda.cfm. Accessed March 9, 2014.
2. Madison AB, Feldman-Winter L, Finkel M, et al. Commentary: consensual adolescent sexual activity with adult partners – conflict between confidentiality and physician reporting requirements under child abuse laws. Pediatrics 2001;107:E16.
3. US Department of Health and Human Services, Administration for Children and Families Child Welfare Information Gateway. Immunity for reporters of child abuse and neglect: summary of state laws. Available at: https://www.childwelfare.gov/ systemwide/laws_policies/statutes/immunity.cfm. Accessed March 9, 2014.
4. Lukefahr JL, Narang SK, Kellogg ND. Medical liability and child abuse. In: Donn SM, McAbee GN, editors. Medicolegal issues in pediatrics. 7th edition. Elk Grove Village (IL): American Academy of Pediatrics; 2012. p. 253–7.
5. US Department of Health and Human Services, Administration for Children and Families Child Welfare Information Gateway. Reporting suspected child abuse and neglect. Available at: https://www.childwelfare.gov/pubs/usermanuals/ childcare/chapterthree.cfm. Accessed March 9, 2014.
6. Kellogg ND, Hiser D. AAP committee on child abuse and neglect. Pediatrics 2010;125:197–201.
7. American Academy of Pediatrics, Committee on Early Childhood, Adoption and Dependent Care. Health care of young children in foster care. Pediatrics 2002; 109(3):536–41.
8. Asnes AG, Leventhal JM. Managing child abuse: general principles. Pediatr Rev 2010;31:47–55.
9. American Academy of Pediatrics, Committee on Child Abuse and Neglect. When inflicted skin injuries constitute child abuse. Pediatrics 2002;110:644–5.

10. Tirosh E, Shechter SO, Cohen A, et al. Attitudes towards corporal punishment and reporting of abuse. Child Abuse Negl 2003;27:929–37.
11. Gunn VL, Hickson GB, Cooper WO. Factors affecting pediatricians' reporting of suspected child maltreatment. Ambul Pediatr 2005;5:96–101.
12. VanHaeringen AR, Dadds M, Armstrong KL. The child abuse lottery-will the doctor suspect and report? Physician attitudes towards and reporting of suspected child abuse and neglect. Child Abuse Negl 1998;22(3):159–69.
13. Flaherty EG, Sege R, Binns HJ, et al. Health care providers' experience reporting child abuse in the primary care setting. Arch Pediatr Adolesc Med 2000;154: 489–93.
14. Shor R. Pediatricians in Israel: factors which affect the diagnosis and reporting of maltreated children. Child Abuse Negl 1998;22(2):143–53.
15. Flaherty EG, Jones R, Sege R. Telling their stories: primary care practitioners' experience evaluating and reporting injuries caused by child abuse. Child Abuse Negl 2004;28:939–45.
16. Vulliamy AP, Sullivan R. Reporting child abuse: pediatricians' experiences with the child protection system. Child Abuse Negl 2000;24(11):1461–70.
17. Anderst J, Kellogg ND, Jung I. Is the diagnosis of physical abuse changed when child protective services consults a child abuse subspecialty group as a second opinion? Child Abuse Negl 2009;33:481–9.
18. Louwers ECFM, Korfage IJ, Affourtit MJ, et al. Effects of systematic screening and detection of child abuse in emergency departments. Pediatrics 2012;130: 457–64.
19. Benger JR, Pearce V. Simple intervention to improve detection of child abuse in emergency departments. BMJ 2002;324(7340):780–2.
20. Clark KD, Tepper D, Jenny C. Effect of a screening profile on the diagnosis of non accidental burns in children. Pediatr Emerg Care 1997;13:259–61.
21. Guenther E, Olsen C, Keenan H, et al. Randomized prospective study to evaluate child abuse documentation in the emergency department. Acad Emerg Med 2009;16:1–9.
22. Showers J, Laird M. Improving knowledge of emergency physicians about child physical and sexual abuse. Pediatr Emerg Care 1991;7:275–7.
23. Block RW, Palusci VJ. Child abuse pediatrics: a new pediatric subspecialty. J Pediatr 2006;148(6):711–2.

Legal Issues in Child Maltreatment

Sandeep K. Narang, MD, JD[a],*, John D. Melville, MD[b]

KEYWORDS

- Legal issues • Child maltreatment • Medicolegal issues • Expert witness

KEY POINTS

- Discuss the legal duty to report suspicion of child maltreatment.
- Understand processes and duties associated with giving effective and ethical expert witness testimony.
- Obtain appropriate, informed consent for child maltreatment medical evaluations.
- Explore current issues of civil liability exposure related to reporting and evaluating suspected child maltreatment.

INTRODUCTION

Patient advocacy is an integral part of pediatric practice. Few patients require that advocacy as urgently as the child who has been abused or neglected. The pediatrician's opportunity to serve the child, whom other protectors may have failed, necessitates interactions with law enforcement, child protection agencies and the courts: entities unfamiliar to many pediatricians. In this article, four legal issues are discussed that arise when pediatricians report or evaluate children suspected of being abused or neglected: a physician's duty as a mandated reporter; a physician's responsibilities when called to court as an expert witness; informed consent for maltreatment-specific evaluations; and liability confronting providers involved in child maltreatment.

MANDATED REPORTING

For most pediatricians, the first and most frequent interaction with the child protection system is as a mandated reporter. Federal law requires states to have mandated reporting laws regarding child maltreatment.[1] Pursuant to this law, states must require

Disclosure: Dr Narang has been paid as an expert consultant/witness in child maltreatment cases.

[a] Pediatrics, UTHSC-Houston, 6410 Fannin Street, Suite 1425, Houston, TX 77030, USA; [b] Child Advocacy Center, Akron Children's Hospital, 6505 Market Street Building C, Suite 3100, Boardman, OH 44512, USA
* Corresponding author.
E-mail address: Sandeep.Narang@uth.tmc.edu

Pediatr Clin N Am 61 (2014) 1049–1058
http://dx.doi.org/10.1016/j.pcl.2014.06.016
0031-3955/14/$ – see front matter © 2014 Elsevier Inc. All rights reserved.

"mandatory reporting by individuals required to report," and establish a system to respond to such reports. "Individuals required to report" is not defined by federal law, and significant variation exists among the states.[2] Separate, and subtly different, mandated reporting laws exist in all states and territories of the United States.[3] Additionally, a federal statute extends this duty to professionals on federal land or in federal facilities where state law does not apply.

Most states require a report when a mandated reporter, in their professional capacity, "reasonably suspects" or has "reason to believe" that a child has been abused or neglected. Other states enumerate specific professions as mandated reporters but also require all adults to report suspected maltreatment. New Jersey and Wyoming simply require all adults to report without mention of professions. As recent high-profile cases have reminded us,[4–6] many adults fail to report suspicion or even knowledge of child maltreatment.

What constitutes "reasonable suspicion" or a "reasonable cause to believe" is an issue that has perplexed and frustrated physicians for decades. Recent studies have shown that one of the reasons for underreporting child abuse is a misinterpretation of the level of certainty needed before reporting. In CARES (Child Abuse Reporting Experience Study),[7] physicians did not report 27% of the injuries that they determined to be likely or very likely caused by child abuse. Levi and Brown[8] reported that 15% of the physicians whom they studied required 75% or more probability of abuse before they would report. Multiple studies have confirmed that physicians have varying interpretations of what constitutes reasonable suspicion.

The most helpful judicial clarification of "reasonable suspicion" comes not from child abuse reporting cases but from a search and seizure case under the 4th Amendment. The US Supreme Court stated in *Illinois v Wardlow* that "a reasonable, articulable suspicion" equates to something "more than an inchoate and unparticularized suspicion or 'hunch'."[9] Thus, in maltreatment cases, a "reasonable suspicion" is some objective, articulable fact that would lead a reasonable person to suspect that abuse or neglect might have occurred. However, *practitioners should understand that the threshold for reporting maltreatment does not require incontrovertible certainty*. A mandated reporter must report a reasonable suspicion even when the provider cannot prove, or doubts, that abuse or neglect has occurred.

Another reason why pediatricians fail to report is that they do not trust the child protection system to help the patient or family. In a physician focus group study that examined physician perceptions of child maltreatment reporting systems,[10] participants opined that they could help the family without involving child protection authorities. This approach is legally risky. Other reasons that physicians have indicated for not reporting include fear of testifying, increased time demands for these types of cases, and reluctance to get entangled in the legal system.

The Health Insurance Portability and Accountability Act (HIPAA) is, incorrectly, an oft-perceived impediment to reporting abuse and neglect. HIPAA specifically permits disclosures to "a public health authority or other appropriate government authority authorized by law to receive reports of child abuse or neglect."[11] Similarly, most states explicitly exempt mandated reporting of child maltreatment from the physician-patient privilege of confidentiality. Thus, the pediatrician may disclose protected health information to an appropriate investigative agency without parental notification or consent. When the physician is not the reporter of suspected abuse or neglect, the physician may still disclose Protected Health Information to the Child Protection Services or law enforcement when certain conditions are met (eg, when permitted by state law, when deemed necessary to prevent serious harm to a child, and when limited to only information related to the abuse or neglect).

Local reporting procedures vary widely by state. Pediatricians need to be aware of their local procedure. Most states offer a toll-free hotline for child maltreatment reporting. Liability for failing to report is discussed in detail later.

Pediatricians are required to report knowledge or reasonable suspicion of child abuse or neglect to appropriate authorities. HIPAA and other confidentiality laws allow disclosure of patient medical information in mandated reports. Failure to report not only endangers children but exposes the physician to legal and professional consequences.

EXPERT WITNESS TESTIMONY

Although not a common aspect of pediatric practice, practitioners may be called to testify in a variety of legal proceedings related to child maltreatment. In a criminal trial, the state seeks to prove the guilt of a defendant beyond a reasonable doubt and to impose a sentence. In civil proceedings, litigants, including government officials (eg, child protective services), attempt to establish findings by a preponderance of the evidence, so they can obtain orders regarding child custody, visitation, or child support. Pretrial hearings, such as *Frye* and *Daubert* hearings, determine which evidence or witness testimony is permitted at a subsequent trial. Rarely, pediatricians may become involved in governmental administrative hearings (eg, licensure or revocation of licensure) tangent to maltreatment cases.

Although practitioners may feel uncomfortable testifying as an expert in child maltreatment, the definition of "expert" in this context is broad. The Federal Rules of Evidence define an expert as someone with "scientific, technical, or other specialized knowledge" that would assist the judge or jury in deciding the case.[12] One need not be the foremost authority on child maltreatment, nor understand every nuance of the subject, to qualify.[13] Practitioners who are unsure about proper testimony in a child maltreatment case are advised to consult with a physician board certified in the recently established subspecialty of child abuse pediatrics.

A practitioner's first formalized contact with the testimonial process comes in the form of a subpoena. A subpoena is a legal document that notifies a witness that they are needed to present evidence in court. A subpoena might require testimony (*subpoena ad testificandum*), the production of documents (*subpoena duces tecum*), or both. Because a subpoena suspends typical rules regarding medical confidentiality, it is important for the physician to read carefully which disclosures are commanded (and therefore allowed) by the subpoena. A provider receiving a subpoena for a medical record that they did not create should notify the attorney issuing the subpoena of the appropriate custodian instead of disclosing the record. On receiving any subpoena, the wisest course is to call the attorney who issued the subpoena. The attorney should discuss which testimony or documents are required and also the facts or opinions to which the attorney hopes the witness will testify.

The best preparation for any kind of court testimony is to be thoroughly familiar with the medical facts of the case. Although many courts permit a witness to refer to notes during testimony, the witness should be able to recite the basic facts of the case (patient's name, age, dates seen, high points of the history, and injuries found) from memory. The expert should be familiar with the patient's entire chart, because questions may be asked about the patient's medical conditions unrelated to abuse or neglect.

The testimony of an expert witness begins with qualification as an expert witness. The qualification of a witness as an expert is a legal procedure by which the witness shows to the court sufficient training, research, writing, professional activities, or other qualifications to serve as an expert.[12] The official judicial determination of an "expert" comes when an attorney asks the judge to recognize the witness as an expert in a particular subject matter. Being qualified as an expert entitles the expert to offer opinions in court.[14] In answering questions, from either party, the witness should consider themselves an impartial educator of the court about the topic of their expertise. A physician has an ethical obligation to provide accurate, unbiased testimony based on sound scientific principles.[15]

Less commonly, a practitioner may be called as a fact witness, rather than an expert witness. When testifying as a fact witness, the qualification step mentioned earlier is omitted. However, unlike an expert, a fact witness is not allowed to provide an opinion or interpretation of what the witness observed. A fact witness may testify only to the specific facts that the witness has seen, heard, felt, and so forth.

At many steps in the legal process, evidentiary rules, court rulings, or party agreements may limit the content of a witness' testimony. In general, these restrictions are not a concern for the witness; it is the attorney's responsibility to ask questions that elicit admissible testimony. This is another reason that the best strategy is to answer each question as posed, rather than trying to anticipate or manipulate the testimony.

Child protection has long been hindered by physicians who give irresponsible testimony.[16] Irresponsible testimony includes testimony for which the expert is insufficiently qualified, or testimony based on idiosyncratic theories that have either not been substantiated by well-conducted medical studies or have not gained wide acceptance in the medical community. The American Academy of Pediatrics' recommendations for expert witnesses are listed in **Box 1**.[15] The American Medical Association Code of Medical Ethics requires that physicians who testify based on "a theory not widely accepted in the profession" must "characterize the theory as such."[17]

INFORMED CONSENT IN CHILD MALTREATMENT

Although not readily apparent, the detection, diagnosis, and treatment of child maltreatment can raise numerous informed consent issues for physicians and other health care professionals. For example, are medical providers ever required to obtain informed consent from caregivers before conducting child maltreatment evaluations? If so, under which circumstances? If a provider suspects maltreatment, and is required to obtain informed consent, what information must the practitioner provide to the caregiver to obtain informed consent? Must a provider specifically state that they suspect abuse for consent to be truly informed or is more nonspecific language permissible? Are there circumstances under which a child may provide informed consent for a medical evaluation? If so, what are those? Which course of action should a provider take if they are required to obtain informed consent for a nonemergent maltreatment evaluation and the parent/guardian refuses to provide that consent?

Whether informed consent is required before conducting a child maltreatment evaluation depends on 2 factors: (1) the jurisdiction in which a health care professional

---

Box 1
American Academy of Pediatrics recommended qualifications for physician expert witnesses

1. Licensed in the state where the expert practices medicine

2. Board certification in the area relevant to the testimony

3. Actively engaged in clinical practice of medicine relevant to the testimony

4. Unless retired from clinical practice, most of a physician's professional time should not be devoted to expert witness work. If retired, a physician should only testify on cases that occurred when he or she was in active practice

practices; and, (2) whether the evaluation is emergent or not. In some US jurisdictions, a practitioner who assists or participates in an investigation of allegation of maltreatment (ie, conducts a nonemergent evaluation for abuse) is immunized from any civil or criminal liability related to that participation.[18] Thus, in these jurisdictions (eg, Texas), informed consent from anyone (eg, the caregiver, child, child protective services) is not necessary before conducting an evaluation for abuse or neglect. Some jurisdictions have made specific provisions of immunity for actions taken by medical practitioners in connection with making a report of suspected child maltreatment. These actions include[18]:

a. Taking any necessary photographs or radiographs
b. Taking a child into emergency protective custody
c. Performing a medical examination on the child
d. Performing medically relevant tests

The emergency exception to informed consent has been long recognized, and its component elements broadly described in common and statutory law. A provider may presume consent and proceed with appropriate evaluation and treatment if the following four conditions are met[19]:

1. There is a serious and immediate threat to life or health
2. No available option exists for obtaining actual informed consent
3. There is a need for urgent intervention (delay in care is not safe)
4. The professional administers only care and treatment of emergent conditions that pose an immediate threat to the child

The most common child maltreatment scenario in which this exception may arise is in emergent cases of physical or sexual abuse (eg, when a child is brought by ambulance, unconscious or obtunded, with subdural hematomas or severe intra-abdominal trauma; or, when a child is brought to a medical facility with clear findings of violent, penetrative genital or anal trauma). In those circumstances, providers may pursue laboratory testing, radiologic imaging, and treatment that are necessary for the care of the child. In these emergent circumstances in which consent is bypassed, it is prudent for practitioners to document well the conditions present that precipitated the lack of informed consent.

In those jurisdictions in which immunity is not available to a provider who assists or participates in a report of child maltreatment, a practitioner must obtain informed consent for further evaluation or testing. Examples of such "non-emergent" scenarios include an older child or adolescent with nonextensive bruising who appears clinically well, or a child with a remote history [>96 hours] of sexual contact and no signs or symptoms of current genital trauma. If a practitioner is uncertain if consent is necessary in a child maltreatment scenario, it may be prudent to consult a child abuse specialist.

What constitutes full informed consent in child maltreatment cases is nuanced and case specific. The goal of informed consent is to ensure that patients have a "comprehensive understanding of the clinical situation."[20] Courts have long held that informed consent does not require providers to disclose every remote risk associated with a medical procedure or treatment. Thus, in child maltreatment cases, when a practitioner suspects abuse and desires to perform additional testing (eg, a skeletal survey), it is sufficient for a practitioner to provide general statements (such as "the additional imaging is being performed to look for additional skeletal injuries") as justification for those medical procedures. Specific statements, such as "I am looking for abusive injuries," are not necessary.

Although children cannot usually provide legal consent for medical care or treatment, in most states, there are exceptions to this general rule. These exceptions include emancipated minors, mature minors, and special circumstances. The consideration of these exceptions arises when caring for adolescents, especially in circumstances of suspected sexual abuse. "Emancipation" refers to a court process by which a minor shows that they are self-supporting, have assumed adult responsibility for their welfare, and are no longer under the care of their parents. In considering a minor's petition for emancipation, courts assess a multitude of factors: whether the minor is or has been married, has children, is a member of the armed forces, or is financially independent and living separate and apart from the parents.[21] Although a minor may show characteristics of "emancipation," or even declare themselves to be so, a physician should never assume emancipation unless provided clear court documentation affirming so.

As with the emancipation exception, courts consider various factors in assessing a "mature minor," including age, reasoning ability, intellectual capacity, and comprehension of the health issue. But, unlike the emancipation exception, in which indicia of emancipation are usually itemized, courts have found that determination of a child's maturity is case specific.[22] As with emancipation, although a minor child may show characteristics of a mature minor, or even declare themselves to be so, a physician should never assume that mature minor status applies unless they are provided with clear court documentation affirming so.

In furtherance of public policy goals of encouraging adolescents to seek treatment in certain medical scenarios, many states permit a minor to bypass parental consent and seek treatment of certain medical conditions. These scenarios may present directly in child maltreatment cases, or tangent to them[23]:

a. Reproductive health (including contraception, abortion, prenatal care, and pregnancy)
b. Sexually transmitted infections
c. Mental health
d. Substance abuse

Aside from the specific exceptions discussed earlier, the general rule is that parental informed permission is necessary before nonemergent medical intervention on a minor child. However, the consent of only one parent or guardian is required, not both. If a child is in the legal custody of a state protective agency or resides with foster parents, the agency or foster parents, rather than the minor's biological parents, have the authority to make medical decisions and should provide appropriate documentation showing that authority. If the parent or legal guardian refuses to consent to evaluation or treatment that the provider thinks is necessary, the provider or others (eg, state protective services) should petition a court to intervene or to compel parental compliance. All medical providers, especially those routinely involved in the care of maltreated children, should be knowledgeable of their state-specific conditions.

LIABILITY

A practitioner's liability risk in child maltreatment cases stems from three areas: reporting abuse and neglect, expert testimony, and diagnosing maltreatment (eg, malpractice and deprivation of constitutional rights). Although all US jurisdictions provide some form of immunity from liability for persons making reports of suspected maltreatment in good faith, statutory immunity for participating in other aspects of child protection cases (eg, providing testimony in a judicial proceeding, performing case reviews, or providing care/treatment to a child) is variable from jurisdiction to jurisdiction. For example, 36 States and the District of Columbia provide immunity to reporters who participate in any judicial proceedings that may arise from a child maltreatment report.[18] As mentioned earlier, only 26 states provide immunity to reporters who assist with or participate in a child maltreatment investigation.[18] *Thus, given the variable jurisdictional protections, health care providers should become familiar with the governing statute in their jurisdiction.* Recognizing the loopholes in reporting immunity, the Secretary of Health and Human Services has recently made recommendations to Congress for strengthening immunity in child maltreatment cases.[24]

Practitioners should be aware that reporter immunity attaches only if the report is made in "good faith." "Good faith" implies that the reporter, to the best of their knowledge, genuinely suspects that a child may have been abused or neglected.[25] Some state statutes specify a presumption of good faith, meaning that the good faith of the reporter is assumed until it is disproved. Conversely, many jurisdictions deny or revoke immunity for reporters who make false or malicious reports. More than half of the jurisdictions specify either civil or criminal penalties for false reporting.[18]

As immunity comprises one edge of the reporting sword, liability comprises the other. Almost all states list penalties for mandatory reporters who fail to report suspected abuse or neglect, with Wyoming, Maryland, and North Carolina being the excepted jurisdictions.[18] These penalties may be in the form of fines or imprisonment. In 39 jurisdictions, they are classified as misdemeanors. However, some states regard repeat failures to report or failure to report serious abusive injuries as potential felony offenses. Although uncommon, failure to report can also subject the health care provider to licensure review. Despite the policy intent to encourage reporting, charges against providers for failure to report have been infrequent, even in states in which authorities have been more aggressive in enforcing the reporting laws.[26] When charges were brought, court records show that most cases were thrown out.

Practitioners who provide expert testimony in child maltreatment cases are exposed to liability in a variety of ways. Aside from the statutory immunity afforded for participating in judicial proceedings in 36 jurisdictions, practitioners must still be aware of potential liability from the unlicensed practice of medicine (in certain jurisdictions), professional censure from the provision of unethical or unreliable expert testimony, and liability from the commission of perjury. Although professional organizations[27] and some courts[28] have deemed the provision of expert testimony as the practice of medicine, this also is jurisdiction specific. Florida, for example, requires any physician providing testimony within that jurisdiction to attain an expert witness certificate before providing that testimony.[29] Thus, in child maltreatment cases, an out-of-state expert witness must first attain a limited measure of Florida licensure before providing testimony in that state or be subject to liability for the unlawful practice of medicine. Providers should familiarize themselves with the specific statutory provisions that may affect them.

However, as mentioned earlier, health care professionals should always strive to provide expert testimony that is reliable, honest, unbiased, and based on evidence-based scientific principles. Failure to do so opens the practitioner to embarrassment on cross-examination, potential grievance with professional societies or state medical boards, or, more rarely, a malpractice suit. Although not uniform among professional societies, professional societies have become increasingly more active in the regulation of unethical or unreliable expert testimony.[30] Some have published examples of unethical expert testimony; some have censured members; and, some have even expelled members. Such professional society activism, as a means of regulating improper expert testimony, has found favor in the courts.[28] Thus, practitioners should be aware of the mandates of their professional society.

Unbeknown to many practitioners, involvement in child maltreatment cases can result in civil suits known as "1983 actions." These actions are brought by parents under the protections of 42 USC §1983, which affords US citizens civil redress against the State for violations of constitutional rights.[31] These actions allege that providers who assist child protective services in the process of removing children from their custody violate parents' constitutional rights to familial relations and the right to be free from unlawful seizures under the Fourth Amendment of the US Constitution.[32] To date, these actions have been resoundingly unsuccessful in the courts.[32] However, even the successful defeat of these actions is not without costs to providers: loss of time, higher malpractice costs, and significant emotional anguish. Thus, it is prudent for providers to review their malpractice insurance coverage policies to ensure that those policies contain sufficiently broad language so as to provide coverage for expert testimony and other involvement in the child maltreatment evaluation and treatment process.

Practitioner liability in child maltreatment cases can arise from a variety of circumstances. Providers should be well acquainted with the governing laws of reporting and testimony in their jurisdiction, of the specific mandates of their professional society and state medical board, and of the provisions of coverage of their malpractice insurance. If providers have additional or more case-specific questions, it may be prudent to consult with their local child abuse pediatrician or hospital counsel.

SUMMARY

Child maltreatment poses various medicolegal issues and challenges for the health care professional. Because the ways and workings of the legal world are often foreign to the health care professional, this can, understandably, pose some degree of emotional angst. Some of the more common medicolegal issues include reporting child maltreatment, the presentation of ethical and effective expert testimony, informed consent in child maltreatment cases, and various liability risks related to child maltreatment cases. However, the health care professional can minimize medicolegal risk associated with child maltreatment cases by remaining knowledgeable about the laws within their jurisdiction, the mandates of their professional society and state medical board, and the local resources (eg, child abuse pediatrician and hospital counsel) available to them.

REFERENCES

1. 42 USC 5100 et seq.
2. 42 USC 13031.
3. Child Welfare Information Gateway. Mandatory reporters of child abuse and neglect. Washington, DC: US Department of Health and Human Services, Children's Bureau; 2012. Available at: http://www.childwelfare.gov/systemwide/laws_policies/statutes/report.cfm. Accessed March 30, 2014.
4. The Boston Globe. Spotlight on investigation: abuse in the catholic church. Available at: http://www.boston.com/globe/spotlight/abuse/. Accessed March 30, 2014.
5. Freeh L. The Freeh Report on Pennsylvania State University. Available at: http://progress.psu.edu/the-freeh-report. Accessed March 30, 2014.
6. Chase R. Lawsuit involving pedophile pediatrician settles. Available at: http://bigstory.ap.org/article/lawsuit-involving-pedophile-pediatrician-settled. Accessed March 30, 2014.

7. Jones R, Flaherty EG, Binns HJ, et al. Clinicians' description of factors influencing their reporting of suspected child abuse: report of the Child Abuse Reporting Experience Study Research Group. Pediatrics 2008;122:611–9.
8. Levi BH, Brown G. Reasonable suspicion: a study of Pennsylvania pediatricians regarding child abuse. Pediatrics 2005;116(1):e5–12.
9. Illinois v Wardlow, 528 US 119. 2000.
10. Flaherty EG, Jones R, Sege R. Telling their stories: primary care practitioners' experience evaluating and reporting injuries caused by child abuse. Child Abuse Negl 2004;28:939–45.
11. Committee on Child Abuse and Neglect. Policy statement-child abuse, confidentiality, and the health insurance portability and accountability act. Pediatrics 2010; 125:197–201.
12. Federal Rules of Evidence 702. Available at: http://www.law.cornell.edu/rules/fre/rule_702. Accessed March 30, 2014.
13. State v Wakisaka, 78 P3d 317, 333. 2003.
14. Federal Rules of Evidence 703. Available at: http://www.law.cornell.edu/rules/fre/rule_703. Accessed March 30, 2014.
15. Committee on Medical Liability and Risk Management. Policy statement–expert witness participation in civil and criminal proceedings. Pediatrics 2009;109(5): 974–9.
16. Chadwick DL, Krous HF. Irresponsible testimony by medical experts in cases involving the physical abuse and neglect of children. Child Maltreat 1997;2:313–21.
17. American Medical Association. Code of ethics opinion 9.07–medical testimony. Available at: http://www.ama-assn.org/ama/pub/physician-resources/medical-ethics/code-medical-ethics/opinion907.page. Accessed March 30, 2014.
18. Child Welfare Information Gateway. Immunity for reporters of child abuse and neglect. Washington D.C.: U.S. Department of Health and Human Services, Children's Bureau; 2012. Available at: http://www.childwelfare.gov/systemwide/laws_policies/statutes/immunity.pdf. Accessed March 30, 2014.
19. American Academy of Pediatrics Committee on Pediatric Emergency Medicine and Committee on Bioethics. Policy statement–consent for emergency medical services for children and adolescents. Pediatrics 2011;128(2):427–33.
20. American Academy of Pediatrics Committee on Bioethics. Informed consent, parental permission, and assent in pediatric practice. Pediatrics 1995;95(2):314–7.
21. Available at: http://www.law.cornell.edu/wex/table_emancipation. Accessed March 30, 2014.
22. Driggs A. The mature minor doctrine: do adolescents have the right to die? Health Matrix Clevel 2001;11:687–718.
23. Boonstra H, Nash E. Minors and the right to consent to health care. The Guttmacher report on public policy. Available at: http://www.guttmacher.org/pubs/tgr/03/4/gr030404.pdf. Accessed March 30, 2014.
24. Sebilius K. Report to congress on immunity from prosecution for professional consultation in suspected and known instances of child abuse and neglect. 2013. Available at: http://www.acf.hhs.gov/sites/default/files/cb/capta_immunity_rptcongress.pdf. Accessed March 30, 2014.
25. Kellogg N, Lukefahr J, Narang S, American Academy of Pediatrics, Committee on Medical Liability and Child Abuse. Medicolegal issues in pediatrics. 7th edition. Elk Grove Village (IL): American Academy of Pediatrics; 2012.
26. USA Today. Mandatory abuse reporting laws. Available at: http://usatoday30.usatoday.com/news/nation/story/2012-01-02/unreported-child-abuse/51981108/1. Accessed March 30, 2014.

27. American Medical Association. Expert witness testimony: Policy H-265.993. Available at: http://www.aapl.org/AMA_expert_witness.htm. Accessed March 30, 2014.

28. Austin v AANS, 253 F3d 967 (7th Cir 1991); but see Seisinger v Siebel, 220 Ariz. 85; 203 P3d 483 (where the court deemed testimony to not be the practice of medicine).

29. Florida Statutes section 766.102(12) (2011) and Florida Statutes section 458.3175(2011). Available at: http://www.flboardofmedicine.gov/licensing/expert-witness-certificate/. Accessed March 30, 2014.

30. American Association of Neurological Surgeons. Professional conduct: witness testimony. AANS Bul 2006;15(2):3–4. Available at: www.aans.org/bulletin/pdfs/summer06.pdf. Accessed March 30, 2014.

31. 42 USC §1983. Available at: http://www.law.cornell.edu/uscode/text/42/1983. Accessed March 30, 2014.

32. Mohil v Glick, 842 F Supp2nd 1072 (ND Ill 2012).

Foster Care and Healing from Complex Childhood Trauma

Heather Forkey, MD[a],*, Moira Szilagyi, MD, PhD[b]

KEYWORDS

- Foster care • Kinship care • Childhood trauma • Adverse childhood experiences
- Maltreatment • Complex trauma • Toxic stress • Resilience

KEY POINTS

- Children enter foster care after experiencing maltreatment, but also multiple other forms of adversity and trauma, that result in toxic stress.
- Toxic stress alters the architecture and function of the brain and adversely impacts physical health, mental health, cognitive abilities, and response to stressors.
- Complex trauma embodies both the toxic stress children have experienced and their subsequent responses to stressors.
- Foster care may exacerbate rather than ameliorate toxic stress and complex trauma.
- Pediatricians and other professionals caring for this population can help children to heal from toxic stress and complex trauma through developmentally appropriate, trauma-informed practices.

INTRODUCTION: FOSTER CARE AND TRAUMA

Annually, about one quarter of a million children are removed from their families and placed in foster care when the child's health and safety are deemed to be at imminent risk because of maltreatment. Removal of children from their family of origin and admission to foster care is and should be a weighty decision. Foster care is intended to be a temporary, healing refuge for children and families. But, because of the stressors that precipitate removal, the uncertainty, upheaval, and losses associated with placement, and the physiologic responses to these traumas, children in foster care often have a significant health burden. These effects are seen in children placed in various foster settings, with unrelated caregivers or with kin. The pediatrician needs

Disclosures: None.

[a] Foster Children Evaluation Service (FaCES), UMass Children's Medical Center, University of Massachusetts Medical School, 55 Lake Avenue North, Worcester, MA 01655, USA; [b] Division of General Pediatrics, Department of Pediatrics, University of Rochester, 601 Elmwood Avenue, Box 777, Rochester, NY 14642, USA

* Corresponding author.

E-mail address: Heather.Forkey@umassmemorial.org

Pediatr Clin N Am 61 (2014) 1059–1072

http://dx.doi.org/10.1016/j.pcl.2014.06.015

to understand complex childhood trauma and how it affects children and families to provide care that promotes healing and improves outcomes.

EXTENT OF THE PROBLEM: OVERVIEW OF FOSTER CARE

Almost all children entering foster care are placed involuntarily by court order, the vast majority for reasons of maltreatment (70%) in the form of neglect (approximately 70%), physical abuse, sexual abuse, emotional abuse, or abandonment. Neglect of basic nutritional, educational, or medical needs, or lack of supervision, is the most commonly cited reason for placement; child physical and sexual abuse have declined in the recent decades.[1,2] Removal may occur urgently after a first-time report to child protective services, or, at the other extreme, after prolonged involvement with child welfare during which preventive strategies have been exhausted. The remaining 30% of admissions are predominantly teens placed by the courts because of their own behaviors or because parents are seeking mental health services, cannot manage their behaviors, or abandon them. However, careful interview with an adolescent often uncovers a history of maltreatment and adversity.

More than half of a million children spend at least some time in foster care annually. In the last decade, there has been an overall decline of 23% in the foster care population. The overall number of children in foster care on a single day (September 30) declined from 523,616 in 2002 to 399,546 in 2012.[3] The average duration of stay has also decreased from 31.3 to 22.4 months. These shifts occurred as child welfare made efforts to preserve families by diverting them from investigation to in-home support services and by engaging extended families as resources for children who could not safely remain at home. Child welfare also focused on shortening the time to permanency, whether through reunification, kinship care, guardianship, or adoption. Interestingly, these declines occurred despite an increase in child abuse reports and the numbers of children in foster care who had experienced multiple forms of maltreatment and were diagnosed as emotionally disturbed.[4]

Although many children (approximately 50%) cycle through foster care in weeks to months, approximately 10% to 20% remain in the system for years. In 2011, about 50% of children were in care for fewer than 12 months; 17% had been in care for more than 3 years.[5] Approximately 50% of children and teens will experience more than 1 foster care placement, with approximately 25% having 3 or more placements. The largest determinant of duration of stay is the biological family's level of cooperation with the individualized case plan for their family, although minority children, older children, children with severe behavioral and developmental disabilities, and children who are part of large sibling groups are almost twice as likely to remain in care longer.[5–7]

The average age of a child in foster care in 2011 was 9.1 years. Most children live either in nonrelative foster homes or kinship homes. Kinship is often broadly defined not just as relatives by blood or marriage, but other adult caregivers who have an established relationship with the child, such as godparents or family friends. Four percent of children reside in preadoptive homes and 16% live in group home or residential care. The race-ethnicity of children in foster care has changed, although minorities remain overrepresented. In 2011, 26% were black/Non-Hispanic, 21% were Hispanic, and 6% were multiracial. Subsets of children in foster care with unique needs and challenges include the intellectually disabled, the severely mentally ill, pregnant or parenting teens, unaccompanied refugee minors, and those abandoned by their families because of the child's mental health or behavioral issues, or because they are gay, lesbian, bisexual, or transgender. Unaccompanied refugee minors have unique trauma histories as they enter foster care from a variety of countries after surviving war, rape, injury, slave labor, trafficking, or the death of family members.

More than 60% of children exit foster care for reunification with parents or relatives; about 20% are adopted. The 9% who emancipate annually usually do so on their 18th birthday, although legislation including the Chaffee Independence Act of 1999 and Fostering Connections to Success and Increasing Adoptions Act of 2008 have expanded funding to states to allow teens who are in school or job training to remain in foster care until age 21.[8] Overall, the outcomes of youth who emancipate are discouraging. Foster care alumni are likely to be underemployed, undereducated, overrepresented among the homeless, and suffer from significant mental health problems.[9,10]

The outcomes for children who reunify or are adopted are even less clear. There is some literature indicating that children who are adopted or remain in long-term stable foster/kinship care fare better than children who return to parents. About 30% of children who are returned to their families reenter care within 1 year.[11] Approximately 9% to 24% of adoptions disrupt (before finalization) or dissolve (after finalization).[12] Failed adoptions are more common for adolescents, with the child's behavior being the most frequently cited reason.[13]

ETIOLOGY: TOXIC STRESS AND COMPLEX TRAUMA

The National Child Traumatic Stress Network defines complex trauma as encompassing both a child's exposure to multiple traumatic events and the broad, pervasive, and predictable impact this exposure has on the individual child.[14] To develop normally, children need an environment in which a responsive, attuned parent or caregiver meets their needs for adequate care, attention, and protection.[15] Children rely on their parents and caregivers to mediate and buffer the world, and life's stressors. When stressors are overwhelming or when parents are unable to help children buffer them, significant adversities, especially in early childhood, can undermine the development of adaptive capacities and coping skills, emotional well-being, learning, and physical health.[15–17]

We have long known that stress leads to a predictable cascade of neuroendocrine changes that enable the individual to deal with a threat, real or perceived. Shonkoff and Garner[17] delineate 3 types of stress that children experience that impact the development of their brains: positive stress, which promotes and is necessary for healthy adaptation and development; tolerable stress, which children are able to manage with help by protective factors, such as an attuned parent; and toxic stress, which causes a chronic or frequent activation of the child's physiologic stress response system and is not adequately buffered.[17,18] Unlike positive or tolerable stress, toxic stress leads, through the excessive or prolonged activation of physiologic stress response systems, to alterations in gene translation, immune response, and neurodevelopment, resulting in predictable behavioral, learning, and health problems. Those areas of the brain involved in cognition, rational thought, emotional regulation, activity level, attention, impulse control, and executive function are particularly vulnerable, especially in the young child. In addition, although genetic predisposition plays some role in the stress response, early and prior experience can magnify the effect.[18,19] Children in foster care have usually experienced chronic, recurrent, or multiple traumas within a chaotic family environment that lacks sufficient buffering and protection, placing them at high risk for complex trauma.[4,14–18,20]

Poverty contributes significantly to complex trauma. Poverty is a pervasive underlying theme for families whose children enter foster care; the poverty extends beyond the financial to a poverty of social supports and parenting skills necessary to create the nurturing and predictable environment children need to thrive (**Box 1**).

SEQUELAE OF THE PROBLEM: HOW TRAUMA IMPACTS THE HEALTH OF CHILDREN IN FOSTER CARE

The interplay of toxic stress, physiologic response, and behavioral adaptations to stress impact the health of children in childhood and over the life course.[16,18,20–22] In the 1990s, the Adverse Childhood Experience studies began to make the link between childhood toxic stress and poor adult health outcomes, including cardiovascular and pulmonary disease, cancer, asthma, autoimmune disease, and depression.[20,21,23] Exposure to drugs in utero, insufficient prenatal care, prematurity, exposure to environmental toxins, and exposure to HIV, hepatitis, tuberculosis, and other communicable diseases, in addition to chronic neglect, physical, and sexual and emotional abuse, have previously been linked with poor health outcomes for children in foster care, both in the short term and into adulthood.[20] Growing literature has begun to elucidate how toxic stress takes its toll. Immune response, as influenced by the neuroendocrine stress response, leads to biologic changes and adaptations that can acutely and chronically lead to poor health outcomes.

Physical Health

Physical health seems to be impacted by both the toxic stressors and the individual child's physiologic response to stress. In fact, studies over the last 3 decades document that children in foster care have much higher rates of acute and chronic illness than same-aged peers,[24–27] including higher rates of infection, asthma, and obesity. Some problems are the direct result of physical trauma (eg, neurologic sequelae of head trauma), whereas other problems are rooted in complex childhood trauma, the impact on the immune response, and chronic inflammation.

Mental Health

Mental health is the most significant health concern for children in foster placement. Prior studies have described the litany and severity of mental health diagnoses and outcomes for children in foster placement. Two thirds of children in foster placement have mental health problems, and children in foster care use a disproportionate amount of mental health resources, but are probably still underserved in terms of

---

Box 1
Types of poverty experienced by children who enter foster care

Financial poverty: Parents unemployed, underemployed, food insecurity, limited access to health care

Poverty of social supports: Families often from poor neighborhoods, limited community resources, single parent families, lack of extended family

Poverty of parenting skills: Parents with mental illness (46%), active substance abuse (48%), cognitive impairment (10%), parents with history of maltreatment, parenting chaotic and unpredictable

Poverty of education: Little stimulation at home, inadequate daycare and early education options, limited support with school work, inadequate attention to possible special education needs, frequent school changes

Poverty of safety: Exposure to violence (84%), including homes with domestic violence, neighborhoods violent with criminal activity common, schools unsafe

needs [28–33] Diagnoses of attention deficit hyperactivity disorder, oppositional defiant disorder, anxiety, and depression are common, and more than 25% of adolescents leaving foster care have posttraumatic stress disorder (a rate higher than war veterans).[34,35]

The high prevalence of mental health issues makes sense when considered in the context of toxic stress, brain development, and neuroscience. Complex childhood trauma may go inadequately diagnosed and treated. Entry into foster care, instead of ameliorating symptoms, may exacerbate them. The child may confront multiple stressors that reinforce their physiologic stress response (**Box 2**). Trauma symptoms may be confused with other mental health disorders and treated with psychotropic medications (PTMs) that may be ineffective; teens in foster may also abuse drugs as a form of self-medication.[35] Accurate diagnosis and treatment requires that we understand the child's behaviors in the context of how trauma has impacted the developing brain, and that we educate and support their caregivers (**Table 1**).[18]

Cognitive Development and Educational Success

Cognitive development and educational success are also adversely impacted by complex childhood trauma. Children in foster care demonstrate developmental and educational delays at higher rates than their peers, with nearly 60% of children younger than 5 years having delays in communication, problem-solving, and social skills and more than 40% of school-age children in special education for cognitive and/or emotional issues.[36,37] Children enter foster care undereducated, although some children make gains while in the system.[38] Only about one third of teens in foster care graduate from high school by the time they age out of foster care. Fewer than 2% go on to higher education.[9]

CLINICAL ASSESSMENT: PEDIATRIC CARE OF THE TRAUMATIZED CHILD IN FOSTER CARE

Recommendations have been published by the American Academy of Pediatrics to guide health evaluations and health care for children in foster care.[39] These standards provide the framework for the frequency and content of health evaluations. For children whose health has been impacted by complex childhood trauma and caregivers who may be unfamiliar with the physiologic impact these stressors can have on children, interaction with a trauma-informed health care provider can be transformative.

Box 2
Stressors for children in foster care

Changes in placement

Separation from parents, neighborhoods, siblings, friends, and extended family

Change of caseworkers, therapists, and health care providers

Change of school, daycare, church/house of worship

Unrealistic goals on the part of the court or child welfare

Promises the biologic parent cannot keep (ie, promises child will be home soon when timeline is determined by court)

Expectations of foster/kinship parents

Vague and difficult to understand timelines for reunification (ie, "when mom is better")

Capricious nature of changes and decisions

Table 1
Glucocorticoid effect on brain from toxic stress

Brain Area	Function	Neuronal Impact of Excess Glucocorticoid in Toxic Stress	Behavioral Consequence from Toxic Stress
Amygdala	Brain "alarm" Responsible for emotional memory Generates aggressive or impulsive behaviors to protect the body	Amygdala hypertrophy	Aggressive behavior with minimal threat Impulsivity that can mimic ADHD
Hippocampus	Brain "search engine" Allows brain to access information from other brain centers Role in learning and memory	Limits neuronal formation (normally, neuron formation in hippocampus occurs throughout lifespan)	Protective effect of some amnesia about prior trauma Limits learning Negatively impacts educational achievement
Prefrontal cortex	Suppresses impulses and emotion generated by limbic system Executive function: Impulse control, working memory, and cognitive flexibility	Slows synaptic connectivity	Limited ability to suppress aggression Limits ability to think through consequences of actions Can look like ADHD, aggression or oppositional defiant disorder

Abbreviation: ADHD, attention deficit hyperactivity disorder.

These practitioners need to be skilled in recognizing, assessing, managing, treating, and explaining the impact of trauma on the child or teen. Caregivers benefit from information on how to help the child in their home heal. Despite documented histories of complex trauma, physical and behavioral diagnoses have often been applied to children in foster care without much consideration of the impact of that trauma. Even when a complete trauma history is not available for a child or teen, pediatricians and mental health professionals should take the opportunity to reassess previous diagnoses through a trauma lens.

Pediatric providers may experience frustration in caring for children in foster care. They are often accompanied to health appointments by caregivers or caseworkers who are unfamiliar with their health histories, yet they often have tremendous health needs and benefit from longer visits. Coordination of health care services and communication among health providers and with child welfare and caregivers can be improved through the use of an electronic, or, if this is not possible, a paper, health "passport" or summary.

A Physical Health Screen

A physical health screen should be performed at the time of placement in foster care, with a comprehensive health evaluation within 1 month of placement.[33] The initial health screen is important to assess children for evidence of maltreatment, including physical and sexual abuse. A compete examination including the anogenital region should be completed. The documentation of findings at placement assists in appropriate medical treatment and informs foster parents and child welfare about possible injury; the latter may decrease subsequent confusion about the origin of injuries noted after placement. The initial health screen allows for the early identification of acute and contagious illnesses and infestations in need of treatment, thus reducing caregiver distress. The comprehensive health evaluation allows for more detailed assessment of physical, mental, and developmental health, as well as an assessment of the adjustment of the child and caregiver.

Chronic conditions such as asthma, eczema, or allergies[40] are common and the practitioner should factor in the impact of glucocorticoid released in response to toxic stress on the inflammatory response, in addition to smoke exposure, allergens, and insufficient use of preventive medication. It is not uncommon for children to have an acute asthma exacerbation or flare up of other illness at placement or with later transitions.[33] Children also enter foster care with incomplete health histories and without their medications and medical equipment; caseworkers and foster/kinship parents need help understanding a child's medical needs.

Providers should inquire about sleeping, eating, and toileting, because difficulties in these areas are common (**Table 2**). Educating caregivers and children that these are expected responses to trauma should facilitate understanding and an empathic approach to such problems. Discussing routines, teaching simple relaxation techniques, and encouraging nonpunitive caregiver responses may reduce child and caregiver anxiety and help to avoid inappropriate medication use. However, the temporary use of medications such as diphenhydramine or melatonin to promote sleep, when there are significant sleep problems or safety concerns such as night wandering, provides foster/kinship parents time to transition the child to a good sleep hygiene routine while reassuring them that they are safe in their current home. Constipation may need to be medically managed during the transition into foster care while the caregiver introduces an appropriate diet and toileting practices. Describing the use of these medications as temporary supports to assist children in getting past trauma responses enables foster/kinship parents to view them as part of the healing process as children adjust to foster care, rather than ongoing health problems.

Mental Health and Trauma Screening

Mental health and trauma screening can be conducted in the pediatric office but comprehensive evaluations, including a full trauma assessment, are recommended for all children and should be conducted within 30 to 60 days of placement, ideally by a trauma-informed mental health professional. Pediatricians may wish to utilize a validated mental health screen and/or a trauma-specific screening tool to more accurately identify symptoms and those in need of urgent referral.[41,42] Caregivers and caseworkers seldom have much history about children, and birth parents may not be available or forthcoming. The accuracy of extant mental health diagnoses may need to be reassessed in the context of a child's trauma experiences and symptoms; some

Table 2		
Review of systems: Findings common in children exposed to trauma		
Function	**Central Cause**	**Symptom**
Sleep	Stimulation of reticular activating system	Difficulty falling asleep, difficulty staying asleep, nightmares
Eating	Inhibition of satiety center, anxiety	Rapid eating, lack of satiety, food hoarding, not eating
Toileting	Increased sympathetic tone, increased catecholamines	Constipation, encopresis, enuresis

symptoms may be proxies for trauma (eg, attention deficit hyperactivity disorder),[43] although comorbid conditions certainly exist. Assessment for childhood trauma as the cause of symptoms, especially when current treatment is not helpful, allows for consideration of a different, and perhaps more beneficial, treatment plan. Even children who do not seem to need mental health intervention benefit from periodic reassessment of their mental health needs given the uncertainties and losses endemic in foster care.

PTM use is more prevalent in foster care than among other children enrolled in Medicaid. PTMs are often prescribed off-label and in combinations for which there are no indications, leading to concern that many children are receiving these medications inappropriately.[44,45] Although there are well-defined diagnoses for which PTMs can be helpful, medication should be 1 part, when indicated, of a robust mental health treatment plan developed by a mental health professional with expertise in complex childhood trauma. There are several guidelines available to the pediatrician regarding PTM use in the foster care population.[46,47] In general, PTMs are best prescribed by a mental health professional for a specific mental health diagnosis for which it is appropriate treatment; it should then be used in the lowest possible dose with close monitoring for effectiveness and side effects. Polypharmacy is all too common, and should be avoided. If medication is used in the short term to manage severe trauma symptoms, the child's need for medication should be carefully monitored.

Developmental and Educational Assessments

Developmental and educational assessments are recommended because of the adverse impact of complex trauma on learning and memory. The child younger than 6 years in foster care should receive formal developmental screening at admission and at regular intervals thereafter. The use of a validated developmental screener doubles the identification of children at risk for developmental delays and in need of referral.[48,49] Under federal law, children under age 36 months with an adjudicated finding of child abuse or neglect are automatically eligible for Early Intervention evaluation.[50] Likewise, school-aged children in foster care should be referred for educational evaluation, unless there is compelling evidence that they are thriving in school. Federal law now requires child welfare to maintain children in their school of origin, which is advantageous to most children in minimizing school disruption.[51]

APPROACH/MANAGEMENT: TRAUMA-INFORMED CARE
Caregiver and Caseworker Education and Support

Caregiver and caseworker education and support is essential when caring for the child in foster care, because translating knowledge about trauma into the daily care of a specific child is challenging, especially when there are unrealistic expectations about how quickly children will respond. Children exposed to multiple traumas, such as abuse, neglect, and domestic violence, often come to foster care with overwhelming negative beliefs and expectations about themselves as powerless, unlovable, and worthless, and about caregivers as unreliable, unresponsive, and rejecting. These feelings can sabotage new relationships. Caregivers may, in turn, express their own frustration or anger in ways that "prove" the negative expectations children have of themselves and caregivers. By reenacting old relationships, the child may evoke familiar negative reactions from new caregivers, confirming their worldview and reinforcing their behaviors.[52] Children and caregivers may thus escalate into a set of negative interactions that become increasingly more intense and frustrating, and threaten the placement.

To avoid this negative spiral, caregivers are encouraged to remain calm in teaching and parenting the traumatized child. Responding with equanimity and reassurance when the child is overwhelmed can ameliorate the child's view of the world as a hostile place, and, through modeling, promote self-regulation skills. The pediatrician can offer advice about positive parenting strategies, including interactive play, routines, reasonable expectations, gentle reminders, distraction techniques, catching the child being good, reading, attentive listening, teaching, and role modeling. These strategies form the foundations of healing for the traumatized child. Caregivers may need advice on helping children manage transitions, especially around visitation with birth parents. It is normal for a child in foster care to express anger toward the birth parent, to displace that onto foster/kinship parents, to experience conflicted loyalties, and to have an unrealistic desire for reunification with an idealized parent. Caregivers who listen calmly, validate children's emotions without reinforcing them, and reassure the child of the caregiver's commitment and affection are helping children to learn and heal.[53]

Referral to Community Resources

Referral to community resources for mental health, behavioral management, educational support, and developmental services can be helpful to children and families. Child welfare is responsible for helping children and birth parents access services, including mental health, trauma therapy, and parenting education. Good communication with child welfare can ensure a coordinated approach to planning. Respite services are helpful to foster parents, but, without appropriate planning and preparation, may be perceived by the child as another rejection and change in caregivers. Resources are also available through the American Academy of Pediatrics and the National Child Traumatic Stress Network and others to help physicians to guide caregivers (**Table 3**).

Referral of the child (and sometimes the whole family) to appropriate trauma-informed services can provide further support and education for caregivers. A list of evidence-based mental health treatments for traumatized children is available.[54] Evidence-based therapies that help to build caregiver attunement and trust with young children include Parent Child Psychotherapy and Parent-Child Interactive Therapy. When family reunification is the permanency plan for the child, these services are ideally offered to birth parents and their appropriately aged children. Trauma-specific therapy for children over age 5 years includes Trauma Focused Cognitive Behavioral Therapy. For children exposed to multiple types of or frequent or extreme toxic stressors, complex trauma therapies such as Attachment, Self-regulation and Competency Therapy are recommended.

Table 3
Resources for clinicians

Resource	Website
AAP Healthy Foster Care America	www.aap.org/fostercare
National Child Traumatic Stress Network	www.nctsn.org
Center on the Developing Child at Harvard University	www.developingchild.harvard.edu
AAP Medical Home for Children and Adolescents Exposed to Violence	www.aap.org/medhomecev
Child Trauma Academy	www.childtrauma.org
SAMHSA National Center for Trauma-Informed Care	www.samhsa.gov/nctic

Abbreviations: AAP, American Academy of Pediatrics; SAMHSA, Substance Abuse and Mental Health Services Administration.

OUTCOMES: RESILIENCE AND STABILITY

Studies on resiliency and recovery from traumatic experiences are just now accumulating, but early data indicate that children need stability in nurturing and responsive families and communities for healing. Stable families are characterized by mentally healthy caregivers who engage in positive parenting practices and who are constant, consistent, and connected to children over time; the stable family is cohesive, supportive, and flexible, and provides a nurturing and stimulating home environment.[55] The characteristics of stability in foster/kinship families also include respect for a child's sense of belonging in their family of origin and being aware and accepting of and celebrating a child's racial/ethnic heritage. Safety and permanency are fundamental to well-being, but insufficient by themselves. Stability, as described, is also necessary and best achieved through a focus on promoting healthy developmental outcomes and well-being at all ages, because this drives appropriate decisions regarding permanency and safety.

Adolescents are the least likely group in foster care to achieve stability. They have often missed the grounding provided by a healthy childhood that enables them to form a stable identity rooted in self-esteem, a sense of autonomy rooted in self-efficacy, and a larger sense of commitment and comfort in relatedness to peers. However, there is hope even for adolescents in foster care; recent studies concluded that one half of adolescents in foster care can form a secure attachment to a foster parent despite ongoing, insecure attachment to their birth parent[56] and that mentoring relationships can promote better outcomes.[57]

SUMMARY

Understanding the effects of multiple adversities and trauma on the health and development of children is fundamental to helping their foster, kinship, and birth parents to deal constructively with children's grief responses and behaviors. Foster and kinship parents are the major therapeutic intervention available to children in foster care and it is incumbent that child welfare, mental health, and pediatric professionals provide appropriate trauma-informed education, guidance, and support to them. To improve outcomes, we all need to provide care that is trauma informed and developmentally driven, across the age spectrum, to children in foster care.[55,56,58]

REFERENCES

1. Finkelhor D, Turner H, Ormrod R, et al. Trends in childhood violence and abuse exposure: evidence from 2 national surveys. Arch Pediatr Adolesc Med 2010; 164(3):238–42.
2. Finkelhor D, Turner HA, Shattuck A, et al. Violence, crime, and abuse exposure in a national sample of children and youth: an update. JAMA Pediatr 2013; 167(7):614–21.
3. US Department of Health and Human Services Administration on Children Youth and Families. Recent trends in foster care. In: Data brief 2013-1. Available at: http://www.acf.hhs.gov/program/cb/resource/data-brief-trends-in-foster-care-1. Accessed January 6, 2014.
4. Conn AM, Szilagyi MA, Franke TM, et al. Trends in child protection and out-of-home care. Pediatrics 2013;132(4):712–9.
5. US Department of Health and Human Services Administration on Children Youth and Families, Children's Bureau. The AFCARS report; preliminary 2011.

Available at: http://www.acf.hhs.gov/sites/default/files/cb/afcarsreport19.pdf. Accessed January 14, 2014.

6. Szilagyi M. The pediatric role in the care of children in foster and kinship care. Pediatr Rev 2012;33(11):496–507.

7. Child Welfare Information Gateway. Major federal legislation concerned with child protection, child welfare and adoption. In: Adoption and Safe Families Act of 1997: Public Law 105–89: H. R. 867. Available at: https://www.child welfare.gov/systemwide/mentalhealth/common/grief.cfm. Accessed January 6, 2014.

8. Pergamit M, McDaniel M, Hawkins A. Housing assistance for youth who have aged out of foster care: the role of the Chaffee Foster Care Independence Program. In: Education Urban Institute for the U. S. Department of Health and Human Services, Office of the Assistant Secretary for Planning and Evaluation. 2012. Available at: http://aspe.hhs.gov/hsp/12/chafeefostercare/rpt.shtml. Accessed February 25, 2014.

9. Pecora PJ, Kessler RC, O'Brien K, et al. Educational and employment outcomes of adults formerly placed in foster care: Results from the Northwest Foster Care Alumni Study. Child Youth Serv Rev 2006;28:1459–81.

10. Thoma R. A critical look at the foster care system: foster care outcomes. Available at: http://www.liftingtheveil.org/foster14.htm. Accessed January 22, 2014.

11. Wulczyn F. Family reunification. Future Child 2004;14(1):95–113.

12. Child Welfare Information Gateway. Adoption disruption and dissolution. Washington, DC: U. S. Department of Health and Human Services, Children's Bureau; 2012. Available at: https://www.childwelfare.gov/pubs/s_disrup.pdf. Accessed February 25, 2014.

13. Rushton A, Dance C. The adoption of children from public care: a prospective study of outcome in adolescence. J Am Acad Child Adolesc Psychiatry 2006; 45(7):877–83.

14. National Child Traumatic Stress Network. Complex trauma. Available at: http://www.nctsn.org/trauma-types/complex-trauma. Accessed January 17, 2014.

15. Center on the Developing Child. Science of early childhood. Available at: http://developingchild.harvard.edu/topics/science_of_early_childhood/. Accessed January 22, 2014.

16. Garner AS, Shonkoff JP. Early childhood adversity, toxic stress, and the role of the pediatrician: translating developmental science into lifelong health. Pediatrics 2012;129(1):e224–31.

17. Shonkoff JP, Garner AS. The lifelong effects of early childhood adversity and toxic stress. Pediatrics 2012;129(1):e232–46.

18. Garner AS. Home visiting and the biology of toxic stress: opportunities to address early childhood adversity. Pediatrics 2013;132(2 Suppl):S65–73.

19. Ouellet-Morin I, Boivin M, Dionne G, et al. Variations in heritability of cortisol reactivity to stress as a function of early familial adversity among 19-month-old twins. Arch Gen Psychiatry 2008;65(2):211–8.

20. Anda RF, Felitti VJ, Bremner JD, et al. The enduring effects of abuse and related adverse experiences in childhood - a convergence of evidence from neurobiology and epidemiology. Eur Arch Psychiatry Clin Neurosci 2006;256(3): 174–86.

21. Felitti VJ, Anda RF, Nordenberg D, et al. Relationship of childhood abuse and household dysfunction to many of the leading causes of death in adults. The Adverse Childhood Experiences (ACE) study. Am J Prev Med 1998;14(4): 245–58.

22. Johnson SB, Riley AW, Granger DA, et al. The science of early life toxic stress for pediatric practice and advocacy. Pediatrics 2013;131(2):319–27.
23. Felitti VJ. Adverse childhood experiences and adult health. Acad Pediatr 2009; 9(3):131–2.
24. Steele JS, Buchi KF. Medical and mental health of children entering the Utah foster care system. Pediatrics 2008;122(3):e703–9.
25. Halfon N, Mendonca A, Berkowitz G. Health status of children in foster care. The experience of the center for the vulnerable child. Arch Pediatr Adolesc Med 1995;149(4):386–92.
26. Simms MD. The foster care clinic: a community program to identify treatment needs of children in foster care. J Dev Behav Pediatriatr 1989;10(3):121–8.
27. Chernoff R, Combs-Orme T, Risley-Curtiss C, et al. Assessing the health status of children entering foster care. Pediatrics 1994;93(4):594–601.
28. dosReis S, Zito JM, Safer DJ, et al. Mental health services for youths in foster care and disabled youths. Am J Public Health 2001;91(7):1094–9.
29. Harman JS, Childs GE, Kelleher KJ. Mental health care utilization and expenditures by children in foster care. Arch Pediatr Adolesc Med 2000;154(11): 1114–7.
30. Heneghan A, Stein RE, Hurlburt MS, et al. Mental health problems in teens investigated by U.S. child welfare agencies. J Adolesc Health 2013;52(5):634–40.
31. Horwitz SM, Hurlburt MS, Goldhaber-Fiebert JD, et al. Mental health services use by children investigated by child welfare agencies. Pediatrics 2012; 130(5):861–9.
32. McCue Horwitz S, Hurlburt MS, Heneghan A, et al. Mental health problems in young children investigated by U.S. child welfare agencies. J Am Acad Child Adolesc Psychiatry 2012;51(6):572–81.
33. Takayama JI, Wolfe E, Coulter KP. Relationship between reason for placement and medical findings among children in foster care. Pediatrics 1998;101(2):201–7.
34. Pecora PJ, Kessler RC, Williams J, et al. Improving family foster care: findings from the Northwest Foster Care Alumni Study. 2005. Available at: http://www.casey.org/Resources/Publications/pdf/ImprovingFamilyFosterCare_FR.pdf. Accessed January 19, 2014.
35. Courtney M, Dworsky A. Midwest evaluation of the adult functioning of former foster youth. Outcomes at age 19. In: Executive summary. 2005. Available at: http://www.chapinhall.org/sites/default/files/ChapinHallDocument_3.pdf.   Accessed January 17, 2014.
36. Jee SH, Conn AM, Szilagyi PG, et al. Identification of social-emotional problems among young children in foster care. J Child Psychol Psychiatry 2010;51(12): 1351–8.
37. Jee SH, Conn KM, Nilsen WJ, et al. Learning difficulties among children separated from a parent. Ambul Pediatr 2008;8(3):163–8.
38. Simms MD, Dubowitz H, Szilagyi MA. Health care needs of children in the foster care system. Pediatrics 2000;106(4 Suppl):909–18.
39. American Academy of Pediatrics. Healthy Foster Care America: health issues and needs. Available at: http://www.aap.org/en-us/advocacy-and-policy/aap-health-initiatives/healthy-foster-care-america/Pages/Health-Issues.aspx.   Accessed January 22, 2014.
40. Jee SH, Barth RP, Szilagyi MA, et al. Factors associated with chronic conditions among children in foster care. J Health Care Poor Underserved 2006;17(2): 328–41.

41. Jee SH, Halterman JS, Szilagyi M, et al. Use of a brief standardized screening instrument in a primary care setting to enhance detection of social-emotional problems among youth in foster care. Acad Pediatr 2011;11(5):409–13.
42. Forkey H, Morgan W, Schwartz K, et al. Trauma screening in a pediatric health clinic for foster children. Presented at: American Academy of Pediatrics National Conference and Exhibition. New Orleans, LA, October 20–23, 2012.
43. Webb E. Poverty, maltreatment and attention deficit hyperactivity disorder. Arch Dis Child 2013;98(6):397–400.
44. Raghavan R, McMillen JC. Use of multiple psychotropic medications among adolescents aging out of foster care. Psychiatr Serv 2008;59(9):1052–5.
45. Zito JM, Safer DJ, Sai D, et al. Psychotropic medication patterns among youth in foster care. Pediatrics 2008;121(1):e157–63.
46. Child Welfare Information Gateway, U.S. Department of Health and Human Services, Children's Bureau. Use of psychotropic mediations: state and local examples. Available at: https://www.childwelfare.gov/systemwide/mentalhealth/effectiveness/pmslexamples.cfm. Accessed January 20, 2014.
47. American Academy of Child and Adolescent Psychiatry. A guide for community child serving agencies on psychotropic medications for children and adolescents. 2012. Available at: http://www.aacap.org/App_Themes/AACAP/docs/Advocacy/policy_resources/Psychopharm_in_SOC_Feb_2012.pdf. Accessed February 17, 2014.
48. American Academy of Pediatrics. Committee on Early Childhood and Adoption and Dependent Care. Developmental issues for young children in foster care. Pediatrics 2000;106(5):1145–50.
49. Leslie LK, Gordon JN, Lambros K, et al. Addressing the developmental and mental health needs of young children in foster care. J Dev Behav Pediatr 2005;26(2):140–51.
50. US Department of Health and Human Services, Administration on Children Youth and Families, Children's Bureau. The Child Abuse Prevention and Treatment Act (CAPTA). 2010. Available at: http://www.acf.hhs.gov/sites/default/files/cb/capta2010.pdf. Accessed January 5, 2014.
51. US Department of Education. McKinney-Vento Homeless Education Assistance Improvements Act of 2001. Available at: http://www2.ed.gov/policy/elsec/leg/esea02/pg116.html. Accessed January 24, 2014.
52. National Child Traumatic Stress Network. Child welfare trauma training toolkit: the invisible suitcase. 2008. Available at: http://www.nctsnet.org/nctsn_assets/pdfs/CWT3_SHO_Suitcase.pdf. Accessed January 4, 2014.
53. American Academy of Pediatrics. Helping foster and adoptive families cope with trauma. 2013. Available at: http://www.aap.org/en-us/advocacy-and-policy/aap-health-initiatives/healthy-foster-care-america/Pages/Trauma-Guide.aspx. Accessed January 23, 2014.
54. National Child Traumatic Stress Network. National child traumatic stress network empirically supported treatments and promising practices. Available at: http://www.nctsn.org/resources/topics/treatments-that-work/promising-practices. Accessed January 7, 2014.
55. Harden BJ. Safety and stability for foster children: a developmental perspective. Future Child 2004;14(1):30–47.
56. Joseph MA, O'Connor TG, Briskman JA, et al. The formation of secure new attachments by children who were maltreated: an observational study of adolescents in foster care. Dev Psychopathol 2014;26(1):67–80.

57. Taussig HN, Culhane SE, Hettleman D. Fostering healthy futures: an innovative preventive intervention for preadolescent youth in out-of-home care. Child Welfare 2007;86(5):113–31.

58. Zeanah CH, Shauffer C, Dozier M. Foster care for young children: why it must be developmentally informed. J Am Acad Child Adolesc Psychiatry 2011;50(12): 1199–201.

Advocacy Opportunities for Pediatricians Caring for Maltreated Children

James E. Crawford-Jakubiak, MD

KEYWORDS

- Advocacy • Child maltreatment • Expert testimony • Multidisciplinary collaborations
- Education

KEY POINTS

- The many ways that pediatricians educate, support, and provide clinical care for children and families in the course of their clinical practice related to child maltreatment are critical, yet often unrecognized, forms of advocacy.
- Engaging in traditional legislative advocacy to advance policies and programs related to the prevention of or the response to child maltreatment remains a fundamental area for advocacy by pediatricians.
- Pediatricians play a critical role when engaging in collaborative work with community partners related to the prevention of or the response to child maltreatment.
- Pediatricians must be willing to provide expert medical testimony regarding child maltreatment in courtroom settings in a responsible, objective manner.
- Pediatricians must recognize the potential impact of vicarious trauma when working as advocates for maltreated children.

INTRODUCTION

An advocate is often defined as a person who intercedes on behalf of another. Pediatricians, at their core, are essentially advocates for children. Most discussions related to pediatricians engaged in advocacy activities related to child maltreatment focus primarily on work done in the legislative and public policy arenas, with little or no attention paid to other areas in which advocacy occurs. Given that only a relatively small percentage of pediatricians actively participate in the legislative process, one could be left with the false impression that few pediatricians actively engage in activities or behaviors that could be characterized as advocacy.[1] There are many opportunities for pediatricians to act as advocates with regard to the health, safety, and welfare of

Center for Child Protection, UCSF Benioff Children's Hospital Oakland, 747 52nd Street, Oakland, CA 94609, USA
E-mail address: JCrawford@mail.cho.org

Pediatr Clin N Am 61 (2014) 1073–1083
http://dx.doi.org/10.1016/j.pcl.2014.06.017   **pediatric.theclinics.com**

maltreated children that may not have been clearly acknowledged as such in the past. This discussion reviews how general pediatricians can engage in advocacy activities on behalf of maltreated children by

- Recognizing and responding to child maltreatment in a clinical setting
- Appropriately reporting suspicions of child maltreatment
- Working collaboratively with outside agencies as cases of possible child maltreatment are investigated
- Providing support to children and families when child maltreatment is suspected or identified
- Providing education related to issues concerning the maltreatment of children
- Participating in the development of policies and legislation at local, state, and national levels
- Recognizing how pediatricians can be personally affected by the maltreatment their patients experience and how this can impact their ability to provide effective care

Child maltreatment is a diagnosis that can be difficult to make, and responding to it can be even more difficult. It is these fundamental difficulties that make a willingness to consider that any patient, from any family, could potentially be impacted by child maltreatment an act of advocacy in and of itself.

SCOPE OF THE PROBLEM AND WHY ADVOCACY BY PEDIATRICIANS REMAINS ESSENTIAL

The US Department of Health and Human Services reported that in 2012, child protective services (CPS) agencies received an estimated 3.4 million reports of suspected child maltreatment, involving approximately 6.3 million children; 60% of these reports were made by professionals. Most of the reports from professionals come from teachers (approximately 16%); physicians have generally been responsible for approximately 8% of reports.[2] The most common form of maltreatment was neglect, followed by physical abuse, sexual abuse, and psychological maltreatment. Many children experience more than one form of maltreatment, or more than one episode of maltreatment. There were 678,810 children who were substantiated as being maltreated in 2012. It is estimated that at least 1640 children died from abuse during 2012 in the United States, although it is likely that between 50% and 60% of child fatalities due to maltreatment are not recorded as such on death certificates.[2] Child maltreatment has both immediate as well as long-term impacts on children and the adults they become. The cost to individuals, families, communities, and society as a whole is enormous.[3–6] The estimated lifetime economic cost resulting from new cases of child maltreatment from a single year is more than $120 billion.[7]

In addition to their direct contact with children and families, pediatricians work collaboratively with a broad range of medical as well as nonmedical professionals who can impact the health, development, and safety of children. Consequently, pediatricians are in a unique position to affect how children can be protected, and how abuse and neglect are recognized and responded to in a wide range of settings.

ADVOCACY WITHIN A MEDICAL SETTING

The most effective form of advocacy that most pediatricians will engage in with regard to child abuse and neglect is by being highly skilled doctors who are familiar with the resources of their communities, provide excellent clinical care to children and families, and know how to recognize child maltreatment and what to do when they encounter it. The day-to-day, year-to-year relationships that pediatricians develop with children and families allow them to not only see and diagnose maltreatment in the office setting, but also to learn about and respond to problems that are occurring in the home as well as other circumstances that may place a child at risk of abuse or neglect. Additionally, pediatricians work closely with other service providers, both medical and nonmedical, and are in a position to effectively advocate on behalf of children and families so that they can engage with services that can help promote the health and welfare of children.

A willingness to consider that child maltreatment may be an appropriate addition to a particular differential diagnosis is, by definition, necessary to diagnose child maltreatment. By recognizing that any patient could potentially be abused and that pediatricians need to respond appropriately when the problem presents itself, pediatricians are advocating for patients. Making a diagnosis of child abuse can create significant tensions between the family and the pediatrician, consume significant amounts of time and other resources in an office, and may require that the pediatrician communicate with CPS and law enforcement and potentially appear in court. Recognizing the importance of all of these activities, and being willing to engage in them despite the difficulties, are important forms of advocacy. The various forms of child maltreatment manifest from a wide variety of circumstances, risk factors, and events. Each form of maltreatment presents with its own unique management challenges, as well as different ways that pediatricians can advocate for their patients.

PHYSICAL ABUSE

Pediatricians recognize that injuries, including injuries caused by physical abuse, can potentially happen to any child, in any family. With most other types of medical conditions, a diagnosis is made in the context of parents or other care providers who give histories that are as accurate and as truthful as possible. One of the common elements in physical abuse cases is that the historical information provided by caregivers may be compromised: the history may be omitted, modified, or simply be a lie. The diagnosis of physical abuse is often made despite attempts to hide the injury, or the true cause of the injury, from a pediatrician.

Some cases of possible physical abuse may be missed due to the nonspecific nature of the symptoms, whereas others may be missed because the significance of the physical finding may not be recognized due to a lack of history. For example, most infants who present with fussiness and vomiting have some underlying medical problem as the cause of their symptoms, but some have occult trauma.[8,9] A willingness to include and keep child maltreatment on a differential diagnosis allows pediatricians to provide medical care that ensures the fewest missed diagnoses of child abuse.

Advocacy related to assessing for possible physical abuse includes obtaining and documenting a thorough history. Although documentation in medical records regarding the history is often terse, in cases of possible child abuse, it is appropriate to expand on the history that is being recorded. Pediatricians are often the first care providers to evaluate a child who has an abusive injury. The initial history obtained by the pediatrician may prove to be very important as the evaluation for possible abuse unfolds. It is critical to get specific details as to how/when/where an injury reportedly occurred, using follow-up questions as needed. Taking the time to collect the history and document it in the medical record is a critical opportunity to advocate for the child's welfare.

Although focused examinations of patients based on the chief complaint constitute a significant proportion of physical examinations done in a general pediatrician's office, recognition of child abuse often requires a more comprehensive examination. Taking the additional time to fully undress a potentially injured infant who presents with "fussiness and vomiting" might reveal bruising hidden under clothes or a diaper, or point tenderness on an extremity overlying an undiagnosed fracture. Certain areas of the body, such as the front and back of the pinnae, the inside of the mouth, and inner aspects of the lips, may be injured but are unlikely to be recognized as such without specifically looking for injury at those sites. Injuries at these sites would raise a concern of possible abuse, especially in young/nonambulatory children.

In situations in which a concern for occult trauma is present, or when trauma has been recognized, but the history provided is troubling for some reason, it is often appropriate to obtain additional imaging studies or laboratory tests. Pediatricians are sometimes reluctant to order such studies. A skeletal survey in a child younger than 2 years who has a concerning injury or presentation has great value, as it may reveal occult injury.[10,11] Obtaining a repeat skeletal survey 2 or 3 weeks after the initial study can potentially identify injuries that had not been recognized on the initial study.[12] Skeletal surveys also can assist in identifying previously unrecognized bone abnormalities related to metabolic disease, dysplasia, and so forth. Pediatricians should get confirmation from the radiologists who are reading the skeletal survey that "babygrams" or other limited surveys are not being done, and that the recommended imaging studies from the American College of Radiology are being obtained. This is particularly important if the study is being conducted at a location that conducts primarily adult imaging studies.[13,14]

Children will sometimes present with unintentional injuries that may for some reason (eg, severity, unusual nature) raise strong concerns for abuse. Ensuring that such mimics of child abuse are recognized as such is a vital role of the pediatrician. A complete history of the events that reportedly resulted in injury may reveal information that assists in recognizing that an injury occurred due to a previously unacknowledged accidental event. A comprehensive evaluation looking for an underlying medical issue that may be causing or contributing to an apparent injury is essential in cases of possible physical abuse. A thorough review of all relevant past medical history and family history should be conducted. Referring a child to a subspecialist, such as a hematologist, endocrinologist, or a child abuse pediatrician, for further evaluation may be very helpful in distinguishing cases of child maltreatment from mimics of abuse.

SEXUAL ABUSE

Few medical diagnoses cause as much anxiety to pediatricians as a diagnosis of sexual abuse. Responding to the needs of children who have been sexually abused can be extremely stressful and take a disproportionate amount of physician and staff time. When children present to a pediatrician's office with a disclosure of sexual abuse, the family typically does not view the pediatrician as their adversary. The family is often specifically seeking out the pediatrician as an advocate, looking to the pediatrician as an ally to assist with the protection of the child and to respond to the crisis the family is facing. In the context of a busy office practice, pediatricians need to conduct their clinical evaluation, assess the child's safety and mental health needs, consider their reporting requirement to CPS and/or law enforcement, and finally, assess whether a forensic examination and/or evidence collection might be indicated. The American Academy of Pediatrics (AAP) provides recommendations regarding the management of suspected sexual abuse in the primary care setting.[15]

The pediatrician plays an instrumental role in determining how, when, and by whom a physical examination should be done on a child who discloses that sexual abuse has occurred. The specific information from the history related to the nature of the abuse, the time frame in which it occurred, and the presence of any other current problems will direct the pediatrician to advocate for the most appropriate medical evaluation. Although most sexually abused children have unremarkable physical examinations,[16] do not contract sexually transmitted infections, or become pregnant, there is still significant benefit for children who disclose sexual abuse to have a formal medical evaluation.

Formal "forensic" or "evidentiary" medical evaluations are often appropriate when children disclose sexual abuse that has happened recently. Many communities have developed clear protocols and teams to which children are referred for these types of examinations.[17] Pediatricians can help to alleviate the anxiety of both children and parents by helping them to understand more about what the examination does and does not entail. Children who disclose nonacute sexual abuse also can benefit from a formal medical assessment. Regardless of when or where the examination occurs, detailed descriptions of the anatomy should be included in the medical record. It is suggested that pediatricians should request a review by an expert clinician of any abnormal finding to ensure that findings are interpreted correctly.[18,19]

Many clinicians use the examination as a "therapeutic examination," as it presents an opportunity to ensure that children hear that regardless of what happened to them, their body still looks "normal" and did not "get changed" by what happened to them. In the relatively uncommon instances in which a child did sustain a significant injury, the pediatrician can specifically address what the injury was, and how it may or may not affect the child in the future. Giving the child some degree of control over what happens during the examination (eg, the order that various parts of the body are examined) can assist in returning to the child a sense of control over what happens to his or her body. Children as well as parents may have questions and fears about infections, pregnancy, or sexual identity that the pediatrician can address. Finally, pediatricians have an opportunity to assess for other needs that the family may have, particularly related to the mental health of parents, siblings, or other family members.

NEGLECT

Neglect is by far the most common substantiated form of child maltreatment in the United States.[2] Neglect involves instances in which a child's basic needs are not met, often with regard to medical care, physical needs, emotional needs, or supervisory needs. The consequences of serious neglect can be devastating, causing both short-term and long-term health consequences, which in some instances can include death. Some forms of neglect can result in impaired brain development, as well as the development of significant emotional and cognitive problems.[20] Most state laws identify parents or legal caregivers as the primary party who is responsible for "omissions of care." Most instances of neglect involve a highly complex interplay between a variety of contributing factors. In instances in which a concern about neglect is identified, pediatricians have an opportunity to act as advocates not only for the child, but also for the parents and family.[21] The heterogeneity of the ways neglect manifests itself requires the pediatrician to be thoughtful and resourceful about both the identification as well as the interventions that are considered.[22] Whether a child experienced potential harm (child left unsupervised in a kitchen with an open flame on the stove) versus actual harm (child sustained a burn injury after playing with fire while unsupervised) is a key determination that a pediatrician needs to make. This will directly impact the reporting decisions that may need to be made, the management, and how best to advocate for the child and family. Pediatricians should make themselves very familiar with the local resources that may be available when various types of neglect are identified. The least intrusive interventions should be tried first. If initial efforts prove to be unsuccessful, or if the immediate risk to the child is too great, it may become necessary to involve CPS.[21,23]

Dr Howard Dubowitz, a leading expert on neglect, summarized the myriad opportunities for advocacy on the part of pediatricians when there is a concern about neglect:

> *Advocacy on behalf of children and families can be to individuals, families, communities and the society. Explaining to a parent that a hyperactive toddler is normal, albeit challenging, and offering alternatives to corporal punishment, illustrates advocacy on behalf of the child. Encouraging a depressed mother to accept treatment is also advocacy. Physicians' efforts to strengthen families, such as encouraging fathers' involvement in childcare, are forms of advocacy. In the community, physicians can be influential advocates for resources for children and families by, for example, supporting parenting programs.[20]*

REPORTING CASES OF SUSPECTED CHILD MALTREATMENT

Pediatricians are legally mandated reporters of suspected abuse and neglect in all states and territories within the United States. The threshold established by the reporting requirement is reasonable suspicion, not certainty. Pediatricians are sometimes reluctant to report suspicions of abuse for a variety of reasons.[24,25] The specific facts of each case need to be thoughtfully assessed when making a decision of whether to report or not. Ensuring the health, welfare, and safety of the child is the primary reason that the reporting mandates have a low threshold. In the United States, mandated reporters who make a report in good faith are protected against liability for having made the report.[26] Disclosures of sexual abuse made by a child do not need "corroboration" (ie, identification of physical findings) to be considered credible or reportable. Pediatricians who adhere to reporting requirements when suspected maltreatment is identified are acting in the best interests of the child.

WORKING COLLABORATIVELY WITH NONMEDICAL PROFESSIONALS

When a report is made in cases of suspected maltreatment, pediatricians often need to interact with investigators from CPS, law enforcement, or other investigative agencies. For many pediatricians, this is an uncommon occurrence, and may be something they have never done before. Some pediatricians may have a very low comfort level about "getting involved" beyond making a mandated report. The ability of investigators to effectively do their jobs is directly impacted by their ability to get necessary medical information from health care providers related to the issue of possible abuse or neglect. Although it is not the role of the physicians to determine who caused an injury, they often have important information to contribute regarding mechanism of injury, timing of injury, developmental issues related to an injury, how commonly a specific injury is or is not seen in accidents, or other types of information that may be known only to the pediatrician. If a pediatrician is not willing to assist an investigator with the medical questions that arise, the child's safety could be at risk. Pediatricians should not feel compelled to offer opinions beyond their level of expertise. If questions arise that a pediatrician feels is beyond his or her level of expertise, the pediatrician should assist in identifying a specialist who can better aid the investigator.

COURTROOM TESTIMONY

Health care providers, pediatricians in particular, are routinely asked to provide medical testimony in a courtroom setting related to the medical aspects of a possible child abuse case. Medical testimony is often essential in child abuse cases, as the children involved may be too young to talk, or incapable of testifying. Medical testimony puts the medical evidence into context so the trier of fact can understand how it is relevant to the case.[27] The pediatrician can enable the trier of fact (judge or jury) to fully understand such issues as the following:

- The extent and nature of the injuries
- The mechanism(s) involved that caused the injuries
- Whether the physical findings identified are consistent with the history that has been provided
- Timing of the injury
- Whether or not an underlying medical problem caused or contributed to the injury
- Relevant child developmental issues

It is the responsibility of each physician who is testifying to ensure that the opinions that he or she is offering are based on "good medicine," are as free from bias as possible, have scientific validity, and provide "balanced objectivity."[28,29] Pediatricians should clearly and completely explain the basis for the opinion being given.[27] Medical witnesses should provide expert medical testimony only on topics that they truly have the training and experience to qualify as experts. Effectively responding to the needs and welfare of a child does not mean that a pediatrician is not able to give objective and accurate medical testimony. Although for many pediatricians the idea of testifying in a courtroom elicits great anxiety, it is essential that pediatricians are willing and prepared to testify in cases of possible child abuse.

EDUCATION

Pediatricians have countless opportunities to engage with others as advocates/educators with regard child abuse and neglect.

- Children: every interaction with patients is an opportunity to engage with them about safety, boundaries, and resources and to remind them that their pediatrician's goal is to make sure that they are safe, well cared for and healthy.
- Parents: visits offer pediatricians an opportunity to educate about problems that may put their children at risk of injury/abuse and resources for services that may be available.
- Families: ask families specifically, "As your pediatrician, what specifically can I do to help you and the family right now?"
- Community agencies: work with relevant community agencies to raise awareness regarding the benefits of multidisciplinary collaboration related to the health and welfare of maltreated children in the community.
- Medical colleagues: engage with colleagues to foster a broader awareness of the issues related to child abuse and neglect to improve recognition, evaluation, and management.
- Self: ensure that the pediatrician participates in educational activities related to child maltreatment. Remain active in the community to stay aware of community programs, as well as other resources for maltreated children or at-risk families.

ADVOCATING FOR YOUTH IN FOSTER CARE

Hundreds of thousands of children in the United States are in foster care at any given time. The AAP's Executive Summary on the health of youth in foster care states, "Youth in foster care have a higher prevalence of physical, developmental, dental, and behavioral health conditions than any other group of children. Typically these health conditions are chronic, underidentified, and undertreated and have an ongoing impact on all aspects of their lives, even long after these children and adolescents have left the foster care system."[30] Few jurisdictions have had the resources to develop formal medical programs to provide services to their youth in foster care. Pediatricians can provide a great service to these children by learning more about how the community's systems function regarding the provision of health care services for children in foster care. The AAP has developed comprehensive recommendations related to the medical needs of these children that are far too detailed to summarize in this section. There are many opportunities for advocacy related to this population of children and adolescents.[30]

ADVOCACY OPPORTUNITIES RELATED TO THE DEVELOPMENT OF POLICY AND LEGISLATION

Pediatricians have many opportunities to impact the health and welfare of maltreated children by becoming involved in the development of policies and/or legislation at local, state, and national levels. All pediatricians can impact their own practices or institutions by ensuring that there are clear policies in place related to the recognition of and response to concerns of child maltreatment. They can ensure that they and their colleagues are familiar with the specific resources that exist in their medical communities before a need to access them arises. Pediatricians can work with their medical and nonmedical colleagues to develop local policies that encourage multidisciplinary approaches to child maltreatment.

Many pediatricians, individually or as part of their local medical society or state chapter of the AAP, have become very involved at the state level as policies and legislation that address child maltreatment are developed. Similarly, pediatricians have the opportunity to effect change at a national level, often by contributing their efforts as part of larger organizations, such as the AAP.

VICARIOUS TRAUMA AND THE DEVELOPMENT OF RESILIENCY

For pediatricians to consistently and effectively engage in the advocacy activities previously discussed, it is essential that they also advocate for themselves. Although providing care for children who have experienced abuse or neglect can be extremely rewarding for pediatricians, the stress, anxiety, and conflict can be challenging and place the pediatrician at risk of vicarious trauma, and over time, symptoms of burnout or compassion fatigue. Vicarious trauma is a phenomenon initially recognized by mental health providers, but is now understood to affect others who provide care to traumatized patients, where the provider becomes adversely affected through their ongoing empathic connections with traumatized patients. Unchecked, this phenomenon can result in responses similar to posttraumatic stress disorder in providers. Problems, such as burnout and compassion fatigue, can occur as well, which can impair or otherwise impact the pediatrician's ability to engage in advocacy activities.[31]

Self-care is necessary to maximize one's ability to continue to provide care in the challenging situations that child abuse cases present. Many health care professionals recommend that providers

- Take care of themselves
- Pay attention to their own needs and feelings
- Establish and maintain connections
- Avoid viewing problems as impossible
- Respond to adverse situations rather than wish they would "go away"
- Maintain a hopeful outlook
- Nurture a positive view of themselves[32]

The concept of resilience involves maintaining flexibility and balance in one's life as one deals with stressful circumstances and traumatic events, including the following:

- Letting one's self experience strong emotions and also realizing when one may need to avoid such experiences to continue functioning
- Spending time with loved ones to gain support and encouragement and also nurturing one's self
- Relying on others and also relying on one's self
- Seeking professional help if the circumstances warrant it[32]

SUMMARY

Pediatricians are advocates for children. It is one of the central elements of the job description. In the course of their work, pediatricians have many opportunities to advocate for abused and neglected children. Advocacy for these children is not limited to legislative advocacy at state and federal levels. The most effective form of advocacy that most pediatricians will engage in with regard to child abuse and neglect is by being highly skilled doctors who provide excellent clinical care to children and families, knowing how to recognize child abuse and what to do when they encounter it, and being familiar with the resources of their communities. The day-to-day, year-after-year relationships pediatricians develop with children and families allow pediatricians to engage in these most critical forms of advocacy.

REFERENCES

1. Bross DC, Krugman RD. Child maltreatment law and policy as a foundation for child advocacy. Pediatr Clin North Am 2009;56:429–39.
2. U.S. Department of Health and Human Services: Administration for Children and Families. Child Maltreatment. 2012. Available at: http://www.acf.hhs.gov/sites/default/files/cb/cm2012.pdf. Accessed January 15, 2014.
3. Libby AM, Sills MR, Thurston NK, et al. Costs of childhood physical abuse: comparing inflicted and unintentional traumatic brain injuries. Pediatrics 2003;112(1):58–65.
4. Johnson SB, Riley AW, Granger DA, et al. The science of early life toxic stress for pediatric practice and advocacy. Pediatrics 2013;131(2):319–27.
5. Bonomi AE, Anderson ML, Rivara FP, et al. Health care utilization and costs associated with childhood abuse. J Gen Intern Med 2008;23(3):294–9.
6. Corwin DL, Keeshin BR. Estimating present and future damages following child maltreatment. Child Adolesc Psychiatr Clin N Am 2011;20(3):505–18.

7. Fang X, Brown DS, Florence CS, et al. The economic burden of child maltreatment in the United States and implications for prevention. Child Abuse Negl 2012;36:156–65.

8. Jenny C, Hymel KP, Ritzen A, et al. Analysis of missed cases of abusive head trauma. JAMA 1999;281(7):621–6.

9. Tilak GS, Pollock AN. Missed opportunities in fatal child abuse. Pediatr Emerg Care 2013;29(5):685–7.

10. American Academy of Pediatrics. Diagnostic imaging of child abuse. Pediatrics 2009;123(5):1430–5.

11. Duffy SO, Squires J, Fromkin JB, et al. Use of skeletal surveys to evaluate for physical abuse: analysis of 703 consecutive skeletal surveys. Pediatrics 2011; 127(1):e47–52.

12. Harper NS, Eddleman S, Lindberg DM, et al. The utility of follow-up skeletal surveys in child abuse. Pediatrics 2013;131(3):e672–8.

13. American College of Radiology. ACR practice guideline for skeletal surveys in children (Res. 54). In: American College of Radiology. ACR standards. Reston (VA): American College of Radiology; 2011. Available at: http://www.acr.org/~/media/ACR/Documents/PGTS/guidelines/Skeletal_Surveys.pdf.

14. Flaherty EG, Perez-Rossello JM, Levine MA, et al. Evaluating children with fractures for child physical abuse. Pediatrics 2014;133(2):e477–89.

15. American Academy of Pediatrics. The evaluation of children in the primary care setting when sexual abuse is suspected. Pediatrics 2013;132(2):e558–67.

16. Anderst J, Kellogg N, Jung I. Reports of repetitive penile-genital penetration often have no definitive evidence of penetration. Pediatrics 2009;124(3):e403–9.

17. Thackeray JD, Hornor G, Benzinger EA, et al. Forensic evidence collection and DNA identification in acute child sexual assault. Pediatrics 2011;128(2):227–32.

18. Adams JA, Kaplan RA, Starling SP, et al. Guidelines for medical care of children who may have been sexually abused. J Pediatr Adolesc Gynecol 2007;20(3): 163–72.

19. Adams JA. Guidelines for medical care of children evaluated for suspected sexual abuse: an update for 2008. Curr Opin Obstet Gynecol 2008;20(5):435–41.

20. Dubowitz H, Bennett S. Physical abuse and neglect of children. Lancet 2007;369: 1891–9.

21. Dubowitz H. Neglect in children. Pediatr Ann 2013;42(4):73–7.

22. Dubowitz H. Understanding and addressing the "neglect of neglect": digging into the molehill. Child Abuse Negl 2007;31:603–6.

23. Keeshin BR, Dubowitz H. Childhood neglect: the role of the pediatrician. Paediatr Child Health 2013;18(8):e39–43.

24. Flaherty EG, Sege RD, Griffith J, et al. From suspicion of physical child abuse to reporting: primary care clinician decision-making. Pediatrics 2008;122(3):611–9.

25. Sege R, Flaherty E, Jones R, et al. To report or not to report: examination of the initial primary care management of suspicious childhood injuries. Acad Pediatr 2011;11(6):460–6.

26. Child Welfare Information Gateway. Mandatory reports of child abuse and neglect. Available at: https://www.childwelfare.gov/systemwide/laws_policies/statutes/manda.pdf. Accessed January 15, 2014.

27. Moreno JA. What do pediatric healthcare experts really need to know about Daubert and the rules of evidence? Pediatr Radiol 2013;43:135–9.

28. Meltzer CC, Sze G, Rommelfanger KS, et al. Guidelines for the ethical use of neuroimages in medical testimony: report of multidisciplinary consensus conference. AJNR Am J Neuroradiol 2014;35(4):632–7.

20. Chadwick DL, Krous HK. Irresponsible testimony by medical experts in cases involving the physical abuse and neglect of children. Child Maltreat 1997;2: 313–21.

30. American Academy of Pediatrics. Fostering health: healthcare for children and adolescents in foster care. 2nd edition. Available at: http://www.aap.org/en-us/advocacy-and-policy/aap-health-initiatives/healthy-foster-care-america/Pages/Fostering-Health.aspx. Accessed January 15, 2014.

31. Flaherty EG, Schwartz K, Jones RD, et al. Child abuse physicians: coping with challenges. Eval Health Prof 2013;36(2):163–73.

32. UCSF: Human Resources Department. A personal strategy for engaging and building your resilience. Available at: http://ucsfhr.ucsf.edu/index.php/assist/article/a-personal-strategy-for-engaging-and-building-your-resilience. Accessed January 10, 2014.

Index

Note: Page numbers of article titles are in **bold face** type.

A

Abuse. *See* Child maltreatment.
Accidental injury, uncertainty about, 1028
Adolescents, informed consent by, 1054
Adverse Childhood Experiences Study, 866, 1062
Advocacy, 883, **1073–1083**
    collaboration in, 1078
    courtroom testimony and, 1079
    definition of, 1073–1074
    education for, 1079
    essential nature of, 1074
    for foster care children, 1080
    for neglect, 1077–1078
    for physical abuse, 1075–1076
    for sexual abuse, 1076–1077
    importance of, 1049
    in medical setting, 1074–1075
    legislation and, 1080
    policy development and, 1080
    reporting and, 1078
    vicarious trauma and, 1080–1081
Affirmations, in motivational interviewing, 915–916
Affordable Care Act, home-visiting program of, 879
Alcohol abuse. *See* Substance abuse.
Alternative healing practices, versus maltreatment, 1012
Anchoring, in child maltreatment decisions, 1001–1002
Anticipatory guidance, for maltreatment prevention, 876–877, 896
Attributions, hostile, in social history, 894, 896

B

Battered children. *See* Child maltreatment.
Beresford model of conceptual uncertainty, 1025
Bias
    in decision making, 998–999, 1002
    in interviewing, 985–986
Body mass index, in nutritional assessment, 941
Bright Futures Project, 867
Bruising, in maltreatment, 926–929

http://dx.doi.org/10.1016/S0031-3955(14)00173-4
0031-3955/14/$ – see front matter © 2014 Elsevier Inc. All rights reserved.

United States Postal Service

Statement of Ownership, Management, and Circulation
(All Periodicals Publications Except Requestor Publications)

1. Publication Title		
Pediatric Clinics of North America		

2. Publication Number	3. Filing Date
4 2 4 - 6 6 0	9/14/14

4. Issue Frequency	5. Number of Issues Published Annually	6. Annual Subscription Price
Feb, Apr, Jun, Aug, Oct, Dec	6	$200.00

7. Complete Mailing Address of Known Office of Publication (Not printer) (Street, city, county, state, and ZIP+4®)

Elsevier Inc.
360 Park Avenue South
New York, NY 10010-1710

Contact Person
Stephen R. Bushing

Telephone (Include area code)
215-239-3688

8. Complete Mailing Address of Headquarters or General Business Office of Publisher (Not printer)

Elsevier Inc., 360 Park Avenue South, New York, NY 10010-1710

9. Full Names and Complete Mailing Addresses of Publisher, Editor, and Managing Editor (Do not leave blank)

Publisher (Name and complete mailing address)

Linda Belfus, Elsevier, Inc., 1600 John F. Kennedy Blvd. Suite 1800, Philadelphia, PA 19103-2899

Editor (Name and complete mailing address)

Kerry Holland, Elsevier, Inc., 1600 John F. Kennedy Blvd. Suite 1800, Philadelphia, PA 19103-2899

Managing Editor (Name and complete mailing address)

Adrianne Brigido, Elsevier, Inc., 1600 John F. Kennedy Blvd. Suite 1800, Philadelphia, PA 19103-2899

10. Owner (Do not leave blank. If the publication is owned by a corporation, give the name and address of the corporation immediately followed by the names and addresses of all stockholders owning or holding 1 percent or more of the total amount of stock. If not owned by a corporation, give the names and addresses of the individual owners. If owned by a partnership or other unincorporated firm, give its name and address as well as those of each individual owner. If the publication is published by a nonprofit organization, give its name and address.)

Full Name	Complete Mailing Address
Wholly owned subsidiary of	1600 John F. Kennedy Blvd, Ste. 1800
Reed/Elsevier, US holdings	Philadelphia, PA 19103-2899

11. Known Bondholders, Mortgagees, and Other Security Holders Owning or Holding 1 Percent or More of Total Amount of Bonds, Mortgages, or Other Securities. If none, check box. ▶ ☐ None

Full Name	Complete Mailing Address
N/A	

12. Tax Status (For completion by nonprofit organizations authorized to mail at nonprofit rates) (Check one)
The purpose, function, and nonprofit status of this organization and the exempt status for federal income tax purposes:
☐ Has Not Changed During Preceding 12 Months
☐ Has Changed During Preceding 12 Months (Publisher must submit explanation of change with this statement)

PS Form 3526, August 2012 (Page 1 of 3 (Instructions Page 3)) PSN 7530-01-000-9931 PRIVACY NOTICE: See our Privacy policy in www.usps.com

---

13. Publication Title		14. Issue Date for Circulation Data Below
Pediatric Clinics of North America		June 2014

15. Extent and Nature of Circulation			Average No. Copies Each Issue During Preceding 12 Months	No. Copies of Single Issue Published Nearest to Filing Date
a. Total Number of Copies (Net press run)			2,224	2,545
b. Paid Circulation (By Mail and Outside the Mail)	(1)	Mailed Outside-County Paid Subscriptions Stated on PS Form 3541. (Include paid distribution above nominal rate, advertiser's proof copies, and exchange copies)	1,286	1,346
	(2)	Mailed In-County Paid Subscriptions Stated on PS Form 3541 (Include paid distribution above nominal rate, advertiser's proof copies, and exchange copies)		
	(3)	Paid Distribution Outside the Mails Including Sales Through Dealers and Carriers, Street Vendors, Counter Sales, and Other Paid Distribution Outside USPS®	564	539
	(4)	Paid Distribution by Other Classes Mailed Through the USPS (e.g. First-Class Mail®)		
c. Total Paid Distribution (Sum of 15b (1), (2), (3), and (4))		▶	1,850	1,885
d. Free or Nominal Rate Distribution (By Mail and Outside the Mail)	(1)	Free or Nominal Rate Outside-County Copies Included on PS Form 3541	82	111
	(2)	Free or Nominal Rate In-County Copies Included on PS Form 3541		
	(3)	Free or Nominal Rate Copies Mailed at Other Classes Through the USPS (e.g. First-Class Mail)		
	(4)	Free or Nominal Rate Distribution Outside the Mail (Carriers or other means)		
e. Total Free or Nominal Rate Distribution (Sum of 15d (1), (2), (3) and (4))		▶	82	111
f. Total Distribution (Sum of 15c and 15e)		▶	1,932	1,996
g. Copies not Distributed (See instructions to publishers #4 (page #3))		▶	510	549
h. Total (Sum of 15f and g)		▶	2,442	2,545
i. Percent Paid (15c divided by 15f times 100)		▶	95.76%	94.44%

16 Total circulation includes electronic copies. Report circulation on PS Form 3526-X worksheet.

17. Publication of Statement of Ownership
If the publication is a general publication, publication of this statement is required. Will be printed in the October 2014 issue of this publication.

18. Signature and Title of Editor, Publisher, Business Manager, or Owner	Date
[signature] Stephen R. Bushing – Inventory Distribution Coordinator	September 14, 2014

I certify that all information furnished on this form is true and complete. I understand that anyone who furnishes false or misleading information on this form or who omits material or information requested on the form may be subject to criminal sanctions (including fines and imprisonment) and/or civil sanctions (including civil penalties).

PS Form 3526, August 2012 (Page 2 of 3)

Moving?

Make sure your subscription moves with you!

To notify us of your new address, find your **Clinics Account Number** (located on your mailing label above your name), and contact customer service at:

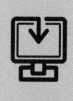

Email: **journalscustomerservice-usa@elsevier.com**

800-654-2452 (subscribers in the U.S. & Canada)
314-447-8871 (subscribers outside of the U.S. & Canada)

Fax number: **314-447-8029**

Elsevier Health Sciences Division
Subscription Customer Service
3251 Riverport Lane
Maryland Heights, MO 63043

*To ensure uninterrupted delivery of your subscription, please notify us at least 4 weeks in advance of move.